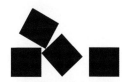

ATLAS OF
ORTHOPEDIC PATHOLOGY

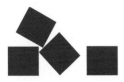

ATLAS OF ORTHOPEDIC PATHOLOGY

Second Edition

Lester E. Wold, MD
Professor and Chairman
Department of Pathology
Mayo Clinic
Rochester, Minnesota

Claus-Peter Adler, MD
Institute of Pathology
University of Freiburg
Freiburg, Germany

Franklin H. Sim, MD
Consultant, Department of Orthopedic Surgery
Chair, Division of Orthopedic Oncology
Mayo Clinic
Rochester, Minnesota

K. Krishnan Unni, MD
Professor and Director, Orthopedic Pathology
Department of Pathology
Mayo Clinic
Rochester, Minnesota

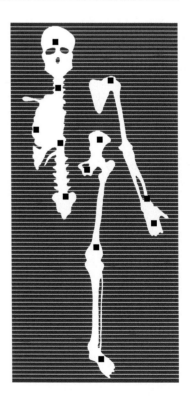

Saunders
An Imprint of Elsevier Science
Philadelphia London Toronto Montreal Sydney Tokyo

SAUNDERS
An Imprint of Elsevier Science

The Curtis Center
Independence Square West
Philadelphia, PA 19106

ATLAS OF ORTHOPEDIC PATHOLOGY, 2/e   ISBN:0-7216-9158-7

Library of Congress Cataloging-in-Publication Data

Wold, Lester E. (Lester Eugene)
    Atlas of orthopedic pathology / Lester E. Wold, K. Krishnan Unni.--2nd ed.
        p. ; cm.
    Rev. ed. of: Atlas of orthopedic pathology / Lester E. Wold ... [et al.]. 1990
    Includes bibliographical references and index.
    ISBN 0-7216-9158-7
        1. Bones--Diseases--Atlases. 2. Orthopedics--Atlases. I. Unni, K. Krishnan, 1941- II.
Title.
        [DNLM: 1. Bone Diseases--pathology--Atlases. WE 17 W852a 2003]
    RC930 .A85 2003
    616.7'107'222--dc21

                                                                    2002070826

Acquisitions Editor: Natasha Andjelkovic

PIT/DNP

Printed in China

Last digit is the print number: 9   8   7   6   5   4   3   2   1

**To our families
who have supported us
through the long gestation and delivery
of this text.**

Atlases in
Diagnostic Surgical Pathology

Consulting Editor:
Gerald M. Bordin, M.D.
Department of Pathology
Scripps Clinic and Research Foundation

Forthcoming Titles:

Fuller, Goodman: Atlas of Neuropathology

Brooks: Atlas of Soft Tissue Pathology

Wenig: Atlas of Head and Neck Pathology, 2E

Smith et al: Atlas of Infectious Disease Pathology

Preface

This atlas of orthopedic tumors and non-tumorous conditions is intended as an introduction to the complex subject of orthopedic pathology. It offers a starting point for pathology residents, orthopedic residents, and radiology residents to learn about the clinical, radiographic, and pathologic features of common and uncommon orthopedic conditions. This atlas is organized into sections of related conditions. Each chapter within a section is organized in a manner to succinctly display data and information.

Clinical signs, symptoms, major radiographic features, radiographic differential diagnosis, gross and microscopic pathologic differential diagnosis, and treatment sections are organized in outline format. Only the major features are presented. For more information the reader is referred to an abbreviated list of references that follows the outlined information. These references are by no means complete, but offer a starting point for a more in-depth review of each condition. This atlas complements many texts that contain abundant information concerning both tumors and tumor-like conditions of bone.

Lester E. Wold, MD
Claus-Peter Adler, MD
Franklin H. Sim, MD
K. Krishnan Unni, MD

Acknowledgments

The authors gratefully acknowledge Drs. David C. Dahlin, John W. Beabout, John C. Ivins, and Richard A. McLeod, without whose helpful encouragement, counsel, and tutelage this book would not have been possible.

Contents

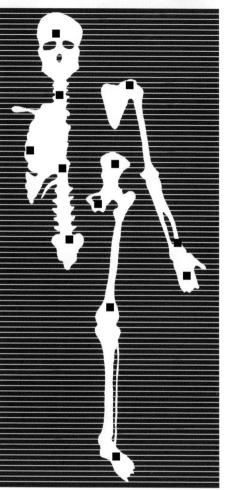

SECTION ■ I

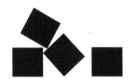

METABOLIC, DEVELOPMENTAL, AND INFLAMMATORY CONDITIONS OF BONE

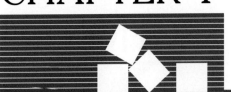

CHAPTER 1

Hyperparathyroidism

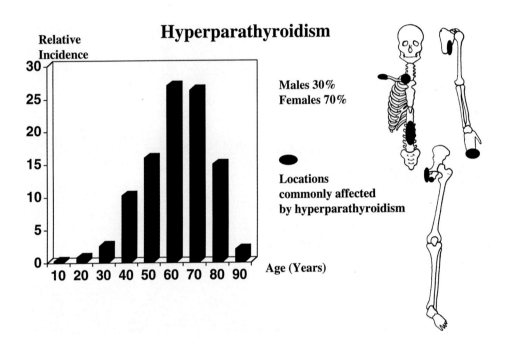

Hyperparathyroidism

Males 30%
Females 70%

Locations
commonly affected
by hyperparathyroidism

CLINICAL SIGNS

1. Most cases are asymptomatic and detected biochemically on screening studies. (Ninety per cent of all cases of hypercalcemia are due to malignancy and hyperparathyroidism, in that order.)
2. Biochemical studies reveal increased serum calcium and decreased serum phosphorus concentrations in cases of primary hyperparathyroidism. (Secondary hyperparathyroidism is initially characterized by increased serum phosphorus concentrations.)
3. Renal stones may be present. (Incidence has decreased from approximately 65 per cent in the mid-1970s to approximately 5 per cent in the mid-1990s.)
4. Hypertension is present in approximately 20 per cent of patients.

5. Depression, psychosis, or severe neurosis is seen in approximately 20 per cent of patients.
6. Osteoporosis is seen in approximately 10 per cent of patients.

CLINICAL SYMPTOMS

1. Bone and joint pain and tenderness are present in about 15 per cent of patients.
2. Flank pain associated with renal stones may occur (present in approximately one third of patients but depends upon the prevalence of screening calcium determinations done in the population).
3. Constipation, indigestion, or ulcer symptoms are present in approximately 30 per cent of patients.

4. Muscle pain is present in approximately 15 per cent of patients.
5. Fatigue is the most common complaint and is mentioned by about half the patients.
6. Polyuria and polydipsia may occur.
7. Nausea and vomiting may be seen in patients with severe hypercalcemia.
8. Approximately 50 per cent of patients are asymptomatic.

MAJOR RADIOGRAPHIC FEATURES

1. Diffuse osteopenia can be seen.
2. Radiographs of the hand show erosion of the tufts of the phalanges and subperiosteal cortical resorption particularly prominent on the radial aspect of the phalangeal shafts.
3. Subperiosteal resorption may be evident in the region of the symphysis pubis, proximal and distal clavicles, ischial tuberosity, scapula, and the plates of the vertebral bodies.
4. Periarticular erosions, particularly of the bones of the hands, wrists, and feet (most commonly involving the distal interphalangeal joint), may be noted.
5. There may be loss of the lamina dura surrounding the tooth roots.
6. Occasionally, patients present with a lytic bony lesion ("brown tumor").
7. Renal calculi may be seen.
8. Bone changes may not be identified in the early stages of the disease.
9. Soft tissue calcification may be present.
10. Decreased cortical bone density may be evident.

RADIOGRAPHIC DIFFERENTIAL DIAGNOSIS

1. Rheumatoid arthritis (periarticular erosions of the small bones).
2. Ankylosing spondylitis (when the disease involves the sacroiliac joints).
3. Primary bone tumor when a brown tumor of hyperparathyroidism is present.
4. Osteomalacia.

MAJOR PATHOLOGIC FEATURES

1. Osteoclasts are increased on the bone surface.
2. In longstanding cases, there is "tunneling" resorption of the trabeculae.
3. With secondary hyperparathyroidism due to renal failure, marrow fibrosis and increased woven bone may be prominent.
4. The brown tumor of hyperparathyroidism is histologically a giant cell reparative granuloma, consisting of numerous multinucleated giant cells lying in a spindle cell, mononuclear cell stroma.

PATHOLOGIC DIFFERENTIAL DIAGNOSIS

1. Giant cell tumor of bone (in cases of brown tumor).
2. Myelofibrosis.
3. Fibrous dysplasia.
4. Paget's disease.

TREATMENT

1. Parathyroid tissue (adenoma or hyperplastic glands) can be surgically removed.
2. New bisphosphonates (pamidronate disodium) are of major value in treating hypercalcemia.
3. Bone disease (osteitis fibrosa cystica) will heal with treatment of the primary parathyroid disease. Occasional large lesions (brown tumors) may require curettage and grafting. Pathologic fractures may require internal fixation.

References

Cohen-Solal M, and Sebert JL: Renal osteodystrophy and hypercalcemia [review]. Curr Opin Rheumatol 5(3):357–362, 1993.
Heath H, Hodgson SF, and Kennedy MA: Primary hyperparathyroidism: incidence, morbidity, and potential economic impact in a community. N Engl J Med 302:189–193, 1980.
Palmer M, Jakobsson S, Akerstrom G, et al: Prevalence of hypercalcaemia in a health survey: a 14-year follow-up study of serum calcium values. Eur J Clin Invest 18:39–46, 1988.
Resnick DL: Erosive arthritis of the hand and wrist in hyperparathyroidism. Radiology 110:263–269, 1974.

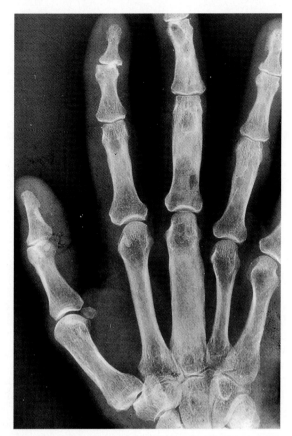

Figure 1-1. Radiograph of the hand illustrating the features of hyperparathyroidism. Note the erosive changes involving the phalangeal tufts and diffuse osteopenia. Subperiosteal resorption of bone is often most prominent on the radial side of the middle and proximal phalanges.

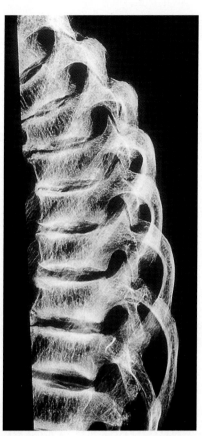

Figure 1-3. Radiograph of the vertebrae and ribs illustrating diffuse osteopenia associated with primary hyperparathyroidism.

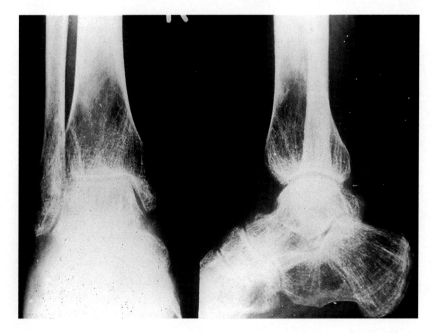

Figure 1-2. Radiograph of the distal tibia illustrating a radiolytic defect. The patient was identified as having primary hyperparathyroidism, and the defect shown is due to a "brown tumor" of hyperparathyroidism. Such lesions may be seen in any skeletal location and may be confused pathologically with a giant cell tumor. If a lesion pathologically resembles a giant cell tumor but is not in an epiphyseal location, then hyperparathyroidism should be excluded.

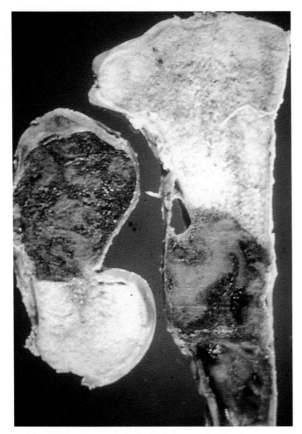

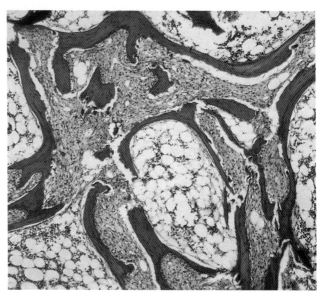

Figure 1–6. The marked dissecting osteitis or "tunneling" associated with longstanding hyperparathyroidism is illustrated in this photomicrograph. The bony trabeculae have been replaced at their center by fibrovascular connective tissue. The marrow in this example remains active but may even be replaced by fibrovascular connective tissue as the disease progresses, particularly in cases of secondary hyperparathyroidism related to renal failure.

Figure 1–4. This gross photograph of the proximal tibia illustrates the appearance of a brown tumor. Although grossly this lesion may resemble a giant cell tumor, its diaphyseal location is helpful in excluding giant cell tumor from the pathologic differential diagnosis. Brown tumors are at present uncommonly seen, as most patients with hyperparathyroidism are identified early in the course of their disease.

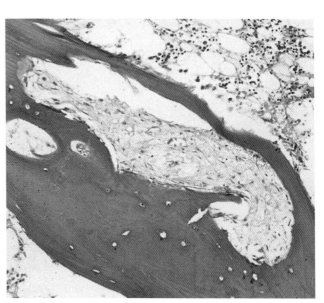

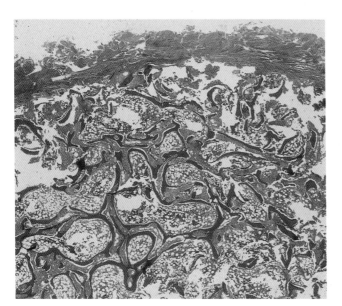

Figure 1–7. Earlier tunneling is shown in this photomicrograph from a patient with primary hyperparathyroidism. Active osteoclastic resorption may be identified in the region of the central trabecular bony destruction.

Figure 1–5. The histologic appearance of well-developed primary hyperparathyroidism is illustrated in this photomicrograph. The low-power histologic pattern shows irregular bony trabeculae that have been significantly remodeled. Figure 1–6 shows the pattern at higher magnification.

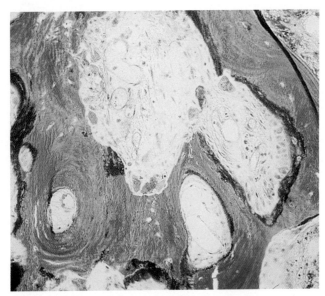

Figure 1–8. Hyperparathyroidism results in greater bony destruction than production. No tunneling is seen in this bone, which shows the earliest effects of changes due to primary hyperparathyroidism.

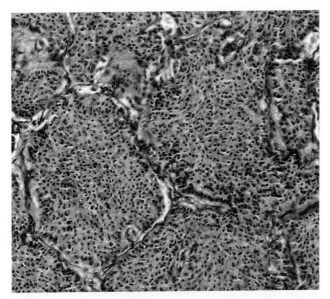

Figure 1–9. Parathyroid adenoma is the most common cause of primary hyperparathyroidism. This photomicrograph illustrates the histologic features of a parathyroid adenoma. Parathyroid hyperplasia is a less common cause of primary hyperparathyroidism, and the pathologist may have trouble distinguishing an adenoma from a hyperplastic gland, as the histologic features of these conditions overlap significantly. Communication with the surgeon to identify how many glands are grossly enlarged is necessary to minimize errors in classification of the parathyroid pathology.

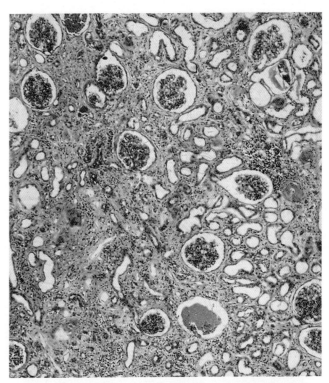

Figure 1–10. This photomicrograph illustrates the histologic appearance of the kidney in a patient with primary hyperparathyroidism.

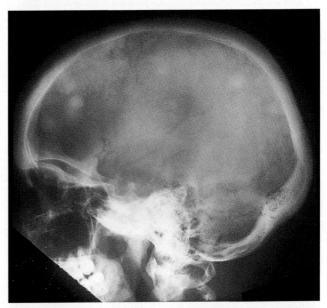

Figure 1–11. This radiograph of the skull is from a patient with renal osteodystrophy. Regions of radiolucency and some regions of increased mineralization are apparent, resulting in a "salt and pepper" appearance. The radiographic features of such examples of secondary hyperparathyroidism may overlap entirely with those seen in patients with primary hyperparathyroidism.

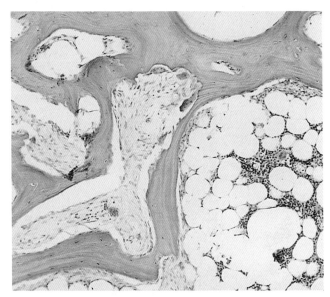

Figure 1–12. This photomocrograph reveals the histologic pattern seen in secondary hyperparathyroidism. Note that the trabecular tunneling previously illustrated in primary hyperparathyroidism (Fig. 1–6) is also evident in this condition. Osteoclastic resorption is also shown.

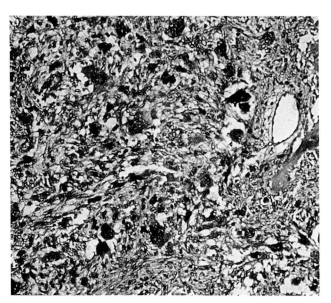

Figure 1–14. At higher magnification, brown tumors show a greater tendency to spindling of the mononuclear stromal cells than is seen giant cell tumors. Reactive new bone may be present in these cases.

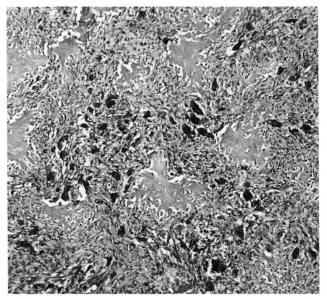

Figure 1–13. This low-power photomicrograph illustrates the features of a brown tumor. Although numerous osteoclast-type giant cells are present, this amount of fibrosis would be uncommon in giant cell tumors of bone. Another feature that helps distinguish such reactive lesions from giant cell tumors is the relative clustering of the giant cells in a brown tumor compared with their more uniform distribution in a giant cell tumor.

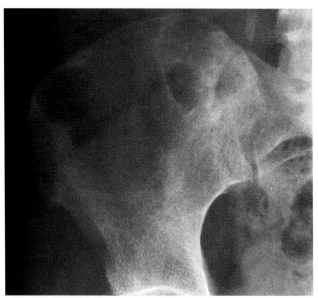

Figure 1–15. This radiograph illustrates a brown tumor of hyperparathyroidism involving the ilium.

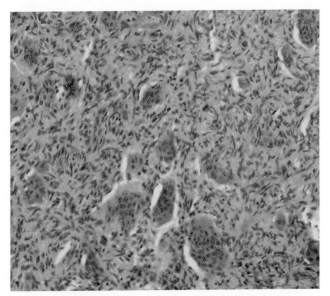

Figure 1–16. This photomicrograph illustrates the histologic pattern of the lesion shown in Figure 1–15. The fibrogenic stroma and greater degree of spindling of the mononuclear cells help differentiate this lesion from a giant cell tumor of the bone.

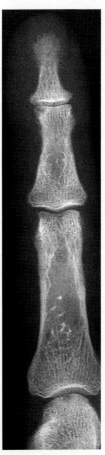

Figure 1–18. AP roentgenogram of the finger in a patient with hyperparathyroidism. Note the subperiosteal resorption of the phalanges. Note also the acro-osteolysis of the tuft and demineralization. Cortical tunneling with coarse trabeculae is present.

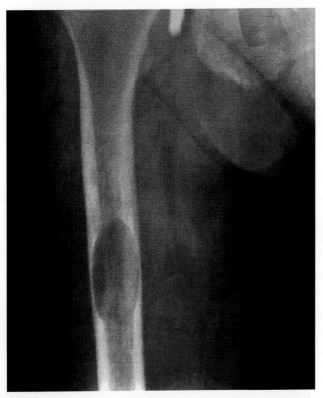

Figure 1–17. Anteroposterior (AP) roentgenogram of the right femur in a 59-year-old male patient with hyperparathyroidism. There is a large, well-defined lytic lesion in the diaphysis, with endosteal erosion and bony expansion.

CHAPTER 2

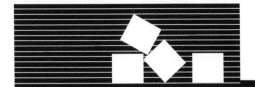

Osteoporosis

CLINICAL SIGNS

1. Osteoporosis occurs most commonly in post-menopausal slender women older than 65 years of age. Other associated clinical features include:
   a. Fair complexion.
   b. Freckles.
   c. Blond hair.
   d. Scoliosis.
2. The hip and forearm fracture with minor trauma.
3. Spasm of the paraspinal musculature is related to pathologic fracture of the vertebrae.
4. Loss of height (related to vertebral collapse) may occur.
5. Dietary intake of calcium is poor.

CLINICAL SYMPTOMS

1. Back pain may be present.
2. Hip pain resulting from hip fracture after minor trauma (e.g., fall) may occur.
3. Osteoporosis may be related to estrogen deficiency, Cushing's syndrome, hyperthyroidism, diabetes mellitus, or immobilization. Clinical symptoms related to these conditions thus may be associated with osteoporosis.

MAJOR RADIOGRAPHIC FEATURES

1. Cortical bone shows thinning.
2. Generalized osteopenia may be seen.
3. In vertebrae, there may be thinning and eventual disappearance of the vertical trabeculae.
4. Thoracic vertebrae may exhibit wedge fractures.
5. Lumbar vertebrae may exhibit crush fractures.
6. Intervertebral disc spaces may show widening.

RADIOGRAPHIC DIFFERENTIAL DIAGNOSIS

1. Systemic mastocytosis.
2. Multiple myeloma.

MAJOR PATHOLOGIC FEATURES

1. Trabecular bone volume is decreased. (Although morphometric studies show a significant difference in the population distribution of trabecular bone volume in osteoporotic and nonosteoporotic individuals, the overlap between the two groups is so great that this measure cannot be used alone to identify osteoporotic patients.)
2. Osteoid volume is decreased.

PATHOLOGIC DIFFERENTIAL DIAGNOSIS

1. Cushing's syndrome.
2. Osteogenesis imperfecta.
3. Homocystinuria.
4. Turner's syndrome.
5. Malabsorption.
6. Immobilization.

TREATMENT

Medical

1. Treatment varies with cause: dietary, supplemental calcium salts.
2. Regular exercise is helpful.
3. Estrogen preparations can be given to postmenopausal women.

4. Bisphosphonates and calcitonin are investigational.
5. Supportive care for vertebral fractures should be provided—analgesics, spinal support, and physical therapy.

Surgical

1. For hip fractures, treatment is internal fixation versus prosthetic replacement.
2. For Colles' fractures, long bone fractures, treatment is closed reduction versus open reduction and internal fixation.

References

Andrew SM, and Freemont AJ: Skeletal mastocytosis. J Clin Pathol 46(11):1033–1035, 1993.

Arnala I: Use of histological methods in studies of osteoporosis. Calcif Tissue Int 49 (Suppl):S31–S32, 1991.

Ashton-Key M, and Gallagher PJ: The value of simple morphometric techniques in the diagnosis of osteoporosis. Pathol Res Pract 188(4–5):616–619, 1992.

Bronner F: Calcium and osteoporosis [review]. Am J Clin Nutr 60(6):831–836, 1994.

Chappard D, Plantard B, and Petitjean M: Alcoholic cirrhosis and osteoporosis in men: a light and scanning electron microscopy study. J Stud Alcohol 52(3):269–274, 1991.

Chines A, Pacifici R, and Avioli LV: Systemic mastocytosis presenting as osteoporosis: a clinical and histomorphometric study. J Clin Endocrinol Metab 72(1):140–144, 1991.

Chines A, Pacifici R, and Avioli LA: Systemic mastocytosis and osteoporosis. Osteoporos Int 3(Suppl 1):147–149, 1993.

Compston JE, and Croucher PI: Histomorphometric assessment of trabecular bone remodelling in osteoporosis [review]. Bone Miner 14(2):91–102, 1991.

Cosman F, Schnitzer MB, and McCann PD: Relationships between quantitative histological measurements and noninvasive assessments of bone mass. Bone 13(3):237–242, 1992.

Croucher PI, Vedi S, and Motley RJ: Reduced bone formation in patients with osteoporosis associated with inflammatory bowel disease. Osteoporos Int 3(5):236–241, 1993.

Diebold J, Batge B, and Stein H: Osteoporosis in longstanding acromegaly: characteristic changes of vertebral trabecular architecture and bone matrix composition. Virchows Arch A Pathol Anat Histopathol 419(3):209–215, 1991.

Jayasinghe JA, Jones SJ, and Boyde A: Scanning electron microscopy of human lumbar vertebral trabecular bone surfaces. Virchows Arch A Pathol Anat Histopathol 422(1):25–34, 1993.

Lane JM, and Vigorita VJ: Osteoporosis. J Bone Joint Surg (Am) 65:274, 1983.

Magaro M, Tricerri A, and Piane D: Generalized osteoporosis in non-steroid treated rheumatoid arthritis. Rheumatol Int 11(2):73–76, 1991.

Motley RJ, Clements D, and Evans WD: A four-year longitudinal study of bone loss in patients with inflammatory bowel disease. Bone Miner 23(2):95–104, 1993.

Ott SM: Clinical effects of bisphosphonates in involutional osteoporosis [review]. J Bone Miner Res 8 (Suppl 2):S597–S606, 1993.

Recker RR: Bone biopsy and histomorphometry in clinical practice. Rheum Dis Clin North Am 20(3):609–627, 1994.

Rillo OL, Di Stefano CA, Bermudez J, et al: Idiopathic osteoporosis during pregnancy. Clin Rheumatol 13(2):299–304, 1994.

Wilkinson JM, Cotton DW, Harris SC, et al: Assessment of osteoporosis at autopsy: mechanical methods compared to radiological and histological techniques. Med Sci Law 31(1):19–24, 1991.

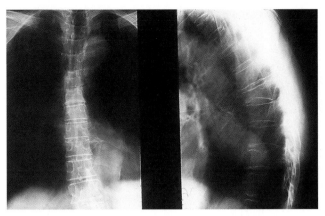

Figure 2–1. Anteroposterior (AP) (left) and lateral (right) radiographs of the thorax in a patient with osteoporosis. Note the diffuse osteopenia and the compression fracture of the thoracic vertebra. Exaggeration of the vertical striations in osteoporotic vertebrae may also be present.

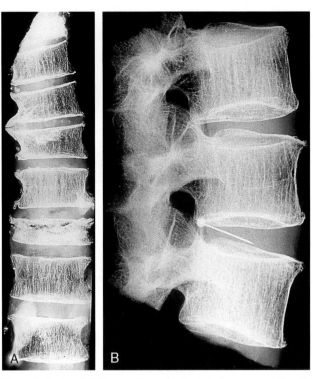

Figure 2–3. *A* and *B,* These radiographs illustrate the exaggerated vertical striations as well as compression fractures commonly seen in osteoporotic vertebrae.

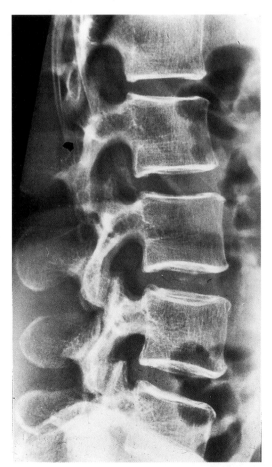

Figure 2–2. This radiograph of the lumbar vertebrae illustrates the exaggerated pattern of vertical striations that can be seen in patients with osteoporosis.

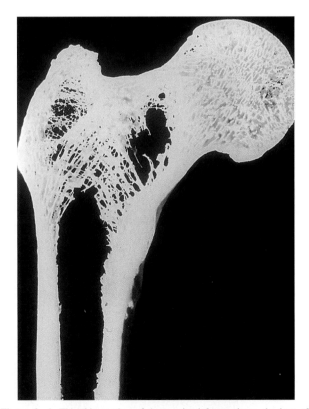

Figure 2–4. This thin section of the proximal femur shows the loss of trabecular bone seen in patients with osteoporosis. Figures 2–5 and 2–6 also illustrate the gross pathologic features seen in osteoporotic bone.

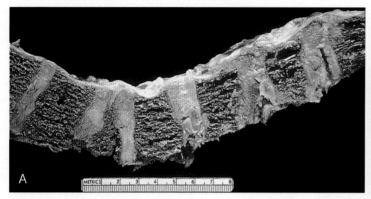

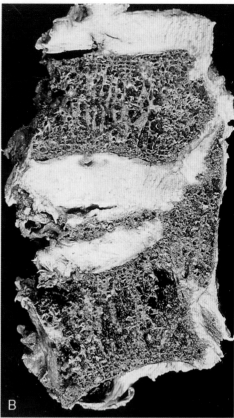

Figure 2–5. *A* and *B* illustrate the gross pathology that results in the radiographic features of osteoporotic vertebrae. Compression fractures are present in both of these specimens.

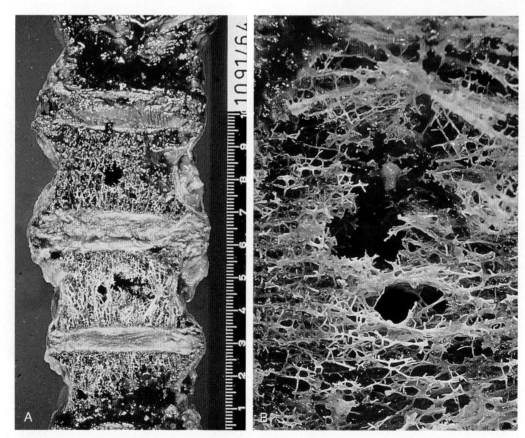

Figure 2–6. *A* and *B,* These two photographs show the loss of trabecular bone in osteoporotic vertebrae. Microfractures of the thinned trabecular bone are common. Histologically, a healing reaction may be present in these regions.

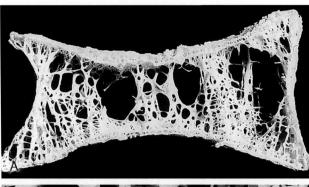

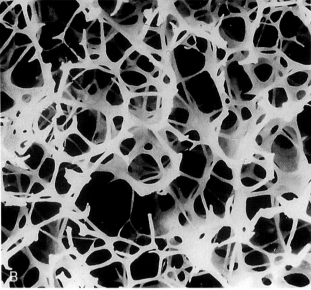

Figure 2–7. *A* and *B,* These two specimens have been carefully prepared to illustrate the marked thinning or loss of trabecular bone in osteoporosis. Compression of the vertebra is also present in this case.

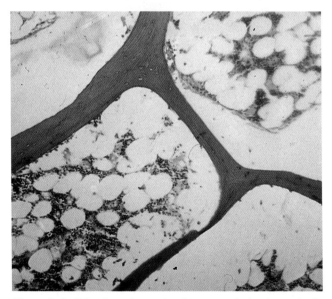

Figure 2–8. This photomicrograph of osteoporotic bone reveals the thinning of trabecular bone without changes in the medullary content. In this case, little osteoblastic or osteoclastic activity is present. Such cases may be described as "inactive."

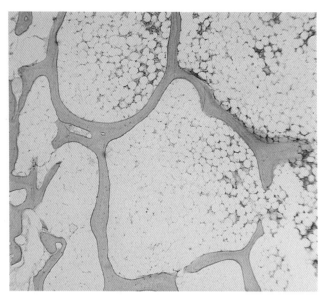

Figure 2–9. Cortical bone loss is a feature of osteoporotic bone, as shown in this photomicrograph. Thinning of the trabecular bone is also present.

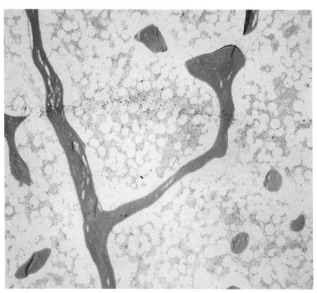

Figure 2–10. This photomicrograph illustrates the features of low turnover or inactive osteoporosis. Little osteoblastic or osteoclastic activity is evident in this biopsy specimen stained with trichrome stain. High turnover or active osteoporosis is characterized by excessive osteoclastic activity in the presence of normal or increased osteoblastic activity.

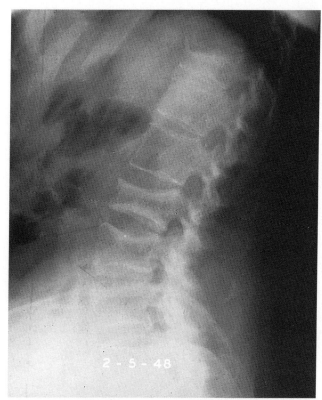

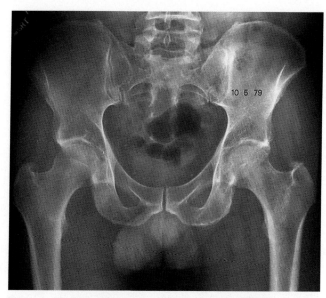

Figure 2–13. Seven months later, the patient shown in Figure 2–12 has experienced resolution of the pain and improvement in the radiograph.

Figure 2–11. Osteoporotic changes in the vertebrae are well illustrated in this x-ray film from a patient with Cushing's disease. Note the widened intervertebral spaces.

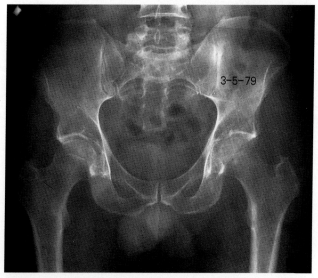

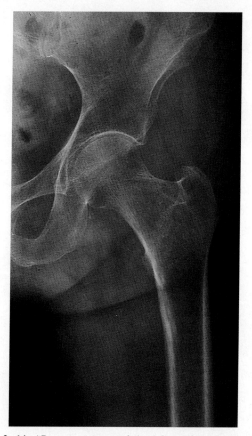

Figure 2–12. AP roentgenogram of the pelvis and proximal femora in a patient with transient osteoporosis. Demineralization of the bone in the proximal femur and acetabulum can be seen.

Figure 2–14. AP roentgenogram of the left proximal femur showing osteoporosis of the hip with diffuse demineralization of the bones and loss of trabeculae. Note the thinning of the cortex.

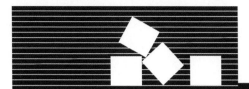

CHAPTER 3

Renal Osteodystrophy

CLINICAL SIGNS

1. The patient is on renal dialysis.
2. The serum phosphate concentration is elevated.
3. The serum ionized calcium concentration is decreased.

CLINICAL SYMPTOMS

1. Bone pain may be present.
2. Muscle weakness may be present.
3. Skeletal deformities may occur.
4. Growth is retarded in children with renal failure.

MAJOR RADIOGRAPHIC FEATURES

1. Generalized bone resorption, may be seen.
2. There may be subperiosteal bone resorption, particularly involving the radial aspect of the proximal and middle phalanges of the hands.
3. Endosteal erosion involving the phalanges (the most sensitive sign of hyperparathyroidism and therefore commonly seen in renal osteodystrophy) and the lateral end of the clavicles may be present.
4. Osteosclerosis of the spine, resulting in a "rugger jersey" pattern, may be evident. (Osteosclerosis may involve the pelvis, ribs, calvaria, and long bones less commonly.)
5. Generalized osteoporosis or osteomalacia may be seen. (Pseudofractures or Looser's zones may be the only evidence of osteomalacia.)
6. Fractures may be present and are more common in the upper ribs in patients with aluminum-associated bone disease.
7. Chondrocalcinosis may be present but is unusual.
8. Vascular calcification may be seen. (Other extraskele-

tal calcium deposits may also be seen in the eye and viscera.)
9. Periarticular calcification may be evident.
10. Rickets may be the presenting feature or first indication of renal failure in children.
11. Slipped epiphyses may be seen in advanced renal failure in children between 11 and 16 years of age. (In general, this represents a fracture through weakened bone adjacent to the growth plate.)

Note: The radiographic features of renal osteodystrophy are a combination of those seen in hyperparathyroidism and osteomalacia due to the impaired ability of the affected patient to convert vitamin D to its active form and the secondary hyperparathyroidism that results.

RADIOGRAPHIC DIFFERENTIAL DIAGNOSIS

1. Hyperparathyroidism.
2. Erosive changes that may be confused with rheumatoid arthritis, infection, or seronegative arthropathies.
3. Neoplasm (if amyloid deposition or a "brown tumor" is present).

MAJOR PATHOLOGIC FEATURES

1. Irregular, thickened, woven trabecular bone is seen.
2. Loose, fibrous connective tissue surrounds the thickened, woven bone.
3. Increased numbers of osteoclasts and osteoblasts are present.
4. Intratrabecular tunnels that are lined by osteoclasts and contain loose fibrovascular connective tissue are present in advanced stages of the disease.

5. The major pathologic features overlap with those of osteomalacia, rickets, osteosclerosis, and osteoporosis.

PATHOLOGIC DIFFERENTIAL DIAGNOSIS

1. Hyperparathyroidism.
2. Vitamin D deficiency.
3. Giant cell tumor (if brown tumor complicates secondary hyperparathyroidism associated with renal failure).
4. Amyloidosis (if amyloid deposits are identified after renal dialysis).

TREATMENT

Medical

1. Treatment of chronic renal failure consists of the following:
   a. Dietary management.
   b. Dialysis.
   c. Renal transplantation.
2. Management of osteodystrophy consists of the following:
   a. Treatment of hyperphosphatemia.
   b. Symptomatic measures for bone pain.

Surgical

1. Subtotal parathyroidectomy can be performed.
2. Fractures and deformities are managed.
3. Manage slipped capital femoral epiphysis.

References

Chazan JA, Libbey NP, London MR, et al: The clinical spectrum of renal osteodystrophy in 57 chronic hemodialysis patients: a correlation between biochemical parameters and bone pathology findings. Clin Nephrol 35(2):78–85, 1991.

Goodman WG, and Duarte ME: Aluminum: effects on bone and role in the pathogenesis of renal osteodystrophy [review]. Miner Electrolyte Metab 17(4):221–232, 1991.

Krpan D, Milutinovic S, Nikolic V, et al: Oxalosis associated with aluminum bone disease: a new type of mixed renal osteodystrophy. Nephron 66(1):99–101, 1994.

Recker RR: Bone biopsy and histomorphometry in clinical practice. Rheum Dis Clin North Am 20(3):609–627, 1994.

Sherrard DJ, Hercz G, and Pei Y: The spectrum of bone disease in end-stage renal failure—an evolving disorder. Kidney Int 43(2):436–442, 1993.

Shih C, Chen KH, and Chang CY: Articular manifestations of renal osteodystrophy. Zhonghua Yi Xue Za Zhi (Taipei) 52(6):372–377, 1993.

Sundaram M: Renal osteodystrophy. Skeletal Radiol 18:415–426, 1989.

Tigges S, Nance EP, Carpenter WA, and Erb R: Renal osteodystrophy: imaging findings that mimic those of other diseases. Am J Roentgenol 165(1):143–148, 1995.

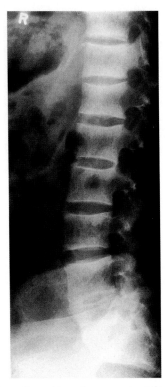

Figure 3–1. The radiographic pattern seen in patients with renal osteodystrophy is variable and contains features of osteomalacia and secondary hyperparathyroidism. This radiograph illustrates the "rugger jersey" spine pattern due to sclerosis adjacent to the vertebral end plates in a patient with renal osteodystrophy.

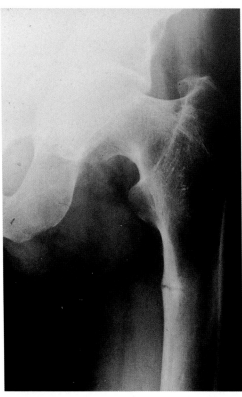

Figure 3–2. Radiograph of the proximal femur in a patient with renal osteodystrophy showing a Looser's zone in the medial cortex. Rachitic changes are common in renal osteodystrophy, particularly when the patient is young and growing.

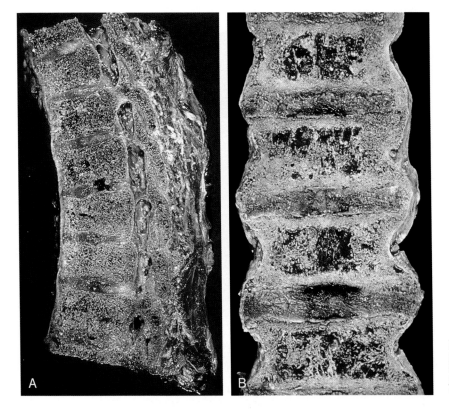

Figure 3–3. These gross specimens are transverse (A) and longitudinal (B) sections through the vertebrae. Loss of trabecular bone and bony sclerosis adjacent to the vertebral discs are commonly seen in well-developed renal osteodystrophy.

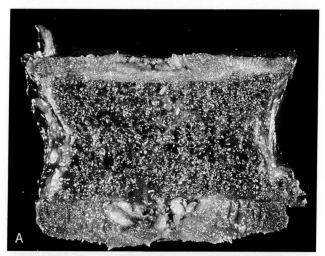

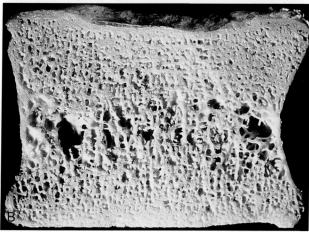

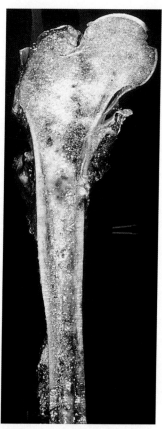

Figure 3–5. This gross section of the proximal femur demonstrates changes seen in renal osteodystrophy. The disorganization of bony architecture mimics that seen in Paget's disease.

Figure 3–4. These two gross photographs contrast the appearance of the vertebrae in the fresh state *(A)* and after processing *(B)*. Both illustrate the loss of trabecular bone, and the processed specimen shows the bony sclerosis adjacent to the vertebral discs.

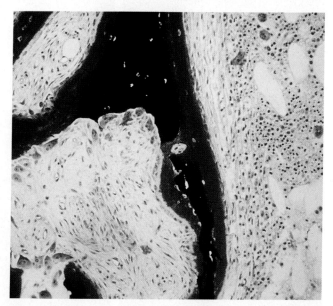

Figure 3–6. This photomicrograph reveals the microscopic features of renal osteodystrophy. Marked osteoclastic activity is evident, and there is deficient mineralization of the bone. Osteoclastic "tunneling" into the bony trabeculae can be seen in advanced renal osteodystrophy (von Kossa stain).

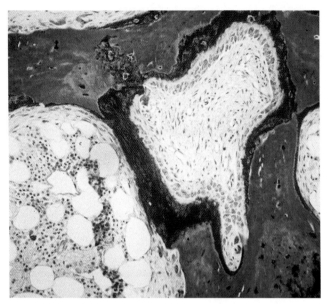

Figure 3–7. Osteoclastic resorption and osteoblastic deposition of new bone are seen in this example of renal osteodystrophy. Bony tunneling is also present (van Giessen stain).

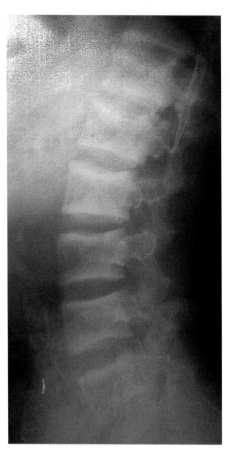

Figure 3–9. This radiograph of the spine illustrates the vertebral end plate sclerosis associated with renal osteodystrophy in a 41-year-old man with renal failure.

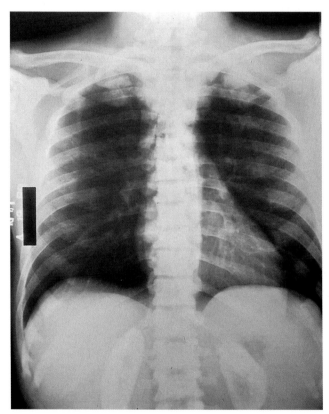

Figure 3–8. This chest radiograph illustrates the radiographic features of renal osteodystrophy in a 33-year-old man with renal failure secondary to hereditary oxalosis (note the dense mineralization of the kidneys bilaterally).

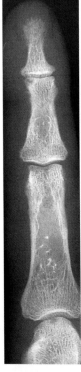

Figure 3–10. Subperiosteal bone resorption, particularly prominent in the phalangeal tufts, is characteristic of renal osteodystrophy.

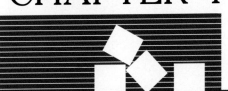

CHAPTER 4

Rickets

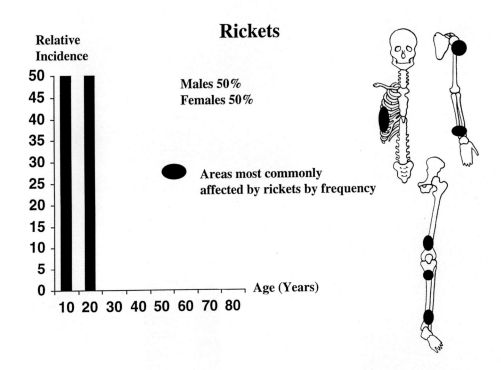

Rickets

Relative
Incidence

Males 50%
Females 50%

● Areas most commonly
affected by rickets by frequency

Age (Years)

CLINICAL SIGNS

1. Widespread skeletal deformities in a child are present. (Rachitic abnormalities result from disturbances in the orderly mineralization and development of the growth plate; these disturbances are seen only prior to closure of the growth plates.)
2. The fontanelles bulge in patients during the first year of life. (During the first months of life, the skull is most severely affected.)
3. "Beading" of the costochondral junction (rachitic rosary) is seen.
4. Depression along the line of the diaphragmatic attachment to the ribs (Harrison's groove) is evident.

5. Wrists and ankles are enlarged secondary to flaring of the epiphyses.
6. The long bones exhibit anterior curvature. (During infancy and early childhood, the long bones show the greatest abnormality.)
7. Spinal abnormalities include dorsal kyphosis, scoliosis, and lumbar lordosis. (These are the result of upright weight bearing and thus are more common in older children.)
8. Muscle weakness is present.
9. Waddling gait is seen.
10. The serum phosphate concentration is decreased.

11. Some common signs by age of the affected child include
    a. Infant: frontal bossing and flattening of the occipital portion of the skull.
    b. Young child: thickening of the forearm at the wrist, rachitic rosary, and Harrison's groove.
    c. Older child: bowing of the tibia and fibula.

CLINICAL SYMPTOMS

1. Bone pain may occur.
2. Growth failure may be exhibited.
3. Lethargy may be experienced.
4. Muscle weakness may be present.

MAJOR RADIOGRAPHIC FEATURES

1. A wide and irregular growth plate (slight widening of the growth plate is an early sign of rickets) is best identified in those most active growth regions.
2. The metaphyseal end of the bone may flare.
3. Bone density is diminished (particularly in the metaphyseal region adjacent to affected growth plates).
4. Widening and cupping of the growth plate may be seen.
5. Cortical thinning may be evident.
6. Pseudofractures (Looser zones) may be seen.
7. Coarse trabeculae may be present.
8. The calvarium in neonates may show posterior flattening.
9. The frontal and parietal bones in neonates may have a squared configuration.
10. The intervertebral discs may expand, with resultant concavity of the vertebrae.
11. Basilar invagination of the skull may be evident.
12. The horizontal orientation of the sacrum is greater than normal.
13. Scoliosis and long bone bowing deformity occur in later childhood.

RADIOGRAPHIC DIFFERENTIAL DIAGNOSIS

1. Fanconi's syndrome.
2. Secondary hyperparathyroidism.
3. In patients less than one year of age: biliary atresia and hypophosphatasia.

4. In patients resistant to the usual vitamin D therapy: renal disease, hypophosphatasia, and tumor-associated rickets (oncogenic osteomalacia).

MAJOR PATHOLOGIC FEATURES

1. Disorganization of the growth plate (disorderly columns of proliferating cartilage) and adjacent metaphysis is evident.
2. The growth plate exhibits widening.
3. Defective mineralization of the bone may be seen immediately subjacent to the growth plate.
4. Pseudofractures may occur.
5. Large amounts of nonmineralized bone are present.

PATHOLOGIC DIFFERENTIAL DIAGNOSIS

1. Osteomalacia.

PATHOGENESIS

1. Abnormalities of vitamin D metabolism:
    a. Vitamin D deficiency: nutritional, malabsorption, lack of sun exposure for conversion of vitamin D to active metabolites. (In the United States, vitamin D deficiency is most commonly related to malabsorption.)
    b. Deficient dermal vitamin D conversion: renal failure, aging.
    c. Deficient hepatic synthesis: primary biliary cirrhosis, biliary atresia.
    d. Defective renal synthesis: hypoparathyroidism, renal failure, oncogenic osteomalacia.
2. Phosphate deficiency:
    a. Deficient intake: excess aluminum hydroxide ingestion.
    b. Impaired renal resorption of phosphate.
3. Defects in mineralization:
    a. Enzyme deficiencies: hypophosphatasia.
    b. Circulating inhibitors of bone mineralization: drugs, bisphosphonates, fluoride, aluminum.
4. States of rapid bone formation: osteopetrosis, renal bone disease (osteitis fibrosa cystica).
5. Other conditions: parenteral hyperalimentation.

TREATMENT

1. Treatment depends upon the underlying cause but may include both medical and surgical approaches.
2. Medical approaches include
   a. Nutritional: ergocalciferol, vitamin D.
   b. Vitamin D supplemented with phosphates for vitamin D–resistant disease.
3. Surgical approaches are individualized depending upon the type of fracture or deformity present but may include
   a. Protected weight bearing for painful stress fracture.
   b. Closed versus open treatment of fracture.
   c. Corrective osteotomies for skeletal deformity.
   d. Epiphysiodesis in selected cases.

References

Gazit D, Tieder M, and Liberman UA: Osteomalacia in hereditary hypophosphatemic rickets with hypercalciuria: a correlative clinical-histomorphometric study. J Clin Endocrinol Metab. 72(1):229–235, 1991.

Kaplan FS, August CS, and Fallon MD: Osteopetrorickets. The paradox of plenty. Pathophysiology and treatment. Clin Orthop Rel Res 294:64–78, 1993.

Klein GL, and Simmons DJ: Nutritional rickets: thoughts about pathogenesis. Ann Med 25(4):379–384, 1993.

Pitt MJ: Rickets and osteomalacia are still around [review]. Radiol Clin North Am 29(1):97–118, 1991.

Sullivan W, Carpenter T, and Glorieux F: A prospective trial of phosphate and 1,25-dihydroxyvitamin D_3 therapy in symptomatic adults with X-linked hypophosphatemic rickets. J Clin Endocrinol Metab 75(3):879–885, 1992.

Weidner N: Review and update: oncogenic osteomalacia-rickets [review]. Ultrastruct Pathol 15(4–5):317–333, 1991.

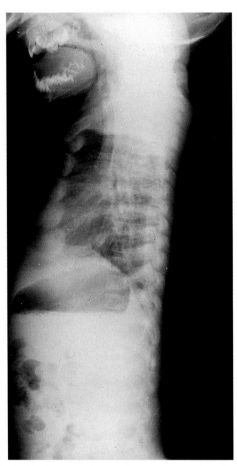

Figure 4–1. This lateral radiograph from a young child with rickets illustrates poor mineralization of the ribs, particularly in the region of the costochondral junction.

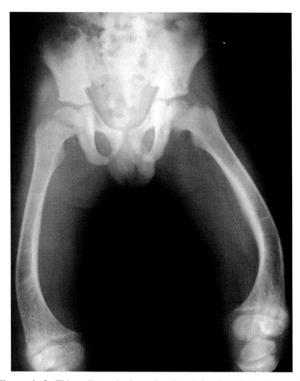

Figure 4–3. This radiograph shows bowing deformity of the femora in a six-year-old patient with rickets. Some metaphyseal flaring is evident in the distal femora, and a thickened bony cortex is present on the concave side of the bony deformity.

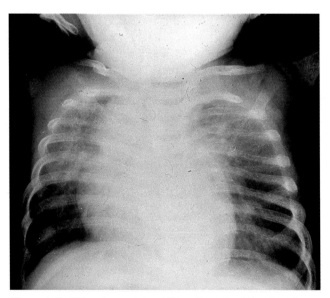

Figure 4–2. This anteroposterior (AP) radiograph of the chest from a young patient with rickets illustrates the irregular and poor mineralization of the ribs seen in this condition. In longstanding cases, the ribs may be deformed in the region of the diaphragmatic attachment, resulting in a groove (Harrison's groove).

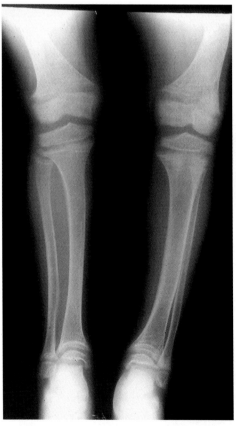

Figure 4–4. This radiograph illustrates widened growth plates and metaphyseal flaring in the distal femora and proximal tibiae bilaterally. Slight bowing of the tibia is evident in this eight-year-old girl with vitamin D–resistant rickets.

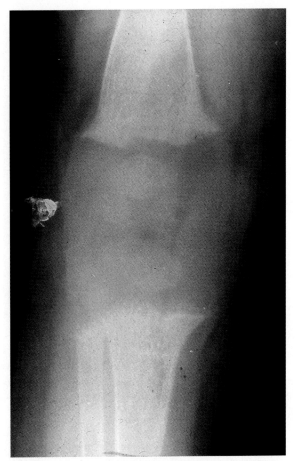

Figure 4–5. Marked rachitic changes are evident in this radiograph of the knee of a three-year-old patient. Metaphyseal flaring and some cupping deformity are present. The irregular appearance of the metaphyseal bone may be the result of irregularly shaped penetrations of the epiphyseal cartilage into the metaphyseal bone.

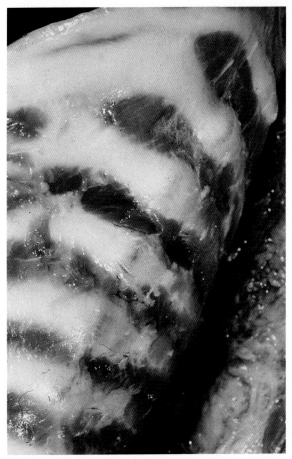

Figure 4–7. This photograph shows at higher magnification the enlargement of the costochondral cartilage that produces the characteristic rachitic rosary.

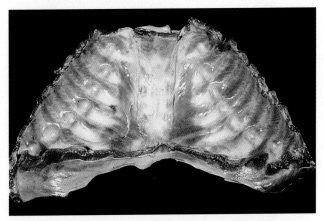

Figure 4–6. This photograph of the rib cage of a young patient who died with rickets illustrates the bilaterally symmetric enlargement of the costochondral cartilage that produces the so-called rachitic rosary.

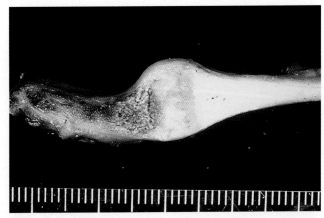

Figure 4–8. A cross-section of rib illustrates an abundance of cartilage forming an ellipsoid mass at the costochondral junction.

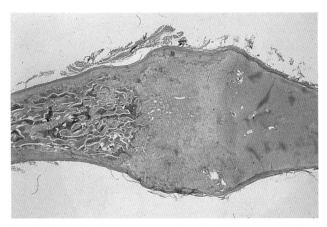

Figure 4–9. This histologic cross-section of a rib from the costochondral region shows an irregular proliferation of cartilage forming an enlarged mass of uncalcified cartilage.

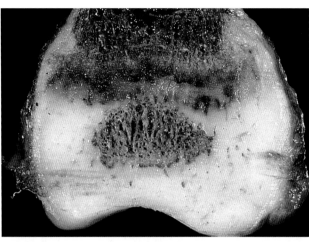

Figure 4–11. This cross-section of the distal femur in a young child who suffered from rickets shows widening of the epiphyseal growth plate as well as irregular masses of cartilage extending into the metaphyseal portion of the bone. These changes are typical of rickets.

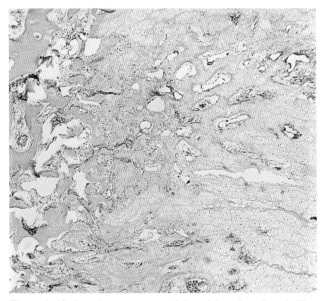

Figure 4–10. Irregular arrangement of the epiphyseal cartilage is illustrated in this photomicrograph. Note the absence of normal calcification of the cartilage.

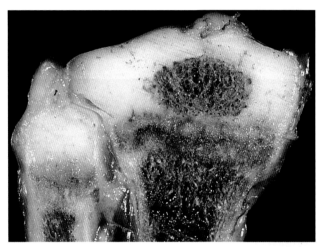

Figure 4–12. This cross-section of the proximal tibia and fibula illustrates features similar to those shown in Figure 4–11.

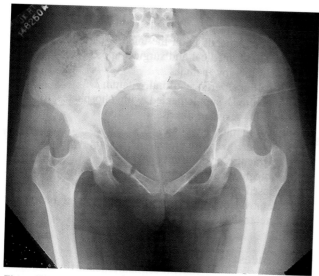

Figure 5–1. Pelvic radiograph of a patient with osteomalacia showing generalized osteopenia. Pelvic pseudofracture is also evident. Similar fractures may occur in the small bones of the feet; however, the axial skeleton is more commonly involved than the appendicular skeleton. Pseudofractures represent zones of nonmineralized osteoid commonly found in regions where vessels cross near the bone.

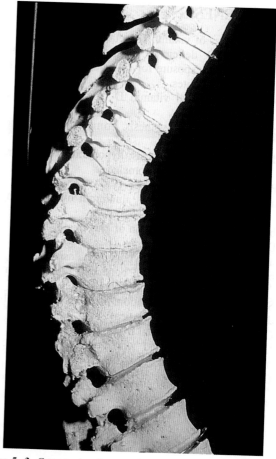

Figure 5–3. Compression fractures, illustrated in this gross pathologic specimen, are commonly identified in patients with longstanding osteomalacia. Radiographically, the osteomalacic vertebrae may bear a superficial resemblance to vertebrae affected by Paget's disease of bone.

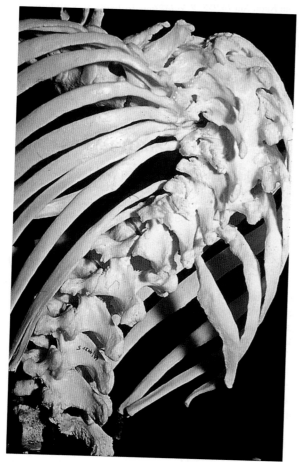

Figure 5–2. This photograph of a gross pathologic specimen illustrates the deformation associated with longstanding osteomalacia. Such bowing is commonly seen in long bones.

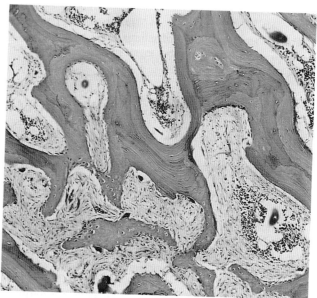

Figure 5–4. This photomicrograph illustrates the histologic features of osteomalacia in a patient suffering from sprue. The biopsy specimen is from the ilium and shows apparent irregular mineralization of the bony trabeculae reflective of poor mineralization of the osteoid. Osteomalacia is difficult to diagnose without the use of non-decalcified specimens or tetracycline labeling prior to bone biopsy.

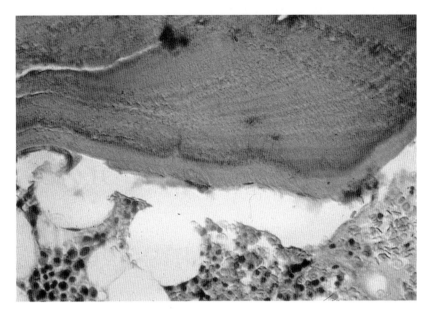

Figure 5-5. This photomicrograph shows the wide layer of nonmineralized osteoid that characterizes osteomalacia. Von Kossa or trichrome stains (see Figures 5-6 and 5-7) more dramatically demonstrate the absence of calcification; however, the same feature is subtly noticeable in well-developed cases of osteomalacia when evaluated with hematoxylin and eosin-stained sections.

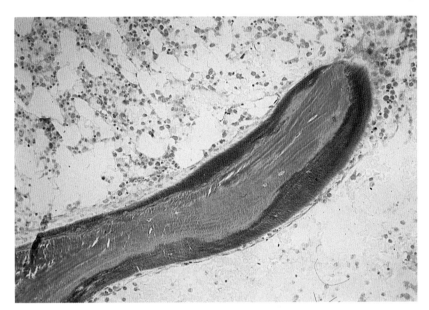

Figure 5-6. This trichrome stain dramatically demonstrates the increased nonmineralized bone in patients with osteomalacia. Morphometric analysis typically reveals that such nonmineralized bony matrix represents more than 10 per cent of the bone mass.

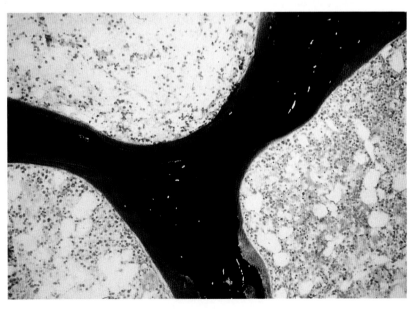

Figure 5-7. This von Kossa stain also illustrates the thick layer of osteoid covering mineralized bone in a patient with osteomalacia. The black staining corresponds to regions of calcified matrix in the biopsy specimen.

CHAPTER 6

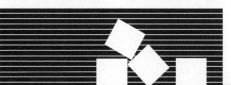

Tumor-Associated Rickets and Osteomalacia (Oncogenic Osteomalacia)

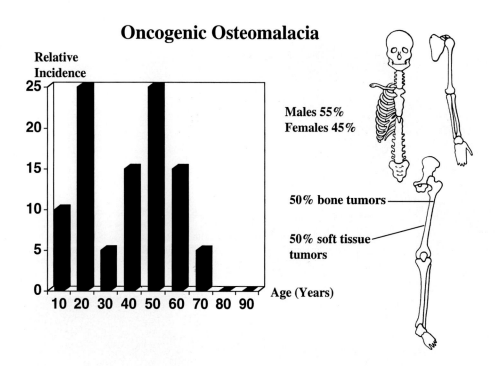

Oncogenic Osteomalacia

Males 55%
Females 45%

50% bone tumors

50% soft tissue tumors

CLINICAL SIGNS

1. Generalized muscle weakness may be present.
2. Hypophosphatemia is the major biochemical abnormality.
3. Serum calcium concentrations are normal to slightly decreased.
4. Serum alkaline phophatase concentrations are variably elevated.
5. Serum concentrations of 1,25-dihydroxyvitamin D are decreased or undetectable.
6. Parathyroid hormone concentrations are increased in approximately half the patients.

Oncogenic Osteomalacia

Relative Incidence

Age Distribution for Patients with Bone Tumors

Males 55%
Females 45%

Most common location for bone tumors resulting in oncogenic osteomalacia

Age (Years)

CLINICAL SYMPTOMS

1. There is a gradual onset of pain in the lower back, lower legs, hips, and/or ankles.
2. Pain is frequently accompanied by generalized muscular weakness and easy fatigability.
3. Patients may be so debilitated as to be bedridden.
4. Symptoms may precede the identification of the tumor by months to years (approximately 60 per cent of patients have had symptoms for one to five years and 20 per cent for five to ten years).
5. Joint pain may be present.
6. An affected bone may fracture with minor trauma.

MAJOR RADIOGRAPHIC FEATURES

Bone Findings Apart from Tumor

1. Generalized osteopenia may be present.
2. Multiple bilaterally symmetric cortical lucent areas may be seen.
3. Pseudofractures or cortical lucent areas may show increased uptake on isotope bone scan (in approximately 20 per cent of cases), particularly of the long bones and wrists.
4. Bone scan may be more sensitive in identifying multiple abnormal areas of increased isotope uptake.

Tumor

1. The radiographic features of the bone tumor are those of
   a. Fibrous dysplasia.
   b. Osteosarcoma.
   c. Chondroblastoma.
   d. Chondromyxoid fibroma.
   e. Giant cell tumor.
   f. Metaphyseal fibrous defect.
   g. Hemangioma.
   h. Other.
2. Tumors associated with osteomalacia may also be of soft tissue origin.

RADIOGRAPHIC DIFFERENTIAL DIAGNOSIS

1. Rickets not associated with a tumor.
2. Osteomalacia not associated with a tumor.
3. Hypophosphatemic rickets and osteomalacia associated with ifosfamide chemotherapy.

MAJOR PATHOLOGIC FEATURES

1. Tumors associated with oncogenic osteomalacia (approximately half are primary soft tissue tumors, and half are primary bone tumors) include
   a. Vascular tumors (approximately half of all tumors show a vascular histologic pattern):
      i. Hemangiopericytoma.
      ii. Hemangioma.
      iii. "Fibrovascular" lesions.
   b. Giant cell lesions:
      i. Giant cell tumor of bone.
      ii. Soft tissue giant cell tumors.
      iii. Other (e.g., pigmented villonodular synovitis [PVNS], malignant fibrous histiocytoma [MFH]).
   c. Metaphyseal fibrous defect.
   d. Osteoblastoma.
   e. Fibrous dysplasia.
   f. Phosphaturic mesenchymal tumor.
   g. Other.

2. The pathologic features of the osteomalacia are identical to those of osteomalacia not associated with a tumor.

PATHOLOGIC DIFFERENTIAL DIAGNOSIS

1. Osteomalacia (apart from the tumor that is causing the osteomalacia, the histologic features are identical to those of osteomalacia not associated with a tumor).
2. Rickets not associated with a tumor.
3. Histologic features of fibrous dysplasia, osteosarcoma, chondroblastoma, chondromyxoid fibroma, malignant fibrous histiocytoma, giant cell tumor, metaphyseal fibrous defect, hemangioma, or a soft tissue tumor—revealed by biopsy of the lesion causing the osteomalacia.

TREATMENT

1. Any patient with nondietary hypophosphatemic osteomalacia or rickets should be evaluated for a tumor.
2. If no tumor is found, then the patient should be treated with phosphate salts and vitamin D.
3. If the urinary phosphate concentration does not decrease and the serum phosphate concentration increases after tumor removal, then incomplete tumor removal should be suspected.

References

Cotton GE, and Van Puffelen P: Hypophosphatemic osteomalacia secondary to neoplasia. J Bone Joint Surg (Am) 68:129–133, 1986.
McClure J, and Smith PS: Oncogenic osteomalacia. J Clin Pathol 40:446–453, 1987.
Park YK, Unni KK, Beabout JW, et al: Oncogenic osteomalacia: a clinicopathologic study of 17 bone lesions. J Korean Med Sci 9:289–298, 1994.
Salassa RM, Jowsey J, and Arnaud CD: Hypophosphatemic osteomalacia associated with "non-endocrine" tumors. N Engl J Med 283:65–70, 1970.
Weidner N, and Santa Cruz D: Phosphaturic mesenchymal tumors: a polymorphous group causing osteomalacia or rickets. Cancer 59:1442, 1987.

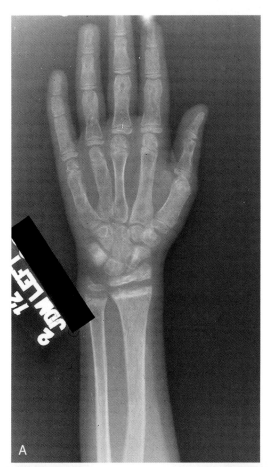

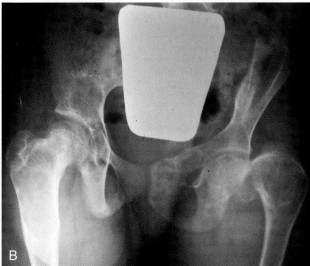

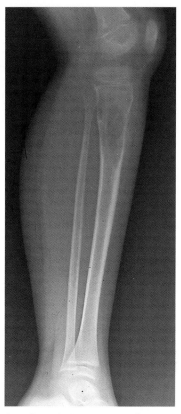

Figure 6–2. This radiograph shows a case of oncogenic osteomalacia associated with an osteosarcoma of the proximal tibia. The physes are widened, and flaring of the metaphyseal region of the distal tibia is also evident.

Figure 6–1. *A*, This radiograph illustrates changes of polyostotic fibrous dysplasia in the small bones. The growth plates of the distal radius and ulna are widened, showing radiographic features of osteomalacia. *B*, Characteristic radiographic features of fibrous dysplasia are evident in this pelvic radiograph of the seven-year-old female patient whose fibrous dysplasia was associated with osteomalacia (*A*).

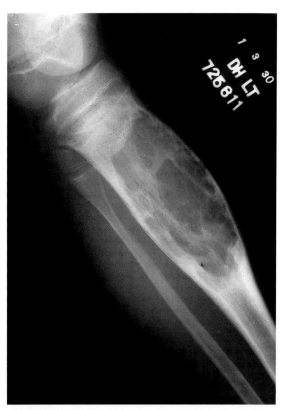

Figure 6–3. This radiograph illustrates a case of tumor-associated osteomalacia. The proximal fibial tumor is a chondromyxoid fibroma that occurred in a 13-year-old patient.

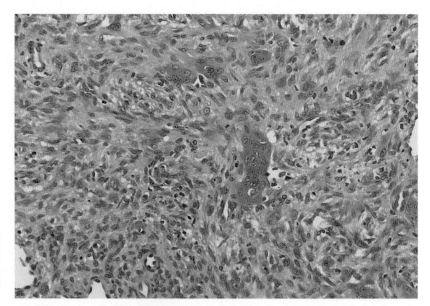

Figure 6–4. This photomicrograph illustrates the histologic features of a phosphaturic mesenchymal tumor. Lesions such as this may be of bone or soft tissue origin. This tumor was a soft tissue tumor in the leg. The tumors may be very small and difficult to localize clinically.

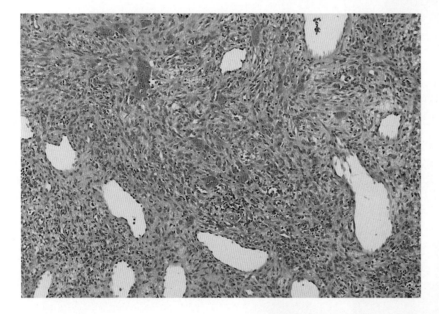

Figure 6–5. This photomicrograph demonstrates a tumor with hemangiopericytomatous histology that was associated with osteomalacia. Many of the neoplasms associated with osteomalacia have a prominent vascular pattern.

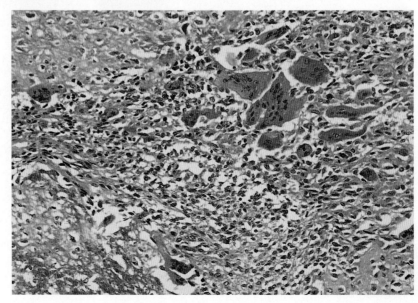

Figure 6–6. Phosphaturic mesenchymal tumors may show diffuse, fine, lacelike calcification. Multinucleated giant cells may also be present, as illustrated in this tumor involving the navicular bone.

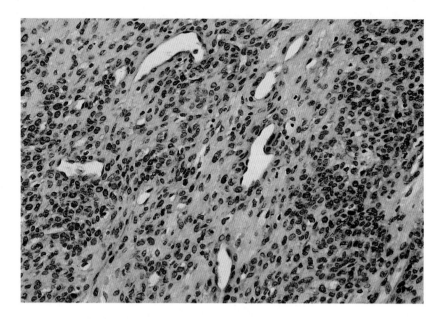

Figure 6–7. This tumor from the humerus was associated with osteomalacia. A hemangiopericytomatous pattern of growth is evident. Excision of the tumor resulted in resolution of the osteomalacia.

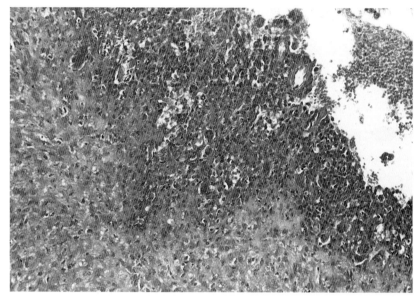

Figure 6–8. This photomicrograph illustrates the histologic pattern of giant cell tumor with secondary aneurysmal bone cyst changes. This tumor of the ilium in a 41-year-old woman was associated with osteomalacia.

CHAPTER 7

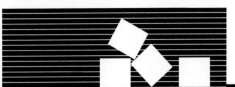

Paget's Disease

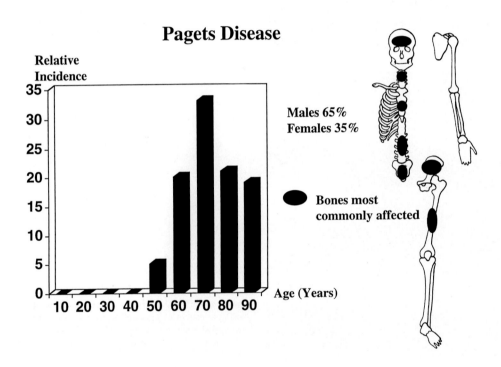

Pagets Disease

Relative Incidence

Males 65%
Females 35%

● Bones most commonly affected

Age (Years)

INCIDENCE

1. Paget's disease is most common in individuals of Northern European origin (approximately 33 per cent of the European population).
2. The male-to-female ratio is approximately 2:1.
3. The most common locations are the innominate bone and femur.
4. Based upon routine radiographic evaluation of the pelvis and lumbar vertebrae, the incidence has been estimated to rise from approximately 3.5 per 1000 to greater than 90 per 1000 between the fourth and ninth decades of life in Northern European countries.

5. Autopsy studies indicate an incidence of approximately 3.5 per cent in patients older than 40 years of age. (Approximately 90 per cent of symptomatic patients are over 40 years of age.)

CLINICAL SIGNS

1. Fracture may occur.
2. Arthritis may be present.
3. Heart failure may occur.
4. The serum alkaline phosphatase concentration is elevated.

5. Serum calcium and phosphorus concentrations are within normal limits.
6. The serum calcium concentration increases with prolonged bed rest.
7. Bone deformity is present in approximately 25 per cent of patients (e.g., forehead prominence, bowing of long bones).
8. Bone pain or periosteal tenderness may be present.
9. An extremity may show increased warmth.
10. Paget's sarcoma is characterized by
    a. A painful mass felt in the region of the affected bone.
    b. Rapidly progressive symptoms.

CLINICAL SYMPTOMS

1. Pain—constant, aching, and diffuse in nature—is felt in the affected region and is the presenting complaint in approximately half the patients. Increased pain in one bone in a patient with Paget's disease should arouse suspicion of the development of a sarcoma.
2. Hearing impairment may be present.
3. Dentures may be ill-fitting.
4. There may be difficulties with mastication.

Note: Approximately only one third of the sites of pagetic bone disease result in clinical symptoms.

MAJOR RADIOGRAPHIC FEATURES

1. There is a propensity to involve the lumbar spine, pelvis, skull, femur, and tibia.
2. The skull shows the following features:
    a. Early changes: well-marginated radiolucent defects (osteoporosis circumscripta).
    b. Late changes: bone thickened and of increased density (radiodense foci with a cotton-wool appearance).
3. The vertebral bodies have a "picture frame" appearance, showing increased width.
4. In long bones the lucent defect extends to the end of the affected bone, with sharp demarcation from uninvolved bone; the junction between affected and unaffected bone is wedge-shaped ("flame" sign or "blade of grass" sign).

5. Fractures that occur through pagetoid long bones are characteristically transverse ("banana" fracture).
6. Fractures are frequently associated with excessive callus formation.
7. The bone scan shows more pagetic sites of osseous involvement than are identified using routine radiographic evaluation, however, once the disease is in the inactive sclerotic phase, the bone scan may not yield positive findings.
8. The computed tomographic (CT) scan is particularly helpful in excluding the possibility of sarcomatous transformation in Paget's disease (examination of the cortex for cortical destruction).
9. There is a high incidence of arthritis and joint narrowing adjacent to the involved bone or bones.
10. Paget's sarcoma is characterized by:
    a. The bone of origin usually showing the changes of Paget's disease.
    b. Extension of the tumor into the surrounding soft tissue (magnetic resonance imaging [MRI] may show this best).
    c. A pattern of geographic bone destruction.
    d. A predilection for the humerus, the tumor only rarely arising in the spine (in comparison with the location of uncomplicated Paget's disease).

Note: Although most cases of Paget's disease progress through the active osteolytic phase to the osteosclerotic stage and remain relatively stable, reversion from the sclerotic to the osteolytic phase can occur. In general, however, if a lytic region is identified within a region of pagetoid bone that has previously been osteosclerotic radiographically, then sarcomatous degeneration should be excluded.

RADIOGRAPHIC DIFFERENTIAL DIAGNOSIS

1. Metastatic carcinoma.
2. Fibrous dysplasia.
3. Malignant lymphoma.
4. Hyperparathyroidism (if vertebral disease presents in a "rugger jersey" pattern).
5. Vertebral hemangioma.

6. Malignant lymphoma (when the spine is involved).

MAJOR PATHOLOGIC FEATURES

1. The disease is arbitrarily divided into three phases:
   a. Osteolytic phase: marrow space replaced by highly vascular fibrous connective tissue; active osteoclastic resorption; prominent osteoblastic new bone formation.
   b. Osteoblastic phase: trabecular plates widened but in a haphazard manner, leading to the mosaic pattern (increased number of cement lines).
   c. "Burnt-out" phase: less cellularity and reduced vascularity of the marrow space.
2. Histologic features include
   a. Mosaic bone with accentuation of cement lines.
   b. Active bone remodeling early and quiescence late.
   c. Cancellous bone replaced by a network of disorganized-appearing thick bone trabeculae.
   d. Extremely vascular fibrous connective tissue occupying the intertrabecular space.
3. Paget's sarcoma is characterized by the following:
   a. Gross:
      i. A destructive lesion involves the bone and extends into the soft tissue.
      ii. The soft, fleshy tumor generally is whitish to brown.
   b. Microscopic:
      i. At low magnification, the tumor is highly cellular.
      ii. The tumor generally is composed of spindle cells.
      iii. At higher magnification, the spindle cells show significant pleomorphism and cytologic atypia.
      iv. The specific diagnosis may be that of osteosarcoma, fibrosarcoma, or malignant fibrous histiocytoma.

PATHOLOGIC DIFFERENTIAL DIAGNOSIS

1. Hyperparathyroidism.
2. Fibrous dysplasia.
3. Osteofibrous dysplasia.
4. Paget's sarcoma (if the lesion is in the florid lytic phase).

TREATMENT

Medical

1. Calcitonin is given.
2. Bisphosphonates (etidronate/pamidronate) are administered.

Surgical

1. Pathologic fracture is treated with closed versus open reduction.
2. Osteotomy is performed to correct deformity.
3. Arthroplasty is performed for advanced joint disease.

References

Bone HG, and Kleerekoper M: Clinical review 39: Paget's disease of bone [review]. J Clin Endocrinol Metab 75(5):1179–1182, 1992.

Bowerman JW, Altman J, Hughes JL, Zadek RE: Pseudo-malignant lesions in Paget's disease of bone. Am J Roentgenol Radium Ther Nucl Med 124:57–61, 1975.

Chapman GK: The diagnosis of Paget's disease of bone [review]. Aust N Z J Surg 62(1):24–32, 1992.

Gallacher SJ: Paget's disease of bone [review]. Curr Opin Rheumatol 5(3):351–356, 1993.

Greenspan A: A review of Paget's disease: radiologic imaging, differential diagnosis, and treatment [review]. Bull Hosp Jt Dis Orthop Inst 51(1):22–33, 1991.

Griffiths HJ: Radiology of Paget's disease [review]. Curr Opin Rheumatol 4(6):124–128, 1992.

Haibach H, Farrell C, and Dittrich FJ: Neoplasms arising in Paget's disease of bone: a study of 82 cases. Am J Clin Pathol 83:596–600, 1985.

Hamdy RC, Moore S, and LeRoy J: Clinical presentation of Paget's disease of the bone in older patients. South Med J 86(10):1097–1100, 1993.

Milgram JW: Radiographical and pathological assessment of the activity of Paget's disease of bone. Clin Orthop Rel Res 127:43, 1977.

Mirra JM, Brien EW, and Tehranzadeh J: Paget's disease of bone: review with emphasis on radiologic features, Parts I and II. Skeletal Radiol 24:163–171, 1995.

Wick MR, Siegal GP, McLeod RA, et al: Sarcomas of bone-complicating osteitis deformans (Paget's disease): fifty years' experience. Am J Surg Pathol 5:47–59, 1981.

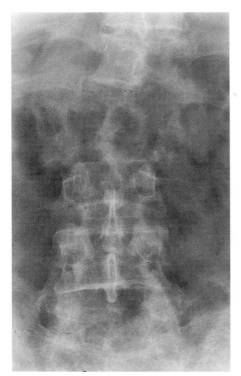

Figure 7–1. The radiographic appearance of Paget's disease involving a vertebra may simulate malignancy, as illustrated in this case. The florid lytic phase of the disease may radiographically simulate sarcoma or metastatic carcinoma. Other vertebral changes associated with Paget's disease include enlargement of the vertebra and peripheral sclerosis, resulting in a "picture frame" appearance of the vertebra.

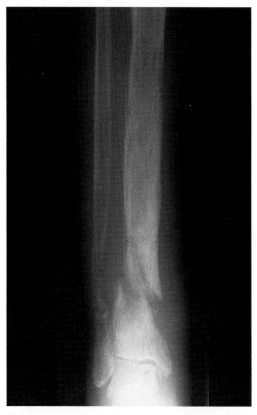

Figure 7–3. A typical fracture through pagetoid bone is illustrated in this radiograph. This "banana"-type transverse fracture most commonly involves the femur or tibia and is often associated with minimal or no trauma.

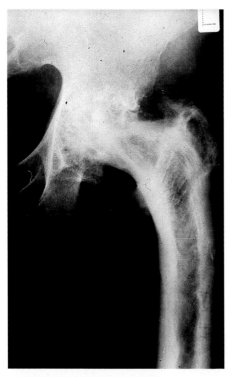

Figure 7–2. This radiograph of the proximal femur demonstrates Paget's disease involving a long bone. Paget's disease always extends to the end of the bone, as illustrated in this example. Other common features include thickening of the cortex, expansion of the bone, and thickened bony trabeculae.

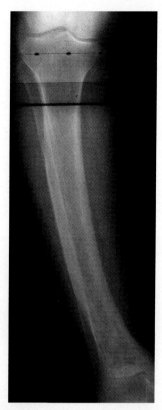

Figure 7–4. This radiograph shows the bowing bony deformity of Paget's disease involving the tibia.

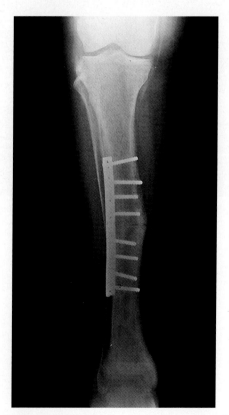

Figure 7–5. This radiograph shows the surgical approach to the correction of the bony deformity in Figure 7–4. Treatment of such bony deformities or fractures is complicated by the altered mechanical properties of pagetoid bone.

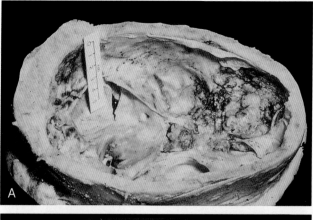

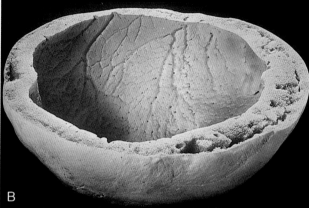

Figure 7–6. *A* and *B*, These two gross specimens illustrate the changes of Paget's disease involving the skull. Thickening of the skull as shown in these examples may compromise the foramina of cranial nerves, resulting in nerve loss. The thickened trabeculae eventually distort the normal diploetic architecture, as illustrated.

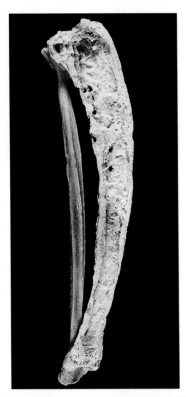

Figure 7–7. This gross specimen of the tibia and fibula shows the changes of Paget's disease involving the proximal tibia. Bowing related to the altered mechanical properties of the pagetoid bone has occurred.

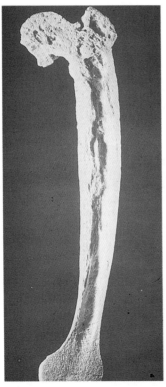

Figure 7–8. Paget's disease of the proximal femur is illustrated in this photograph of a gross specimen. Cortical thickening is evident, and the process extends to the proximal end of the femur. Transition from pagetoid bone to normal bone is usually abrupt unless the disease has been complicated by the development of a sarcoma.

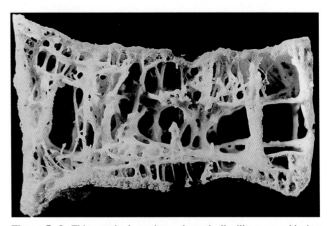

Figure 7–9. This vertebral specimen dramatically illustrates widening of the medullary bony trabeculae from a 72-year-old man with long-standing Paget's disease.

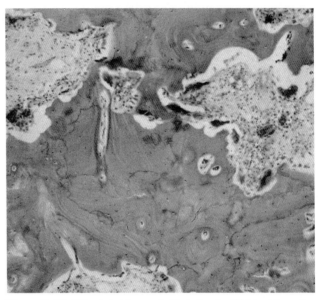

Figure 7–10. This photomicrograph illustrates the thickened bony trabeculae with prominent cement lines characteristic of Paget's disease. Numerous osteoclasts and increased osteoblastic activity are seen in this example as well. The irregular cement lines may be better appreciated in non-decalcified specimens.

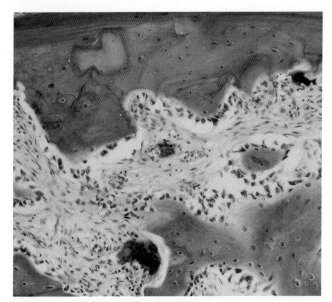

Figure 7–11. Higher magnification of the histologic features of pagetoid bone reveals increased osteoclastic and osteoblastic activity. Osteoclasts may be larger than normal in such cases. The medullary bone is also filled with a loose fibrovascular connective tissue that is frequently seen in Paget's disease.

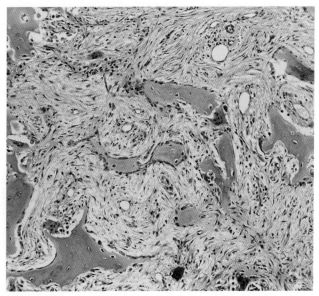

Figure 7–12. This example of well-developed Paget's disease shows the histologic features that can simulate those of fibrous dysplasia. The irregular pattern of pagetoid bone in association with the fibrous tissue replacement of the medullary contents can result in a confusing histologic pattern for the pathologist.

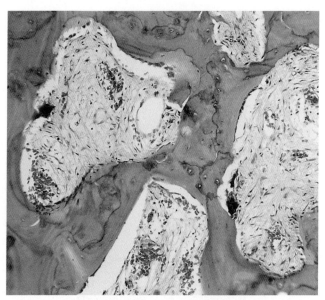

Figure 7–13. Irregular cement lines are often visible in pagetoid bone, even in decalcified specimens such as this one.

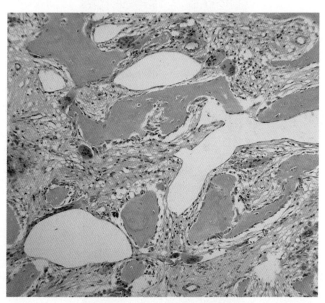

Figure 7–14. Increased vascularity of pagetoid bone is illustrated in this photomicrograph. Such vascularity may become so pronounced as to cause significant changes in the cardiovascular function of the affected patient. When the biopsy shows prominent vascularity in pagetoid bone, the differential diagnosis entertained by the pathologist may even include a vascular tumor.

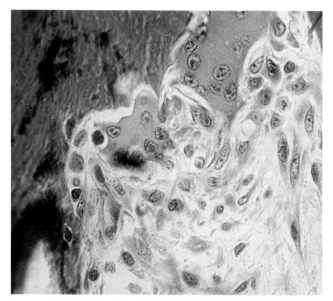

Figure 7–15. This trichrome stained section of pagetoid bone shows osteoclastic resorption of the trabecular bone. Osteoblastic deposition of osteoid is also evident.

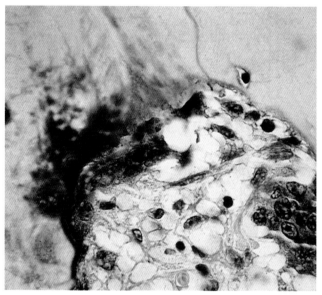

Figure 7–16. This acid phosphatase stain of pagetoid bone illustrates the enzymatic activity of osteoclasts.

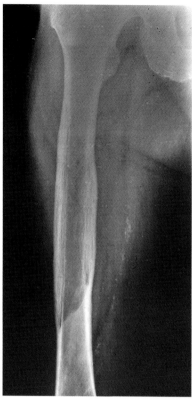

Figure 7–17. This radiograph illustrates the lytic phase of Paget's disease involving the proximal femur. The "blade of grass" appearance is evident in the proximal extent of the lesion.

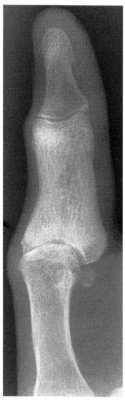

Figure 7–18. This radiograph illustrates sclerosis and expansion of the proximal phalanx of the thumb due to Paget's disease.

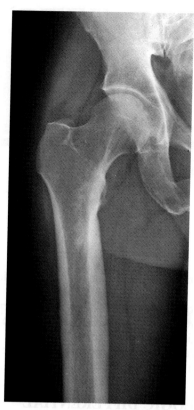

Figure 8–1. This radiograph illustrates the diffuse diaphyseal cortical thickening characteristic of Camurati-Engelmann disease. The patient was a 58-year-old man who presented with bilateral leg pain.

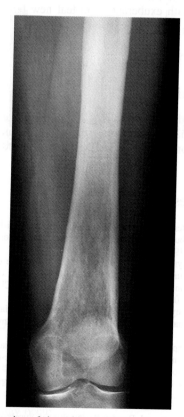

Figure 8–2. Sparing of the epiphyseal region, as shown in this radiograph, is characteristic of Camurati-Engelmann disease.

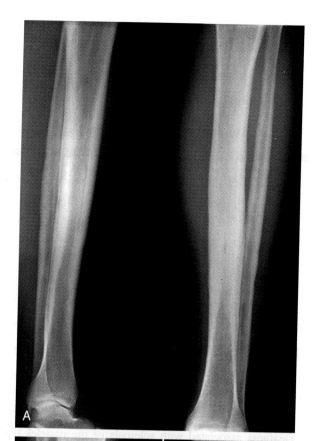

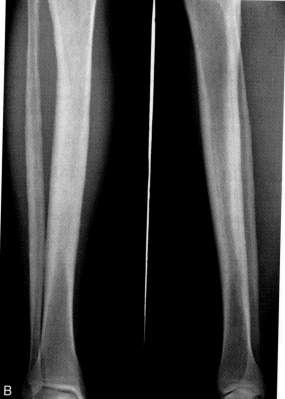

Figure 8–3. The bilateral symmetric nature of progressive diaphyseal dysplasia (Camurati-Engelmann disease) is evident in these radiographs of the right (*A*) and left (*B*) lower extremity.

6.

M

1.

2

3

4

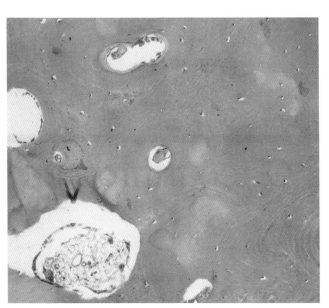

Figure 8–4. This photomicrograph illustrates the thickened cortical bone characteristic of Camurati-Engelmann disease. Increased osteoid may be seen.

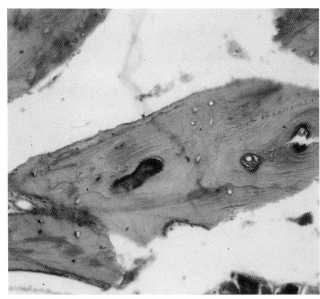

Figure 8–5. Although the bone of Camurati-Engelmann disease lacks the prominent cement lines associated with Paget's disease, this differentiation may be subtle, as shown in this photomicrograph of a specimen from the tibia in a patient with Camurati-Engelmann disease.

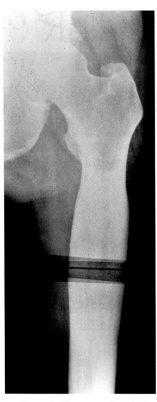

Figure 8–6. This radiograph illustrates the diaphyseal thickening of cortical bone seen in patients with Camurati-Engelmann disease. Although the disease begins early in life, sporadic cases with onset late in adult life have been reported.

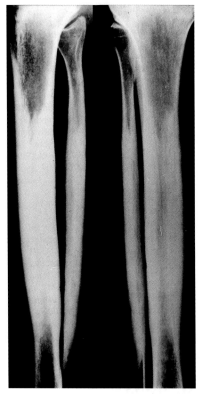

Figure 8–7. This radiograph of the lower extremities illustrates Camurati-Engelmann disease in a 67-year-old man. The skull and, rarely, vertebrae, small bones, clavicle, mandible, and pelvis can also be affected.

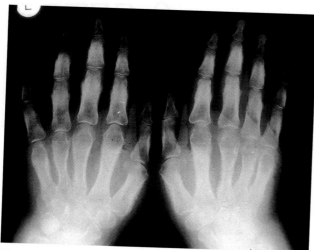

Figure 9–1. This radiograph shows the hands of a 62-year-old man with pulmonary hypertrophic osteoarthropathy. Clubbing of the fingers is due in part to thickening of the subungual soft tissues. Other changes that may be seen involving the small bones include periosteal new bone formation.

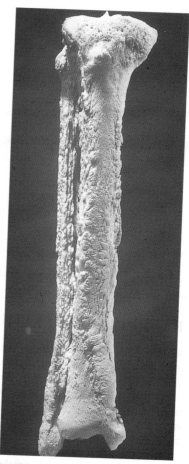

Figure 9–3. This macerated gross specimen of the tibia and fibula from a 58-year-old woman with pulmonary osteoarthropathy illustrates the dramatic thickening and irregularity of the cortical new bone characteristic of the condition.

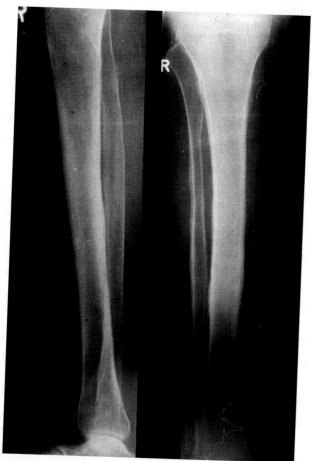

Figure 9–2. Thick periosteal new bone is often seen in the region of painful, swollen joints in pulmonary hypertrophic osteoarthropathy. These features are similar to those in patients with rheumatoid arthritis. This radiograph illustrates periosteal new bone formation in a 77-year-old woman with pulmonary hypertrophic osteoarthropathy.

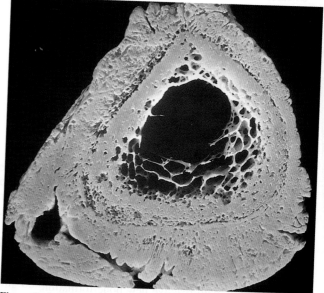

Figure 9–4. This cross-section of macerated tibia is from the specimen illustrated in Figure 9–3. It shows that the new bone is entirely on the periosteal surface, whereas the endosteal surface and medullary bone are relatively preserved.

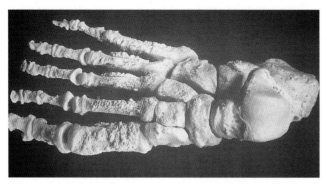

Figure 9–5. This macerated gross specimen illustrates changes in the small bones of the foot. Marked periosteal new bone formation and resultant distortion of the affected bones are evident.

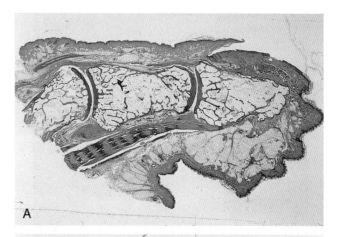

A

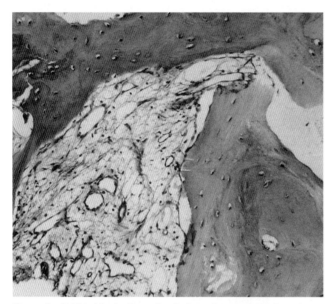

Figure 9–6. This histologic section is from the mature periosteal new bone seen in pulmonary hypertrophic osteoarthropathy. No characteristics of this new bone distinguish it from other conditions that result in periosteal new bone deposition. On occasion, a mononuclear cell infiltrate may also be present, suggesting that the new bone formed is related to inflammation in the adjacent joint.

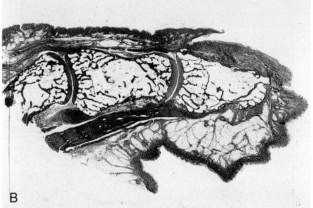

B

Figure 9–7. A and B, These two photomicrographs show the finger of a patient with idiopathic pulmonary fibrosis. Clubbing of the fingers related to soft tissue swelling is evident. The joints are unaffected.

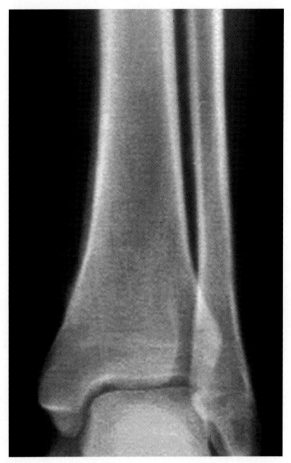

Figure 9–8. Anteroposterior (AP) roentgenogram of the distal tibia and ankle in a patient with pulmonary hypertrophic osteoarthropathy. Note the benign-appearing, laminated periosteal new bone formation of the distal tibial metaphysis. In most instances, bilateral changes are apparent.

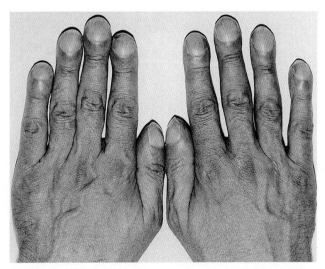

Figure 9–9. This photograph illustrates the clinical appearance of clubbing of the fingers associated with pulmonary hypertrophic osteoarthropathy in a patient with carcinoma of the lung.

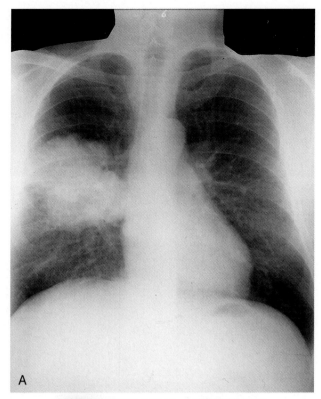

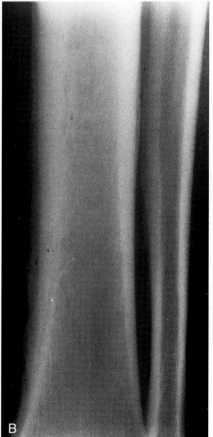

Figure 9–10. The chest radiograph (*A*) reveals a large carcinoma of the lung. The patient had leg pain and radiographic evidence of pulmonary hypertrophic osteoarthropathy involving the tibia and fibula (*B*).

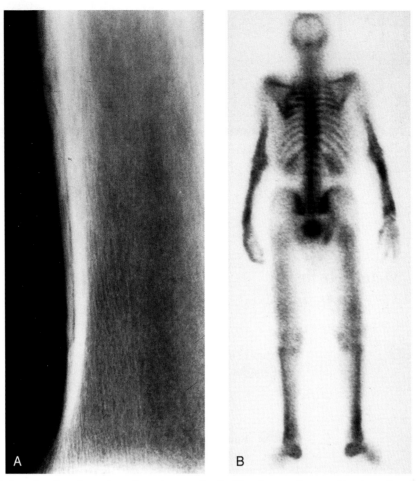

Figure 9–11. *A,* The diaphyseal periosteal new bone formation associated with pulmonary hypertrophic osteoarthropathy is illustrated in this radiograph. *B,* Such regions of periosteal new bone formation are hot on bone scan.

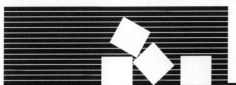

CHAPTER 10

Melorheostosis

Melorheostosis

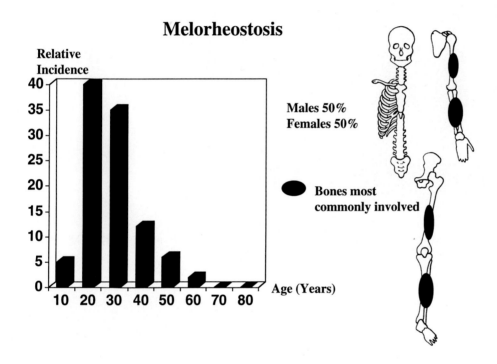

Relative Incidence vs. Age (Years)

Males 50%
Females 50%

● Bones most commonly involved

CLINICAL SIGNS

1. The long bones may exhibit deformity. (The lower limb is more commonly affected than the upper limb.)
2. Joint motion may be limited owing to contracture and fibrosis of the soft tissue in the region of the affected bone or bones.
3. The affected extremity may appear larger in circumference than normal.
4. The affected bone is usually shorter than normal.
5. The skin over the affected bone may be tense or erythematous.
6. Laboratory tests are usually within normal limits.

7. Fibromas, fibrolipomas, and capillary hemangiomas may be seen.

CLINICAL SYMPTOMS

1. Angular joint deviation may be present.
2. Limb length discrepancy may be exhibited.
3. Dull joint pain may be experienced. (Pain may be described as constant and low-grade.)
4. Joint contractures may occur.
5. Para-articular ossifications may be seen.
6. Muscle atrophy and patellar dislocation may occur.
7. Occasionally, the patient may be asymptomatic (more common in children than adults), and the finding is an incidental radiographic abnormality.

MAJOR RADIOGRAPHIC FEATURES

1. Cortical hyperostosis may be seen in a linear or segmental distribution, with sharp demarcation from the unaffected bone.
2. The characteristic appearance is that of melted wax dripping down the side of a candle.
3. The process may be monostotic or polyostotic or, rarely, may involve multiple limbs and the trunk.
4. The process may involve the shoulder or hip as well as the adjacent long bone.
5. When multiple bones are involved, the linear hyperostosis extends from one bone to the next in a nearly continuous manner.
6. If the process involves the lower portion of the leg or the forearm, then usually only one of the two bones is involved.
7. Periarticular soft tissue may also show ossification. (When present, it is usually in association with extensive bony disease.)
8. Dense islands of bone can occur in the epiphysis of the affected bone.
9. Bone scan may show increased uptake in the involved bones and soft tissue.
10. Sites of involvement include the lower limb, upper limb, skull, spine, ribs, and pelvis.
11. In children, the primary radiographic feature is endosteal hyperostosis, as compared with the well-developed features noted previously.
12. Extraosseous soft tissue masses and ossification may be present.

RADIOGRAPHIC DIFFERENTIAL DIAGNOSIS

1. Periostitis ossificans.
2. Myositis ossificans (heterotopic ossification).
3. Periosteal hematoma.

MAJOR PATHOLOGIC FEATURES

1. Hyperostotic bone is densely sclerotic.
2. Thickened lamellar bone may obliterate the haversian system.

3. New bone and cartilage may be present in the cartilage surrounding the affected joints.
4. Osteoclastic activity is not a prominent feature.
5. The marrow space may show some fibrous tissue proliferation.
6. Grossly, the cortex of the affected bone is thickened, with narrowing of the medullary canal.
7. Islands of dense bone may be present in the epiphyses of long bones and in the small bones of the hands and feet.

PATHOLOGIC DIFFERENTIAL DIAGNOSIS

1. Periostitis ossificans.
2. Myositis ossificans.
3. Periosteal hematoma.

TREATMENT

Medical

1. Pain can be controlled with analgesics.
2. Bracing can be used to prevent progressive joint contractures.

Surgical

1. Release of contractures can be accomplished.
2. Leg length inequality can be corrected.
3. Ilizarov gradual distraction may be more effective than traditional osteotomies because of neurovascular stretch injury.

References

Campbell CJ, Papademetriou T, and Bonfiglio M: Melorheostosis. A report of clinical, roentgenographic, and pathological findings in 14 cases. J Bone Joint Surg (Am) 50:1281–1304, 1968.

Dimar JR, and Campion TS: Melorheostosis: two case presentations and review of the literature. Orthop Rev 16:615–621, 1987.

Murray RO, and McCredie J: Melorheostosis and the sclerotomes. A radiological correlation. Skeletal Radiol 4:57–71, 1979.

Yu JS, Resnick D, Vaughan LM, et al: Melorheostosis with an ossified soft tissue mass: MR features. Skeletal Radiol 24:367–370, 1995.

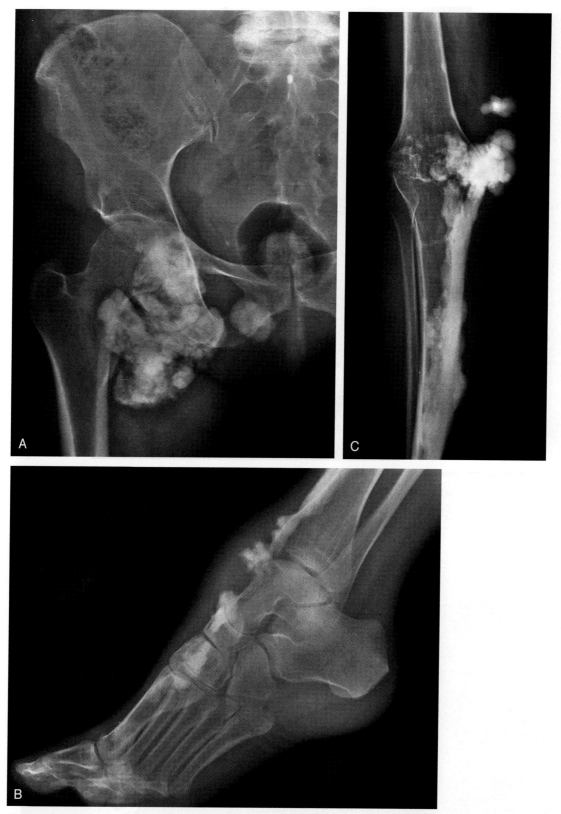

Figure 10–5. *A,* Anteroposterior (AP) roentgenogram of the right hemipelvis and hip in a patient with melorheostosis. Note the tumoral calcinosis with a large lobulated calcified mass adjacent to the right hip. *B,* Lateral roentgenogram of the foot showing cortical thickening and the flowing candle wax type of appearance seen in classic melorheostosis. *C,* AP roentgenogram of the knee and proximal tibia showing similar findings, with both a cortical base and soft tissue involvement.

CHAPTER 11

Osteopetrosis

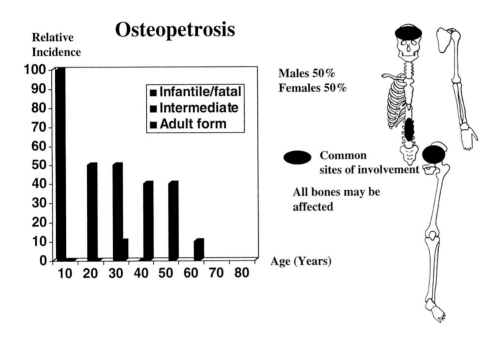

Osteopetrosis

Relative Incidence

■ Infantile/fatal
■ Intermediate
■ Adult form

Age (Years)

Males 50%
Females 50%

Common sites of involvement

All bones may be affected

Synonyms: Osteopetrosis is also called marble bone disease, congenital osteosclerosis, and Albers-Schönberg disease.

CLINICAL SIGNS

1. Clinical signs depend upon the type of disease (mode of inheritance). Autosomal recessive disease may result in intrauterine or early childhood death.

In the Newborn or Infant

1. Anemia or pancytopenia may be present.
2. Hepatosplenomegaly may be seen.
3. Failure to thrive and infections may occur.
4. Early death may occur.

In Childhood (Autosomal Recessive Inheritance)

1. Physical growth may be retarded.
2. Multiple fractures may occur.
3. Osteomyelitis may complicate up to 10 per cent of cases.
4. Cranial nerve palsies are present in approximately 15 per cent of cases, with particular propensity to involve cranial nerves II, III, and VII.

In Adulthood (Autosomal Dominant)

1. Approximately 45 per cent of patients in this group may be asymptomatic.
2. Bone pain is present in approximately 20 per cent of patients in this group.

3. Carpal tunnel syndrome may be seen.
4. Multiple fractures are present in approximately 40 per cent of patients in this group; more than 30 fractures have been seen in a single patient.
5. Osteomyelitis is present in approximately 10 per cent of patients in this group.
6. Cranial nerve palsies are present in approximately 5 per cent of patients in this group.
7. The serum acid phosphatase concentration is elevated in the majority of patients.

CLINICAL SYMPTOMS

1. Loss of hearing may occur.
2. Loss of vision may occur.
3. Multiple fractures are the major symptom in 40 per cent of adult patients.
4. Bone pain is reported in approximately 25 per cent of adults, particularly in the lumbar region.
5. Recurrent infections may be experienced.
6. Spontaneous bruising and bleeding may be seen.

MAJOR RADIOGRAPHIC FEATURES

1. The entire skeleton shows a diffuse marked increase in density.
2. Bones are shortened.
3. Metaphyses may be wider than normal.
4. Loss of corticomedullary differentiation may be seen.
5. In less severe cases, there are alternating areas of affected and apparently normal bone, resulting in a somewhat "striped" appearance.
6. A "bone within a bone" appearance may be seen (particularly in the tarsals, vertebral bodies, phalanges, and iliac wings).
7. In the adult autosomal dominant form of the disease, a "rugger jersey" spine appearance may be present owing to radiodensity of the superior and inferior portions of the vertebral body.
8. Computed tomographic (CT) scan is helpful in assessing the diameter of the auditory and optic canals.
9. Magnetic resonance imaging (MRI) is helpful in assessing the degree of marrow activity in the patient with osteopetrosis. (In the infantile autosomal reces-

sive form of the disease, there is a lack of marrow signal from the vertebral bodies.)
10. Bone scan is helpful in identifying cases complicated by osteomyelitis. (Osteomyelitis in this condition has a propensity to involve the mandible.)
11. Autosomal dominant osteopetrosis may be classified into at least three subtypes based upon radiographic appearance. The following table summarizes the major features of each type.

Radiographic Finding	Type I	Type II	Type III
Generalized	+	+	+
Calvarial sclerosis	+	−	+
Skull base sclerosis	−	+	−
"Rugger jersey" spine	−	+	−
Pelvic "endobones"	−	+	+

Modified from Kovacs, et al.

RADIOGRAPHIC DIFFERENTIAL DIAGNOSIS

1. Widespread osteoblastic metastases.
2. Chronic fluorosis.
3. Myelosclerosis.
4. Idiopathic osteosclerosis.
5. Melorheostosis.
6. Mastocytosis.

MAJOR PATHOLOGIC FEATURES
Gross

1. The metadiaphyseal bone is widened, resulting in an Erlenmeyer flask–like appearance.
2. Bone has increased mass per unit volume.
3. Bone tends to be smaller than normal.
4. Bone is dense when cut in cross-section.

Histologic

1. Irregular bone surrounding a cartilage core may be seen.
2. Osteoclasts may be reduced in number.

3. Marrow space may be diminished or absent.
4. Epiphyseal microfractures may be present.
5. Prominent cement lines may be seen.

PATHOLOGIC DIFFERENTIAL DIAGNOSIS

1. Fracture callus (if the biopsy specimen is from the region of a healing fracture).
2. Other sclerosing bone dysplasias.

TREATMENT

Medical

1. Bone marrow transplantation may be performed.
2. Back pain is treated conservatively (rest, bracing, nonsteroidal anti-inflammatory drugs [NSAIDs]).

Surgical

1. Fractures are treated conventionally. (Healing may be delayed.)
2. Osteotomy is for long bone deformity and coxa vara.

References

Andersen PE Jr, and Bollerslev J: Heterogeneity of autosomal dominant osteopetrosis. Radiology *164*:223–225, 1987.

Coccia P, Krivit W, Cervenka J, et al: Successful bone-marrow transplantation for infantile malignant osteopetrosis. N Engl J Med *302*:701–708, 1980.

El-Tawil T, and Stoker DJ: Benign osteopetrosis: a review of 42 cases showing two different patterns. Skeletal Radiol 22:587–593, 1993.

Greenspan A: Sclerosing bone dysplasias—a target-site approach. Skeletal Radiol *20*:561–583, 1991.

Helfrich MH, Aronson DC, Everts V, et al: Morphologic features of bone in human osteopetrosis. Bone *12(6)*:411–419, 1991.

Kolawole TM, Hawass ND, Patel PJ, and Mahdi AH: Osteopetrosis: some unusual radiological features with a short review. Eur J Radiol *8*:89–95, 1988.

Kovacs CS, Lambert RGW, Lavoie GJ, and Siminoski K: Centrifugal osteopetrosis: appendicular sclerosis with relative sparing of the vertebrae. Skeletal Radiol *24*:27–29, 1995.

Milgram JW, and Jasty M: Osteopetrosis: a morphologic study of twenty-one cases. J Bone Joint Surg (Am) *64*:912–929, 1982.

Shapiro F: Osteopetrosis. Current clinical considerations [review]. Clin Orthop Rel Res *(294)*:34–44, 1993.

Silvestrini G, Ferraccioli GF, Quaini F, et al: Adult osteopetrosis: study of two brothers. Appl Pathol *5*:184–189, 1987.

Singer FR, and Chang SS: Osteopetrosis [review]. Semin in Nephrol *12(2)*:191–199, 1992.

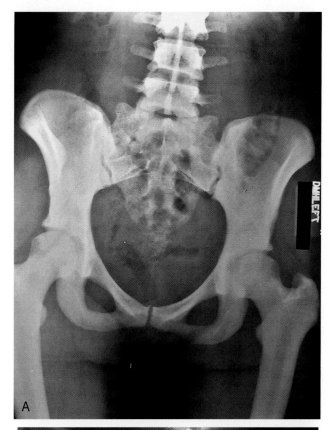

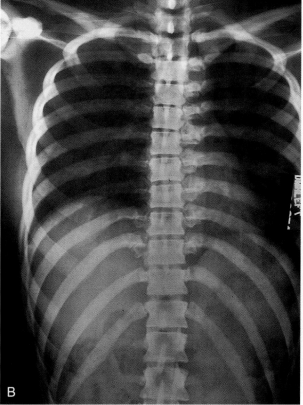

Figure 11–1. *A,* Anteroposterior (AP) roentgenogram of the pelvis and proximal femora in a patient with osteopetrosis. *B,* AP roentgenogram of the chest and thoracic spine. Note the focal cortical thickening of the glenoid and right shoulder.

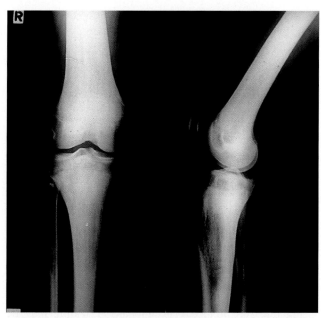

Figure 11–2. This radiograph illustrates the case of a 26-year-old man with osteopetrosis. The distal femur and proximal tibia are densely sclerotic, and some lack of metaphyseal remodeling is evident in the distal femur. Normal corticomedullary differentiation is not seen.

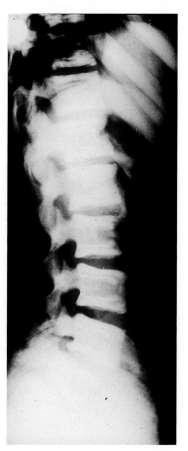

Figure 11–3. Osteopetrotic bone changes are evident in the vertebrae of this 21-year-old man. Increased density of the proximal and distal thirds of the vertebrae results in a striped pattern.

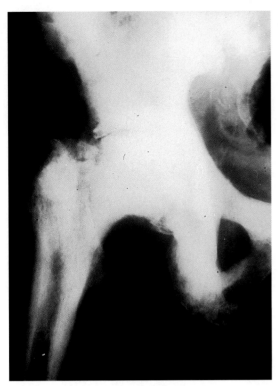

Figure 11–4. This radiograph of the proximal femur shows osteopetrosis in a 65-year-old man. Patients with less severe forms of this disease most commonly present with axial bony lesions or fractures through the mechanically inferior dense bone.

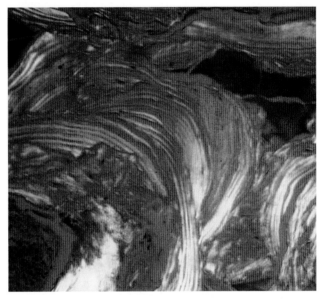

Figure 11–6. As shown in this photomicrograph, osteopetrotic bone, whether formed by endochondral ossification or from membranous bone, is abnormal. In the latter, primitive bone persists and cartilage cores are not seen.

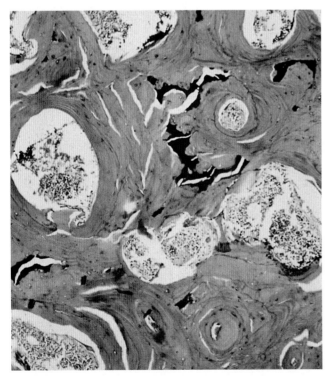

Figure 11–5. This photomicrograph of osteopetrotic bone shows the thickened and disorganized arrangement of the medullary bone. Within the bony trabeculae there are frequently islands of calcified cartilage.

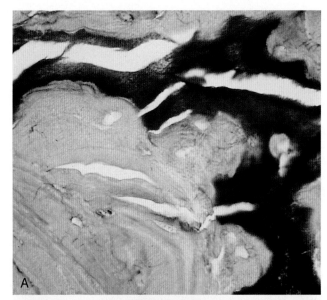

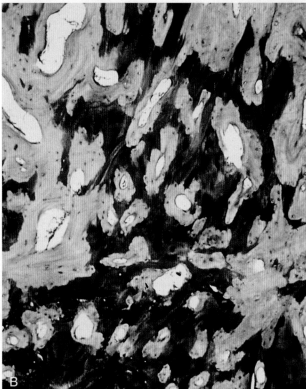

Figure 11–7. *A* and *B*, These two photomicrographs illustrate the histologic features of osteopetrotic bone formed by endochondral ossification. The heavily mineralized cartilage cores are evident in the deep purple–stained regions.

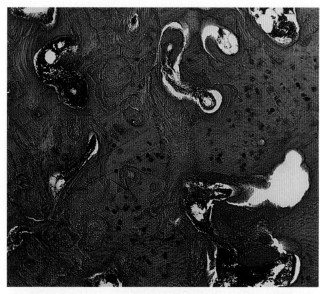

Figure 11–8. This photomicrograph illustrates densely ossified osteopetrotic bone with fewer cartilaginous islands. The histologic pattern of the disease is variable.

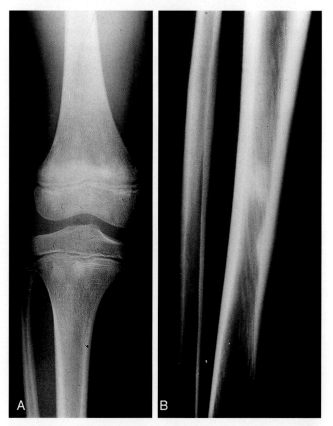

Figure 11–9. *A* and *B*, Densely sclerotic foci may also be radiographically identified in patients with lead poisoning, as shown in these radiographs of the tibia in an eight-year-old male patient.

CHAPTER 12

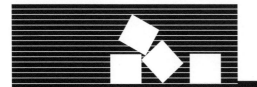

Osteogenesis Imperfecta

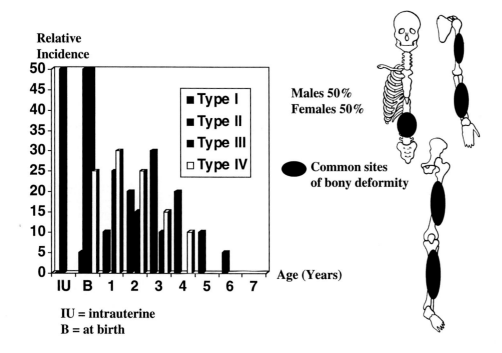

CLASSIFICATION

1. Type I has an autosomal dominant inheritance (approximately 40 per cent of cases).
   Synonyms: Dominantly inherited osteogenesis imperfecta with distinctly blue sclerae, van der Hoeve's syndrome, Eddowes' syndrome.

2. Type II has an autosomal recessive inheritance (approximately 25 per cent of cases).
   Synonyms: lethal perinatal osteogenesis imperfecta, lethal osteogenesis imperfecta congenita, osteogenesis imperfecta letalis type Vrolik.

3. Type III has an autosomal recessive inheritance (approximately 3 per cent of cases).

Synonyms: progressively deforming osteogenesis imperfecta with normal sclerae, osteogenesis imperfecta congenita, osteogenesis imperfecta congenita type Vrolik, osteopsathyrosis idiopathica of Lobstein.

4. Type IV has an autosomal dominant inheritance (approximately 32 per cent of cases).
   Synonyms: dominantly inherited osteogenesis imperfecta with normal sclera, osteopsathyrosis idiopathica of Lobstein, Ekman-Lobstein disease.

CLINICAL SIGNS: GENERAL

1. There is an increased propensity to fracture. (Fractures may be present at birth.)
2. Immobilization of the fracture results in diffuse osteoporosis.
3. Blue sclerae are present in some patients.
4. Poorly formed dentition or early loss of multiple teeth may be seen in some patients.
5. Ligamentous laxity may occur.
6. Short stature may be present.
7. Scoliosis may be present.

CLINICAL SIGNS: TYPE SPECIFIC

Type I

1. Distinctly blue sclerae are present throughout life.
2. Presenile conductive hearing loss occurs in 20 per cent of patients by 20 years of age and nearly 100 per cent by 60 years of age.
3. Kyphoscoliosis occurs in approximately 20 per cent of adults.
4. Joint hyperlaxity is found in approximately 50 per cent of patients.
5. Premature arcus senilis may occur.
6. Dentinogenesis imperfecta may be present. (It occurs in approximately 40 per cent of patients.)
7. Approximately 10 per cent of patients have fractures at birth, but fractures may not commence until infancy or childhood.
8. The majority of patients are two to three standard deviations below the population mean for height.
9. The frequency of fractures decreases at adolescence and increases again in postmenopausal women.

10. Easy bruising may occur in approximately 80 per cent of patients.

Type II

1. Intrauterine death occurs in approximately 50 per cent of cases, and death in early infancy occurs in approximately 50 per cent.
2. The tissues exhibit extreme fragility. (Limbs or head may be macerated during delivery.)
3. The facial and skull bones show extremely poor mineralization.
4. Micrognathia and a small, narrow nose may be present.
5. Girls outnumber boys by approximately 1.4 : 1.0.

Type III

1. Marked bone fragility leads to progressive deformity of the long bones, skull, and spine.
2. Approximately 50 per cent of patients have fractures at birth, and all have fractures by two years of age.
3. Sclerae may be blue at birth but become progressively less so as the patient ages.
4. Growth failure is marked and mortality is high owing to complications of kyphoscoliosis.
5. The skull may be hypoplastic but is not as poorly ossified as in type II.

Type IV

1. Sclerae are normal at birth or become so by adulthood.
2. Approximately 25 per cent of patients have fractures at birth or in the neonatal period.
3. The frequency of fracture peaks in childhood and markedly decreases at adolescence.
4. The opalescent dentin of dentinogenesis imperfecta is often present (approximately 70 per cent of patients).
5. Short stature is common owing to progressive kyphoscoliosis.
6. Approximately 30 per cent of patients over 30 years of age have hearing impairment.

7. Easy bruising is present in approximately 40 per cent of patients.

Note: Babies with osteogenesis imperfecta frequently are delivered by cesarean section owing to a breech presentation.

CLINICAL SYMPTOMS

1. Fractures occur frequently.
2. Hyperplastic callus formation may occur.

MAJOR RADIOGRAPHIC FEATURES

1. Osteopenia may be seen.
2. Fractures may be present. (Occasionally, exuberant callus formation may be confused with osteosarcoma.)
3. Bone deformities, primarily bowing, may be seen.
4. The long bones are small and slender compared with normal bones.
5. Vertebrae may show scoliosis, secondary compression fractures, and wedging of vertebral bodies. Expansion of the intervertebral discs causes so-called codfish vertebrae, characterized by their biconcave shape.
6. The skull exhibits multiple centers of ossification (so-called wormian bone).
7. Scalloped radiolucent areas with sclerotic margins at the epiphyseal end of the bone may be evident; such areas are more common in the lower extremities.

RADIOGRAPHIC DIFFERENTIAL DIAGNOSIS

1. Battered-child syndrome.
2. Multiple fractures.
3. Steroid-induced osteoporosis.
4. Osteosarcoma in cases with hyperplastic callus formation.

MAJOR PATHOLOGIC FEATURES

Gross

1. Egg shell–like thinning of the cortical bone may be seen.
2. Little medullary spongy bone is present.
3. Recent or healed fractures may be seen.
4. The long bones may show angulation and bowing.
5. Epiphyseal changes include
   a. Cartilaginous nodules within secondary centers of ossification.
   b. One or more "indentations" into the metaphysis or complete disruption of the growth plate (corresponding to radiographic epiphyseal lucencies).

MICROSCOPIC

1. The growth plate shows disorganization.
2. The mineralized zone of the growth plate cartilage exhibits decreased thickness.
3. Fragments of growth plate may be seen.

4. Persistence of calcified cartilage into the diaphysis may be present.
5. Metaphyseal microfractures may be evident.
6. Abnormal bony callus formation may be seen.

TREATMENT
Medical

1. Experimental therapy with calcitonin and bisphosphonates has been ineffective.
2. Gene therapy is promising.
3. Supportive care includes exercises, ambulation with bracing, and wheelchair use as necessary.

Surgical

1. Fractures are treated with closed reduction.
2. Intramedullary rod fixation (standard versus elongating rods) is used for recurrent fractures or deformities.
3. Scoliosis is managed with segmental instrumentation and fusion.

References

Byers PH, Wallis GA, and Willing MC: Osteogenesis imperfecta: translation of mutation to phenotype [review]. Am J Med Genet *28(7)*:433–442, 1991.

Cassella JP, Barber P, Catterall AC, et al: A morphometric analysis of osteoid collagen fibril diameter in osteogenesis imperfecta. Bone *15(3)*:329–334, 1994.

Cole WG, Patterson E, Bonadio J, et al: The clinicopathological features of three babies with osteogenesis imperfecta resulting from the substitution of glycine by valine in the pro alpha 1 (I) chain of type I procollagen. Am J Med Genet *29(2)*:112–118, 1992.

Deak SB, Scholz PM, Amenta PS, et al: The substitution of arginine for glycine 85 of the alpha 1(I) procollagen chain results in mild osteogenesis imperfecta. The mutation provides direct evidence for three discrete domains of cooperative melting of intact type I collagen. J Biol Chem *266(32)*:21827–21832, 1991.

Marion MJ, Gannon FH, Fallon MD, et al: Skeletal dysplasia in perinatal lethal osteogenesis imperfecta. A complex disorder of endochondral and intramembranous ossification. Clin Orthop Rel Res *(293)*:327–337, 1993.

Nerlich AG, Brenner RE, Wiest I, et al: Immunohistochemical localization of interstitial collagens in bone tissue from patients with various forms of osteogenesis imperfecta. Am J Med Genet *45(2)*:258–259, 1993.

Sillence D, Butler B, Latham M, Barlow K: Natural history of blue sclerae in osteogenesis imperfecta. Am J Med Genet *45(2)*:183–186, 1993.

Steinmann B, Westerhausen A, Constantinou CD, et al: Substitution of cysteine for glycine-alpha 1-691 in the pro alpha 1(I) chain of type I procollagen in a proband with lethal osteogenesis imperfecta destabilizes the triple helix at a site C-terminal to the substitution. Biochem J *279(Pt 3)*:747–752, 1991.

Stoss H, Pontz B, Vetter U, et al: Osteogenesis imperfecta and hyperplastic callus formation: light- and electron-microscopic findings. Am J Med Genet *45(2)*:260, 1993.

Sztrolovics R, Glorieux FH, Travers R, et al: Osteogenesis imperfecta: comparison of molecular defects with bone histological changes. Bone *15(3)*:321–328, 1994.

Sztrolovics R, Glorieux FH, van der Rest M, and Roughley PJ: Identification of type I collagen gene (COL1A2) mutations in nonlethal osteogenesis imperfecta. Hum Mol Genet *2(8)*:1319–1321, 1993.

Vetter U, Pontz B, Zauner E, et al: Osteogenesis imperfecta: a clinical study of the first ten years of life. Calcif Tissue Int *50(1)*:36–41, 1992.

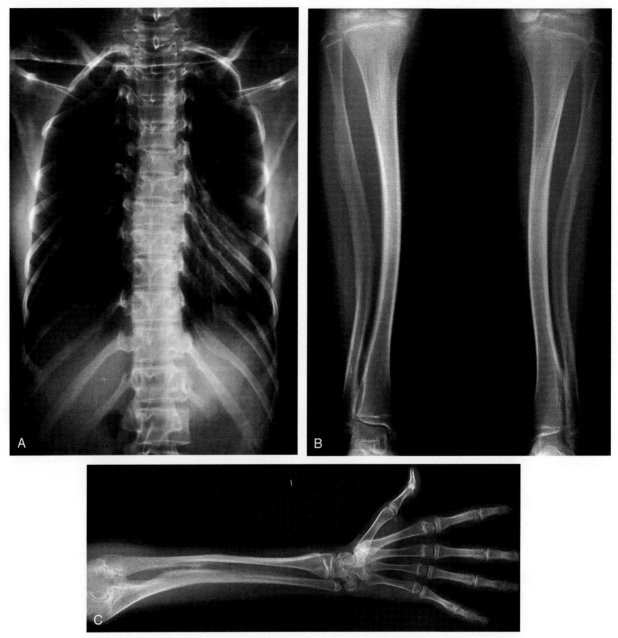

Figure 12–1. *A*, Anteroposterior (AP) roentgenogram of the thoracic spine in a patient with osteogenesis imperfecta. Note the diffuse demineralization of the bones. *B*, AP roentgenogram of both tibiae, showing similar findings. *C*, AP roentgenogram of the forearm and hand. The bones are overconstricted, with a thin, gracile appearance as well as bowing deformity.

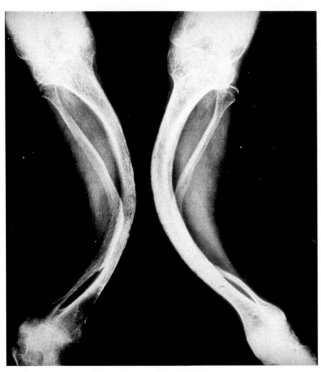

Figure 12–2. Marked deformity of the tibia and fibula is evident in this patient with osteogenesis imperfecta tarda. Such patients are less severely affected than patients who show evidence of the disease at birth, osteogenesis imperfecta congenita. Generalized osteoporosis, multiple fractures, and micromelia may be present at birth in such cases.

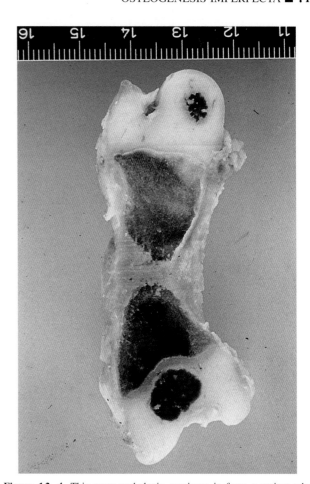

Figure 12–4. This gross pathologic specimen is from a patient who suffered from osteogenesis imperfecta. Fractures treated by immobilization lead to osteoporotic changes that predispose to additional fractures in these patients. This cycle results in marked bony deformity.

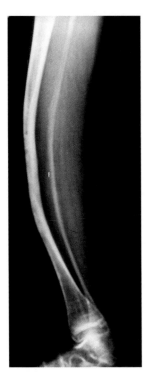

Figure 12–3. This radiograph illustrates the anterior bowing of the tibia seen in a patient with osteogenesis imperfecta tarda. Such bony deformity is more common in the tarda I subgroup of patients, who have deformities usually confined to the lower extremities.

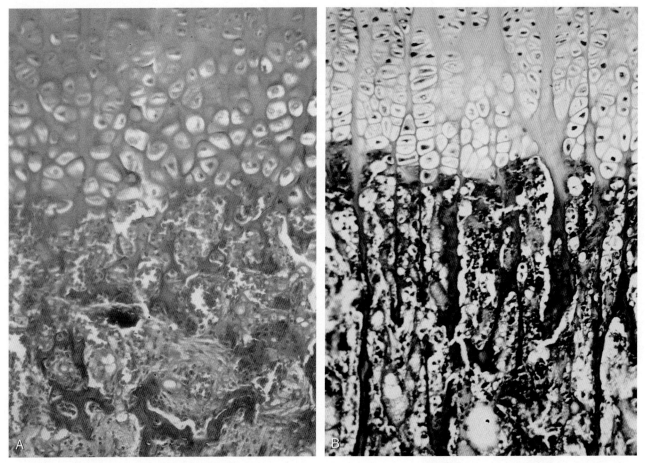

Figure 12–5. *A* and *B*, These two photomicrographs illustrate the histologic features of osteogenesis imperfecta in the region of endochondral ossification. The growth plates are variable in appearance. There is relative preservation of the columns of chondrocytes. Extension of the cartilage into the metaphyseal portion of the bone may be seen. Fragmentation of the growth plate may occur, possibly related to trauma. Islands of cartilage may be seen in the epiphysis and metaphysis when the growth plate has been disrupted.

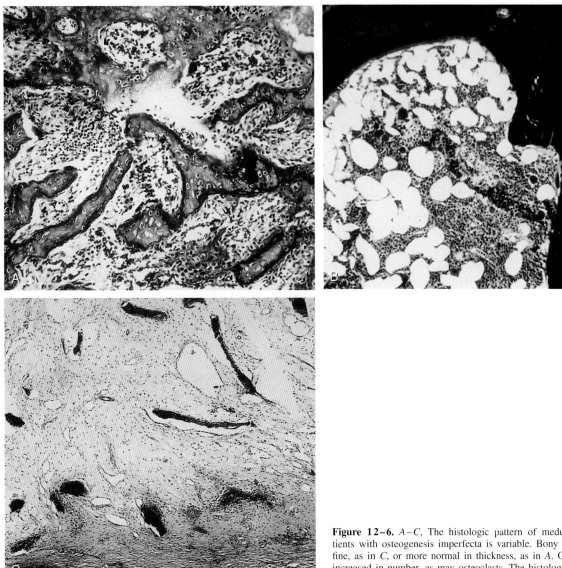

Figure 12–6. *A–C*, The histologic pattern of medullary bone in patients with osteogenesis imperfecta is variable. Bony trabeculae may be fine, as in *C*, or more normal in thickness, as in *A*. Osteoblasts may be increased in number, as may osteoclasts. The histologic appearance may be altered by the healing reaction related to pathologic fractures.

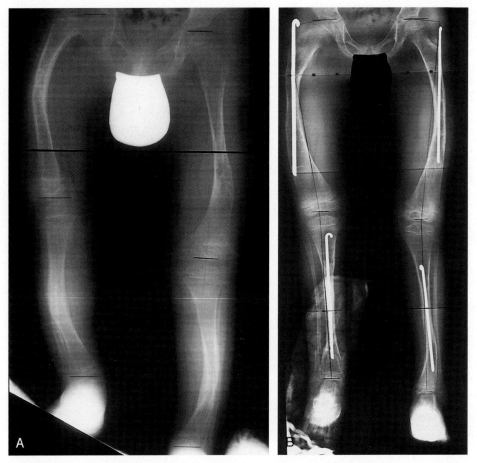

Figure 12–7. Surgical correction of the bony deformities related to multiple fractures in patients with osteogenesis imperfecta can be challenging. One approach is illustrated in *A* and *B*.

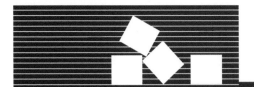

CHAPTER 13

Fluorosis

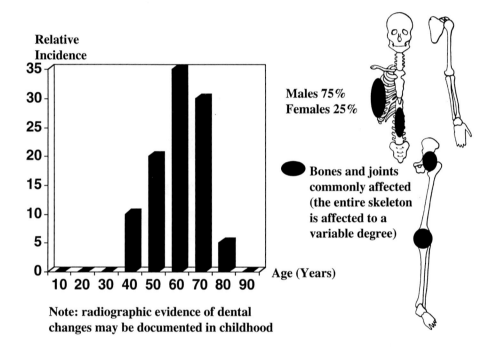

Males 75%
Females 25%

⬬ **Bones and joints commonly affected (the entire skeleton is affected to a variable degree)**

Note: radiographic evidence of dental changes may be documented in childhood

CLINICAL SIGNS

1. Signs depend upon duration and level of exposure to fluoride.
2. Longstanding exposure results in mottling of teeth and anemia.
3. Painful limbs may be present.
4. Joint deformities (knock-knee, limitation of motion) may occur.
5. Kyphosis may be seen.
6. Flexion deformity at the hips may occur.
7. Neurologic symptoms related to compression of the spinal cord and nerve roots may be present.

CLINICAL SYMPTOMS

1. The spinal column may be stiff.
2. Symptoms related to cord compression or compression of nerve roots may be present.
3. Low back pain occurs in 70 per cent of patients.
4. Leg or arm pain occurs in 70 per cent of patients.
5. Loss of appetite occurs in 20 per cent of patients.
6. Joint dysfunction occurs in 50 per cent of patients.
7. Joint deformity occurs in 30 per cent of patients.

MAJOR RADIOGRAPHIC FEATURES

1. Features are variable; osteosclerosis most commonly is present (in approximately 45 per cent of patients), but osteopenia may also be seen (with approximately 20 per cent showing an osteoporotic pattern and 20 per cent showing an osteomalacic pattern).
2. Fluorosis preferentially involves the axial skeleton.
3. Bony osteophytes, particularly vertebral, may be seen.

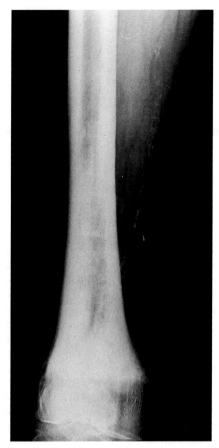

Figure 13-4. Increased bone density is seen in this case of fluorosis involving the femur. The most common radiographic abnormality in patients with endemic fluorosis is calcification or ossification of ligaments, tendons, or soft tissues. Such changes are present in more than 80 per cent of patients with endemic fluorosis. Osteosclerosis and osteopenia are seen with about equal frequency in endemic fluorosis.

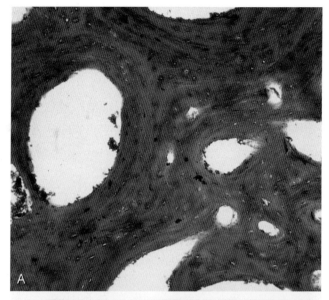

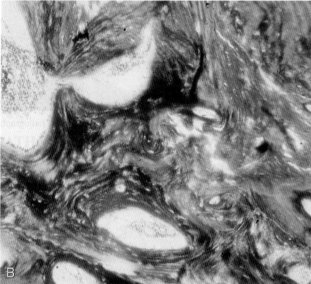

Figure 13-5. *A* and *B*, Fluorotic bone generally exhibits increased trabecular volume. The new bone associated with fluorotic bony trabeculae may show increased osteocytes and altered tinctorial characteristics. Increased osteoblastic and osteoclastic activity may also be present.

CHAPTER 14

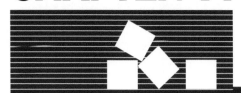

Gaucher's Disease

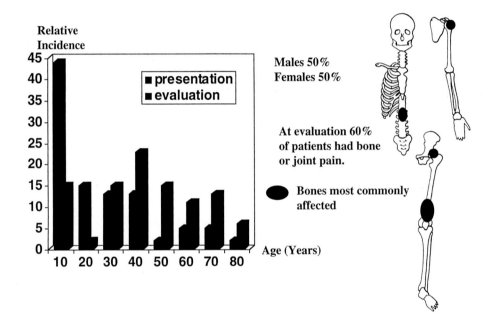

Relative Incidence

- ■ presentation
- ■ evaluation

Age (Years)

Males 50%
Females 50%

At evaluation 60% of patients had bone or joint pain.

● Bones most commonly affected

INHERITANCE PATTERN AND TYPES

1. Inheritance is autosomal recessive.
2. Types are as follows:
   a. Type I: most common (lacks central nervous system involvement).
   b. Type II: rare (involves central nervous system).
   c. Type III: rare (involves central nervous system).

CLINICAL SIGNS

1. Splenomegaly (secondary to accumulation of glucosyl ceramides) may cause abdominal discomfort. Patients with a positive family history of disease may first manifest disease with splenomegaly.
2. Frequency is high in the Ashkenazic Jewish population.
3. The majority of symptomatic patients present with splenomegaly and thrombocytopenia.
4. In children, short stature may be associated with the splenomegaly.
5. Cytopenias include

   a. Thrombocytopenia, the most common, present in approximately 50 per cent of patients.
   b. Anemia, mostly of a mild nature present in approximately 40 per cent of patients.
6. Liver function tests are abnormal.
7. The serum acid phosphatase concentration is elevated.

CLINICAL SYMPTOMS

1. Most patients have a chronic form of the disease with a benign course and may present with fatigue.
2. Abdominal pain (related to splenomegaly) may be present.
3. Weight loss may occur.
4. Rarely, young patients present at younger than three years of age with an acute neuropathic form of the disease.
5. Bony fractures and cord compression related to the associated bone disease can occur.
6. Bone pain is common and may be severe and episodic in nature.

7. The most common presenting symptom is a manifestation of bleeding such as epistaxis, easy bruisability, or prolonged bleeding after a superficial wound.
8. Pulmonary involvement may lead to shortness of breath.

MAJOR RADIOGRAPHIC FEATURES

1. Long bones show irregular cortical thinning.
2. The metadiaphyseal region may expand, producing an Erlenmeyer flask–like deformity particularly of the distal femur, proximal tibia, and proximal humerus.
3. Avascular necrosis of the femoral head is present in approximately 20 per cent of patients.
4. Avascular necrosis of the humeral head is present in approximately 10 per cent of patients.
5. Compression fractures of the thoracic or lumbar vertebrae or both are present in approximately 10 per cent of patients.
6. Endosteal scalloping in the humeri and, less commonly, tibiae is present in approximately 10 per cent of patients.
7. Widening of the humeri, particularly proximally, may be seen.
8. Lytic lesions of the long bones or pelvic bones or both may be evident.
9. Joint space narrowing may be seen.
10. Bone scan may show increased uptake in the region of the proximal humeri, distal femora, and proximal tibiae.
11. Positive bone scan is present in approximately 60 per cent of patients with Gaucher's disease overall. (Bone scan is the most sensitive method for assessing bony involvement in Gaucher's disease.)

RADIOGRAPHIC DIFFERENTIAL DIAGNOSIS

1. Niemann-Pick disease.

MAJOR PATHOLOGIC FEATURES

1. The marrow space is replaced by histiocytes that have abundant crumpled- or wrinkled-appearing cytoplasm.
2. Periodic acid–Schiff (PAS) stains show abundant cytoplasmic positivity in the histiocytes.
3. Infarction may be seen as a secondary change.

PATHOLOGIC DIFFERENTIAL DIAGNOSIS

1. Other storage diseases.

2. Xanthoma.
3. Degenerative change in fibrous dysplasia.

TREATMENT
Medical

1. Enzyme replacement therapy shows promising results.
2. Supportive care is given during an acute crisis (rest and administration of narcotics).
3. Osteomyelitis (often due to anaerobic agents) should be recognized and treated.
4. Back pain may be treated nonoperatively.

Surgical

1. Pathological fractures are treated by closed versus open reduction.
2. Arthroplasty is performed for advanced avascular necrosis and arthritis.

References

Beutler E: Modern diagnosis and treatment of Gaucher's disease [review]. Am J Dis Child *147(11)*:1175–1183, 1993.

Carrington PA, Stevens RF, Lendon M: Pseudo-Gaucher cells. J Clin Pathol *45(4)*:360, 1992.

Chan AC, Wu PC, Ormiston IW, et al: Periosteal Gaucher-like cells in beta-thalassemia major. J Oral Pathol Med *22(7)*:331–333, 1993.

Hainaux B, Christophe C, Hanquinet S, et al: Gaucher's disease. Plain radiography, US, CT and MR diagnosis of lungs, bone and liver lesions. Pediatr Radiol *22(1)*:78–79, 1992.

Hermann G, Shapiro RS, Abdelwahab IF, et al: MR imaging in adults with Gaucher's disease type I: evaluation of marrow involvement and disease activity. Skeletal Radiol *22(4)*:247–251, 1993.

Hermann G, Shapiro R, Abdelwahab IF, et al: Extraosseous extension of Gaucher's cell deposits mimicking malignancy. Skeletal Radiol *23(4)*:253–256, 1994.

Hill SC, Damaska BM, Ling A, et al: Gaucher's disease: abdominal MR imaging findings in 46 patients. Radiology *184(2)*:561–566, 1992.

Horev G, Kornreich L, Hadar H, Katz K: Hemorrhage associated with "bone crisis" in Gaucher's disease identified by magnetic resonance imaging. Skeletal Radiol *20(7)*:479–482, 1991.

Horowitz M, and Zimran A: Mutations causing Gaucher's disease [review]. Hum Mutat *3(1)*:1–11, 1994.

Mistry PK, Smith SJ, Ali M, et al: Genetic diagnosis of Gaucher's disease. Lancet *339(8798)*:889–892, 1992.

Rosenthal DI, Barton NW, McKusick KA, et al: Quantitative imaging of Gaucher's disease. Radiology *185(3)*:841–845, 1992.

Schindelmeiser J, Radzun HJ, Munstermann D: Tartrate-resistant, purple acid phosphatase in Gaucher's cells of the spleen. Immuno- and cytochemical analysis. Pathol Res Pract *187(2–3)*:209–213, 1991.

Zimran A, Kay A, Gelbart T, et al: Gaucher's disease. Clinical, laboratory, radiologic, and genetic features of 53 patients. Medicine *71(6)*:337–353, 1992.

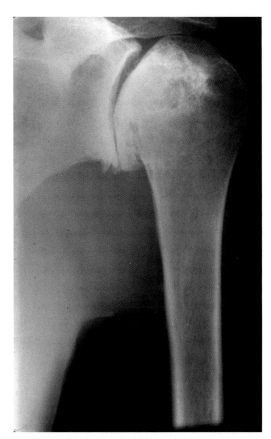

Figure 14–1. This radiograph of the proximal humerus illustrates a common sequela of Gaucher's disease. The accumulation of lipid within histiocytes in the medullary bone interferes with the local circulation, resulting in aseptic necrosis. Other radiographic clues to the diagnosis include abnormal tubulation of the bone, particularly the distal femora.

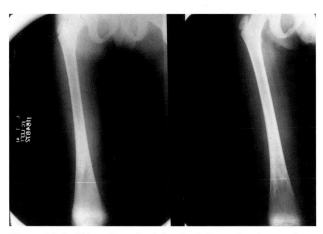

Figure 14–2. This radiograph of the distal femur shows some abnormality of tubulation and associated mineralization of infarcted bone. The characteristic Erlenmeyer flask–type change may also be seen in some cases and is particularly common in the distal femur.

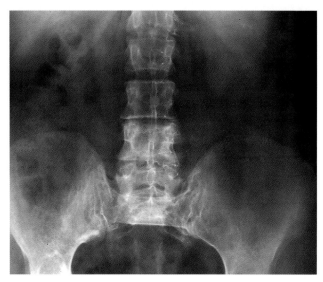

Figure 14–3. Bony sclerosis may be a sign of Gaucher's disease, as illustrated in this case involving the fourth and fifth lumbar vertebrae.

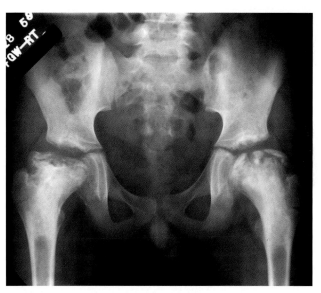

Figure 14–4. In longstanding cases of aseptic necrosis in Gaucher's disease, there may be significant associated bony deformity, as in this case involving the femoral heads bilaterally.

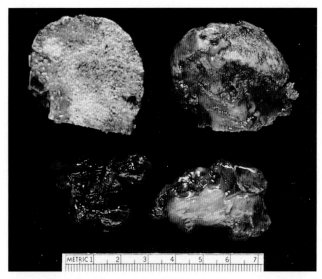

Figure 14–5. Grossly, the femoral head may show only regions of avascular necrosis, as in this example of Gaucher's disease. Areas of yellow discoloration correspond to avascular necrosis as well as to regions with numerous lipid-laden histiocytes. The synovium shown in the lower portion of the photograph is diffusely thickened owing to infiltration by lipid-laden histiocytes.

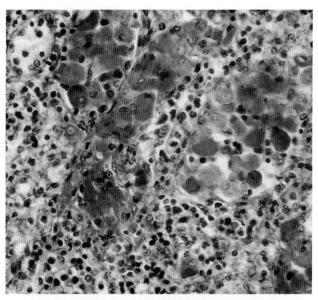

Figure 14–7. This photomicrograph illustrates the periodic acid–Schiff (PAS) positivity of the lipid within the foamy histiocytes in Gaucher's disease involving the marrow. Residual hematopoietic elements are present.

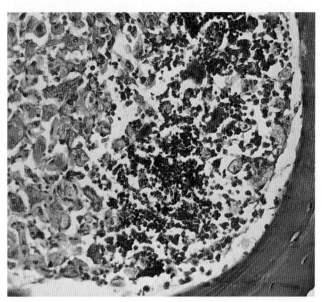

Figure 14–6. This photomicrograph illustrates the abundant cytoplasm of lipid-laden Gaucher's cells. These histiocytes may totally replace the normal fatty and hematopoietic marrow elements.

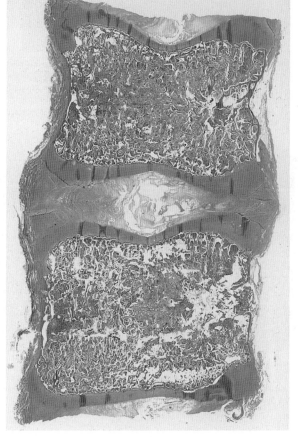

Figure 14–8. This low-magnification photomicrograph of two vertebrae shows multifocal collections of histiocytes in a patient with Gaucher's disease.

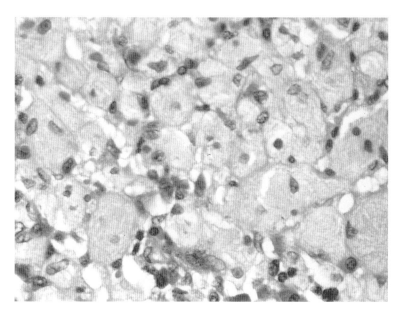

Figure 14–9. The histologic features of the lipid-laden histiocytes of Gaucher's disease involving the rib are illustrated in this photomicrograph. Other storage diseases may show a similar histologic pattern of histiocytes with abundant, clear cytoplasm.

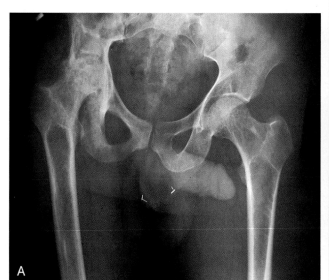

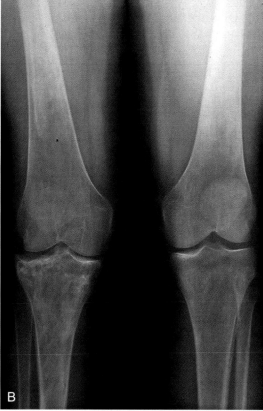

Figure 14–10. *A,* Anteroposterior (AP) roentgenogram of the pelvis and proximal femora in a patient with Gaucher's disease. There is demineralization with cortical thinning and coarse trabeculae. Both medullary canals are expanded in the femoral metaphysis. Note the avascular necrosis with collapse of the right femoral head. *B,* AP roentgenogram of the distal femora and proximal tibiae showing a similar pattern with mixed sclerotic and lucent changes in the medullary canals. On the right, there also appear to be changes of avascular necrosis, with collapse of the lateral tibial plateau.

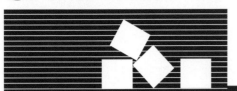
Osteoarthritis

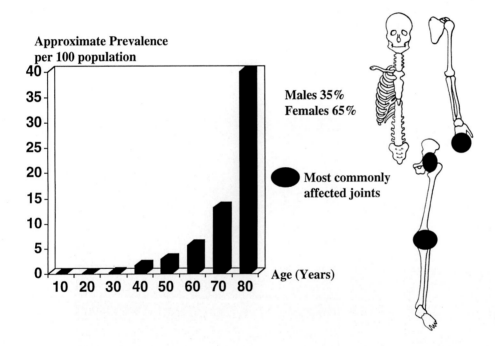

Approximate Prevalence per 100 population

Age (Years)

Males 35%
Females 65%

Most commonly affected joints

CLASSIFICATION

Approximately 20 per cent of patients have an antecedent condition that predisposes to degenerative joint disease. Conditions associated with such secondary osteoarthritis include

1. Congenital dislocation or subluxation of the hip.
2. Joint space infection.
3. Late-stage avascular necrosis.
4. Hip dysplasia.
5. Slipped capital femoral epiphysis.
6. Legg-Perthes disease.
7. Intra-articular fracture.
8. Radiation damage.

CLINICAL SIGNS

1. Pain may occur with motion of the affected joint and is worse at night.
2. Motion may be limited, with lack of full flexion or extension.
3. Heberden's nodes may be seen, mainly in women.
4. Pain subsides later in the course of the disease.
5. Swelling about the affected joint may occur.
6. Crepitus may be present.
7. The affected joint may exhibit instability.
8. The joint may be tender.
9. The erythrocyte sedimentation rate is normal.
10. Synovial fluid analysis shows a noninflammatory pattern.
11. Tests for rheumatoid factor are negative.

CLINICAL SYMPTOMS

1. Pain may occur in the affected joint.
2. Joint dysfunction—e.g., limitation of motion (often of limited duration)—may be experienced.
3. Malalignment and deformity may be present.

MAJOR RADIOGRAPHIC FEATURES

1. The joint space narrows.
2. Osteophytes may be seen at the periphery of the joint.
3. The bone shows increased density.
4. Subchondral cystic change may be evident.
5. In primary generalized osteoarthritis, Heberden's nodes (distal interphalangeal joint) may cause flexion deformities and lateral deviation (index and middle fingers most commonly affected).
6. In magnetic resonance imaging (MRI) studies, the hyaline cartilage shows uniform thinning and varying degrees of signal loss, and osteophytes show a central high signal intensity due to the marrow within the central portion of the osteophyte.

RADIOGRAPHIC DIFFERENTIAL DIAGNOSIS

1. Charcot's joint.
2. Rheumatoid arthritis.

MAJOR PATHOLOGIC FEATURES

Gross

1. The shape of the articular surface of the affected joint may be altered.
2. Cartilage may be absent in the weight-bearing regions of the affected joint.
3. Subchondral bone is polished or eburnated when the articular cartilage is absent.
4. Cystic change is evident; cysts are filled with loose fibromyxoid tissue.
5. Osteophytes are particularly common on the medial surface of the femoral head.

Microscopic

1. Vertical clefting of the articular cartilage may be seen.
2. Villous hyperplasia of the synovium with mild lymphoplasmacytic infiltration may be present.
3. Osteocartilaginous loose body formation may be evident.

4. The articular cartilage may show overgrowth of cells, producing "growth centers."
5. Pannus, although more common in rheumatoid arthritis, may be seen in osteoarthritis.

PATHOLOGIC DIFFERENTIAL DIAGNOSIS

1. Rheumatoid arthritis (although there is generally more inflammation associated with rheumatoid arthritis than osteoarthritis, there is considerable overlap between the two conditions).
2. Other inflammatory arthritides.

TREATMENT

1. Treatment must be individualized depending upon the extent of disease and amount of disability.
2. Medical approaches include
   a. Analgesic agents, e.g., acetaminophen, nonsteroidal anti-inflammatory drugs (NSAIDs).
   b. Relief of joint overstress, i.e., use of walking aid, weight reduction in obese patients, and modification of activities.
   c. Physical therapy to relieve pain, maintain range of motion and strength.
3. Surgical therapy is individualized depending upon location, extent of disease, associated deformity, age, and expectations of the patient:
   a. Arthroscopic techniques for lavage and debridement.
   b. Osteotomy for malalignment of the knee with unicompartmental disease.
   c. Arthrodesis.
   d. Joint arthroplasty for unicompartmental or total joint replacement.

References

Bullough PG: Pathologic changes associated with the common arthritides and their treatment [review]. Pathol Annu 14:69–105, 1979.
Gold RH, Bassett LW, and Seeger LL: The other arthritides. Roentgenologic features of osteoarthritis, erosive osteoarthritis, ankylosing spondylitis, psoriatic arthritis, Reiter's disease, multicentric reticulohistiocytosis, and progressive systemic sclerosis. Radiol Clin North Am 26:1195–1212, 1988.
Hamerman D: Osteoarthritis [review]. Orthop Rev 17:353–360, 1988.
Lane NE, and Kremer LB: Radiographic indices for osteoarthritis. Rheum Dis Clin North Am 21:379–394, 1995.
Martel W, Adler RS, Chan K, et al: Overview: new methods in imaging osteoarthritis. J Rheumatol 18:32–37, 1991.

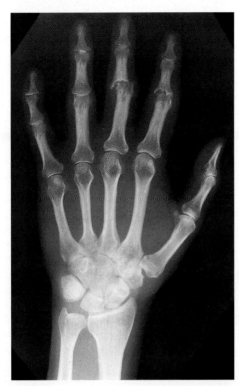

Figure 15–1. This radiograph illustrates osteoarthritic changes in the hand. The interphalangeal joints are commonly involved, with the formation of osteophytes that correspond to clinically identified Heberden's nodes.

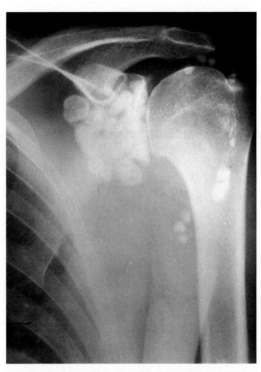

Figure 15–3. This radiograph illustrates degenerative joint disease involving the shoulder joint. Numerous osteocartilaginous loose bodies are present in the joint. Calcification of the cartilaginous component of these bodies, when they are numerous, may even raise a suspicion of chondrosarcoma.

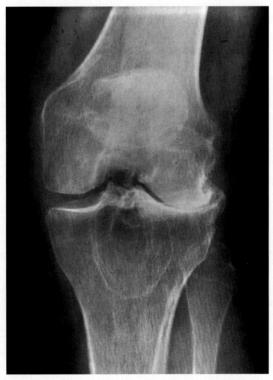

Figure 15–2. This radiograph reveals longstanding changes of osteoarthritis. A subchondral degenerative cyst is present in the proximal tibia. Subchondral sclerosis is identifiable as well. Osteophyte formation also commonly accompanies these two changes.

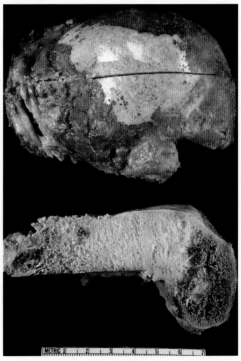

Figure 15–4. This gross specimen of the femoral head is from a patient who suffered from congenital hip dysplasia and subsequent degenerative joint disease. The whitish glistening surface of the femoral head in the upper portion of the photograph corresponds to the region of articular cartilage loss and eburnation of the underlying subchondral bone.

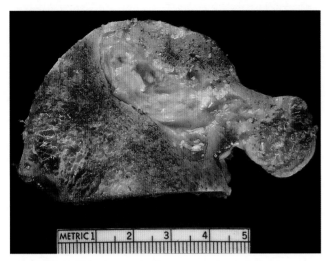

Figure 15–5. This photograph of a gross specimen shows a cross-section of a femoral head with advanced osteoarthritis. A degenerative cyst is present in the subchondral bone to the left of the large osteophyte.

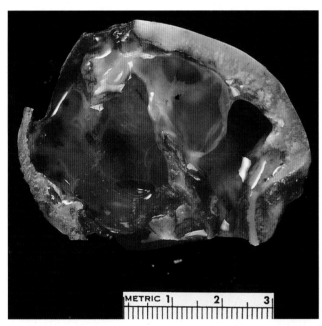

Figure 15–6. This photograph of a gross specimen illustrates advanced degenerative cyst formation nearly replacing the entire femoral head. Clear, glistening synovial fluid is present within the cyst.

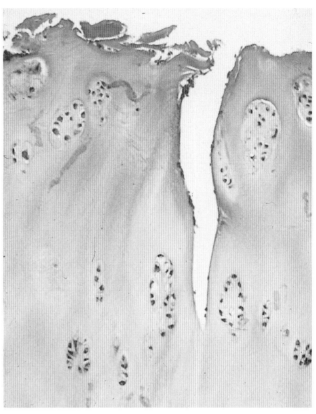

Figure 15–7. This photomicrograph illustrates the first morphologic changes seen in osteoarthritis. Such vertical clefting has been termed "fibrilization." Subsequent softening of the cartilage leads to further degeneration. The process does not uniformly affect the entire articular cartilage surface but is variable from region to region.

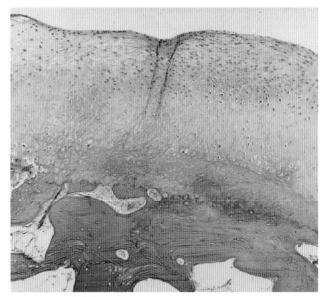

Figure 15–8. Early in the course of the disease, regions of the articular cartilage may be relatively normal histologically, as in this specimen from the femoral head.

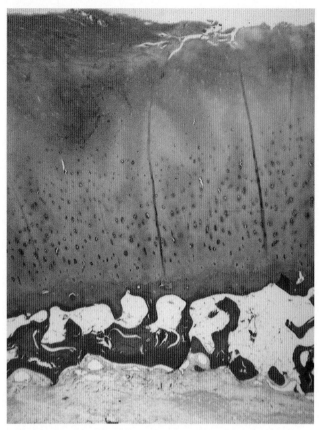

Figure 15–9. This photomicrograph illustrates degenerative clefting of the articular cartilage. In addition, a degenerative cyst is identified in the lower portion of the photomicrograph.

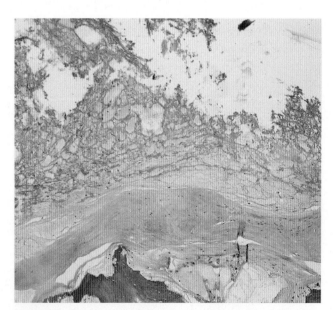

Figure 15–10. This photomicrograph shows the contents of the degenerative cyst at higher magnification. Such cysts are filled with amorphous eosinophilic debris. The cyst wall is generally a hypocellular fibrotic connective tissue.

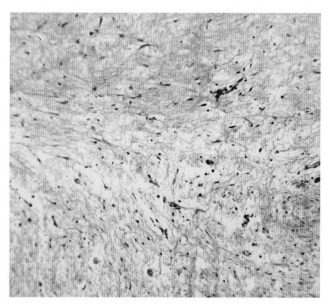

Figure 15–11. This photomicrograph illustrates the histologic appearance of a degenerative cyst of the tibia that contains hypocellular myxoid connective tissue. Radiographically, the appearance of this cyst simulated that of a neoplasm.

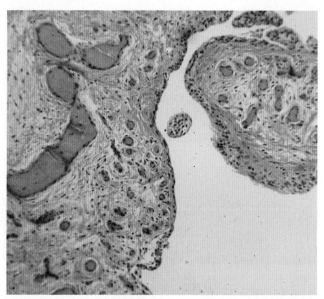

Figure 15–12. This photomicrograph illustrates villous hyperplasia of the synovium from a patient with osteoarthritis. In advanced cases of osteoarthritis, villous hypertrophy of the synovium may be marked and associated with fibrous thickening of the joint capsule.

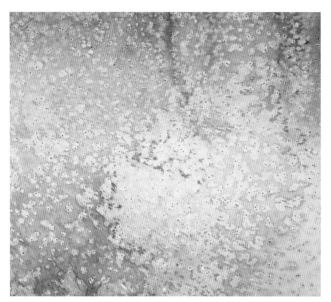

Figure 15–13. This photomicrograph demonstrates the histologic features of an osteocartilaginous loose body from a patient with osteoarthritis of the knee. Such loose bodies may become embedded in the hypertrophic synovium.

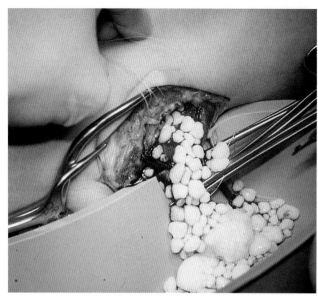

Figure 15–15. Numerous loose bodies may be associated with osteoarthritis, as shown in this intraoperative photograph.

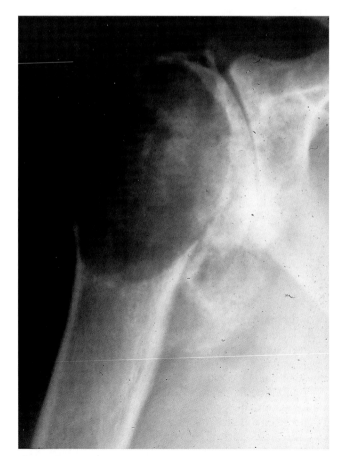

Figure 15–14. This radiograph illustrates osteoarthritis of the shoulder with an associated large degenerative cyst occupying the proximal humerus. Although large, the cyst is well circumscribed with mild peripheral sclerosis.

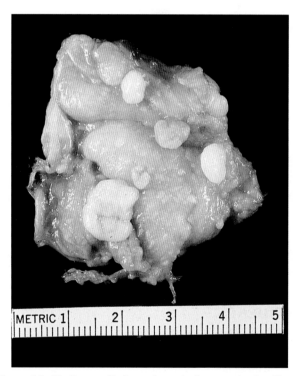

Figure 15–16. Osteocartilaginous loose bodies associated with osteoarthritis may become embedded in the synovium, as shown in this photograph. Such cases may be indistinguishable from synovial chondromatosis.

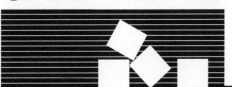

CHAPTER 16

Charcot's Joint

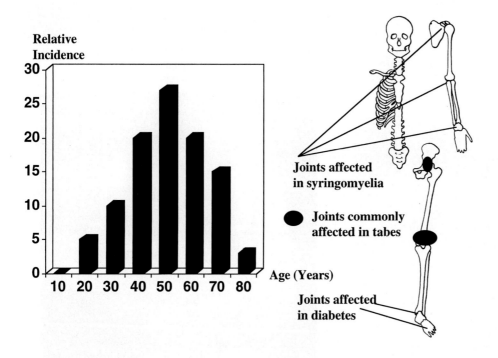

Relative Incidence

Age (Years)

Joints affected in syringomyelia

● **Joints commonly affected in tabes**

Joints affected in diabetes

INCIDENCE

The incidence of Charcot's joint in diabetic patients is approximately 0.4 per cent but rises to 16 per cent in patients with diabetic neuropathy.

CLINICAL SIGNS

1. Charcot's joint is characterized by rapidly destructive arthritis of a single joint in the absence of pain or a history of trauma.
2. Charcot's joint is associated with peripheral neuropathies and spinal cord degenerative diseases, including
   a. Tabes dorsalis.
   b. Syringomyelia.
   c. Advanced diabetes mellitus with peripheral neuropathy.
   d. Congenital insensitivity to pain.
   e. Amyloidosis.
   f. Leprosy.
   g. Residual effect from repeated glucocorticoid injection in the joint.
   h. Transverse myelitis.
   i. Traumatic paralysis.
   j. Spinal dysraphism.
3. Joint crepitation may be present.
4. Loose bodies may be palpated in the joint cavity.
5. The joint changes may precede the identification of a neurologic deficit.
6. Although classically the process is painless, some patients (up to one third in some series) have pain early in the course of the disease.
7. Deep tendon reflexes are absent.
8. Large knee effusions may be seen and may rupture into the surrounding soft tissues and present as Baker's cyst.
9. The affected joint may be swollen and warm, mimicking the appearance of an infected joint.

10. Scoliosis may be seen in patients with spinal causes. (Approximately 50 per cent of patients with syringomyelia have scoliosis.)
11. Synovial fluid analysis shows a clear, straw-colored fluid with a normal white blood cell count.

CLINICAL SYMPTOMS

1. The process is painless.
2. Joint instability may occur.
3. Crepitation in the joint may be present.
4. There is rapid progression of joint abnormality. (It may evolve in a period of weeks.)
5. The ability to ambulate progressively decreases.

MAJOR RADIOGRAPHIC FEATURES

1. Extensive destruction of the joint space may be seen.
2. Extensive destruction of the bone adjacent to the joint may be evident.
3. Osteopenia may be present.
4. The destructive process may show sharp cortical margins.

RADIOGRAPHIC DIFFERENTIAL DIAGNOSIS

1. Osteoarthritis.

MAJOR PATHOLOGIC FEATURES

Gross

1. Synovium may appear rusty brown.
2. Synovium may be hyperplastic.
3. Marked destruction of the normal bony contour.
4. Bony and cartilagenous debris embedded in synovium and soft tissue.

Microsopic

1. Bone and cartilagenous detritus.
2. Synovial hyperplasia.
3. Inflammatory reaction in the synovium and adjacent soft tissues.
4. Giant cell reaction to debris.

Pathologic Differential Diagnosis

1. Post-traumatic osteoarthritis.
2. Rheumatoid arthritis (in general the imflammatory reaction is much less pronounced in Charcot joints than in rapidly destructive rheumatoid arthritis).

TREATMENT
Medical

1. The underlying disorder must be promptly recognized and treated.
2. Decreased weight bearing and walking aids can be used.
3. Bracing and orthosis can be used to decrease stress and retard progression of destruction.

Surgical

1. Arthrodesis is difficult to achieve but may be effective in the knee or ankle.
2. Below-knee amputation may become necessary for distal joints or if concomitant infection complicates the clinical course.
3. Resection arthroplasty may be performed.
4. Total joint arthroplasty is generally not recommended because of its high failure rate.

References

Allman RM, Brower AC, and Kotlyarov EB: Neuropathic bone and joint disease. Radiol Clin North Am 26:1373–1381, 1988.
Helms CA, Chapman S, and Wild JH: Charcot-like joints in calcium pyrophosphate dihydrate deposition disease. Skeletal Radiol 7:55–58, 1981.
Kovacs JP, and Bowen JR: Neurotrophic arthropathy. Contemp Orthop 23:359, 1991.
Park YH, Taylor JA, Szollar SM, and Resnick D: Imaging findings in spinal neuroarthropathy. Spine 19:1499–1504, 1994.
Peh WC, Brockwell J, Chau MT, and Ng MM: Imaging features of dissecting neuropathic joints. Australas Radiol 39:249–253, 1995.
Resnick D: Neuroarthropathy. In Resnick D, and Niwayama G (eds): Diagnosis of Bone and Joint Disorders. 2nd ed. Philadelphia, WB Saunders Company, 1988, pp 3154–3168.
Soudry M, Binazzi R, Johanson NA, et al: Total knee arthroplasty in Charcot and Charcot-like joints. Clin Orthop 208:199–204, 1986.

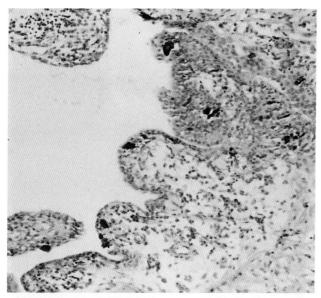

Figure 16–9. This photomicrograph illustrates changes in the synovium from a patient with neuropathic arthropathy. Some villous hypertrophy is evident, and numerous pigment-laden macrophages are present, indicating prior bleeds.

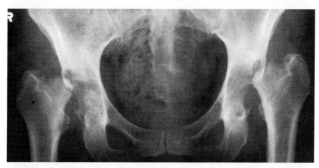

Figure 16–10. This radiograph shows an example of bilateral Charcot's joints of the hip. Destructive changes occurred rapidly over the course of 4 months in this 74-year-old woman.

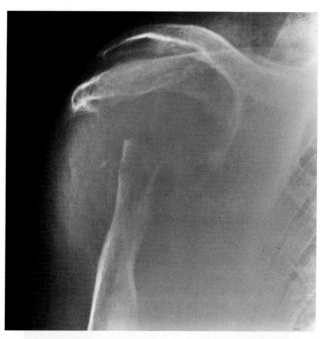

Figure 16–11. This radiograph demonstrates complete destruction of the proximal humerus in a 79-year-old woman. The radiographic differential diagnosis for such a destructive process includes metastatic carcinoma.

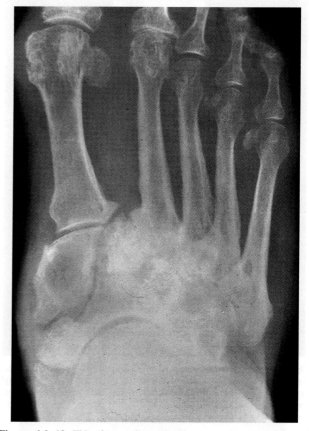

Figure 16–12. This foot radiograph illustrates the appearance of Charcot's joint in a patient with longstanding diabetes mellitus.

CHAPTER 17

Rheumatoid Arthritis

Rheumatoid Arthritis: Prevalence

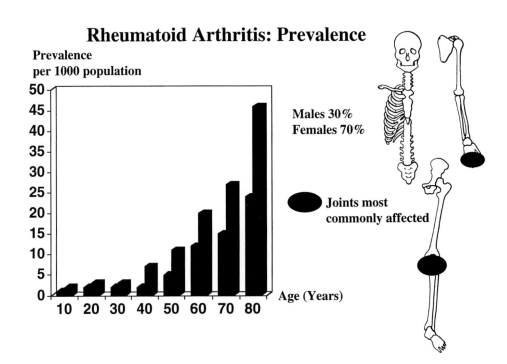

Prevalence
per 1000 population

Males 30%
Females 70%

Joints most
commonly affected

Age (Years)

PREVALENCE

Approximately 1 per cent of the adult population (approximately 6 per 1000 men and 14 per 1000 women) suffers from rheumatoid arthritis; the prevalence increases with age in both men and women (see prevalence graph).

CLINICAL SIGNS

1. Symmetric polyarthritis results in hot, swollen, tender joints.
2. The synovial fluid is milky.
3. Rheumatoid nodules in the skin are present in about one quarter of patients, particularly over the extensor surface of the forearm.
4. Synovial fluid analysis generally shows 20,000 to 50,000 inflammatory cells, with approximately 50 per cent polymorphonuclear leukocytes.
5. Carpal tunnel syndrome may be present.
6. Trigger finger may be present.
7. Tests are positive for rheumatoid factor. (*Note:* Rheumatoid factor is not specific and may be seen in systemic lupus erythematosus, chronic liver disease, Sjögren's syndrome, and other conditions.)
8. The erythrocyte sedimentation rate is elevated.
9. Anemia of chronic disease may be present.

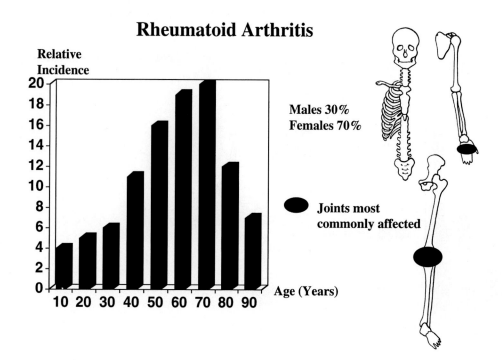

Rheumatoid Arthritis

Males 30%
Females 70%

Joints most
commonly affected

10. Seventy per cent of patients who are positive for rheumatoid factor are positive for HLA-DR4.

CLINICAL SYMPTOMS

1. The course of the disease is characterized by remissions and exacerbations:
   a. Fatigue.
   b. Weight loss.
   c. Fever.
   d. Morning stiffness.
2. Joint pain is present.
3. Skin nodules (rheumatoid nodules) may be seen.
4. Epidemiologic studies show that 50 per cent of patients have symptoms two months to three years prior to diagnosis (similar for both men and women).

MAJOR RADIOGRAPHIC FEATURES

1. Osteopenia of the juxta-articular bone may be seen.
2. The joint space may show narrowing.
3. Juxta-articular bony erosions may be present.
4. Periarticular soft tissue swelling may be evident.
5. Subluxation of the joint may be seen.
6. Marginal bony erosions may be seen.
7. Subchondral cyst formation may be present.
8. Joint effusion may be evident.

RADIOGRAPHIC DIFFERENTIAL DIAGNOSIS

1. Psoriatic arthritis.
2. Osteoarthritis.

3. Septic arthritis.
4. Arthritis associated with ulcerative colitis or lupus.

MAJOR PATHOLOGIC FEATURES

1. The synovium may show the following features:
   a. Synovial papillary hyperplasia with thickening of the villi.
   b. Lymphoplasmacytic infiltration of the synovium.
   c. Subsynovial multinucleated giant cells.
   d. Lymphoid follicle formation in the synovium.
   e. Fibrinous exudate on the surface of the synovium.
   f. Hyperplastic synovium extending over the articular surface (pannus formation).
   g. Fibrinous exudate on the surface and in the substance of the synovium.
   h. Inflamed synovium invading the bone at the articular margin.
2. Bony changes include
   a. Destruction of the articular cartilage by hyperplastic synovium, resulting in "fraying" of the cartilage.
   b. Lymphoplasmacytic infiltration of subchondral bone and even follicle formation.
   c. Infiltration of pannus-like tissue into the articular cartilage from the synovium and subchondral bone.

PATHOLOGIC DIFFERENTIAL DIAGNOSIS

1. Psoriatic arthritis.
2. Arthritis associated with systemic lupus erythematosus.
3. Arthritis associated with ulcerative colitis.

TREATMENT
Medical

Treatment must be individualized. The goal is to relieve pain and inflammation while maintaining joint function and preventing joint deformity.

1. Supportive care—e.g., education, rest, and nutrition—should be instituted.
2. Physical and occupational therapy may be undertaken.
3. Aspirin and other nonsteroidal anti-inflammatory drugs (NSAIDs).
4. Corticosteroids may be beneficial in selected patients.
5. Slow-acting antirheumatic drugs—e.g., gold salts, hydroxychloroquine (Plaquenil), and penicillamine—may be helpful.

Surgical

1. Arthroscopic synovectomy is occasionally indicated in selected cases.
2. Usually, reconstructive joint surgery, i.e., total joint arthroplasty, is performed for advanced destruction.

References

Linos A, Worthington JW, O'Fallon WM, et al: The epidemiology of rheumatoid arthritis in Rochester, Minnesota: a study of incidence, prevalence and mortality. Am J Epidemiol 111:87–98, 1980.

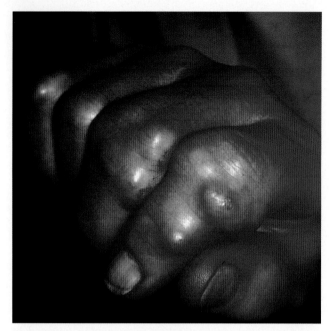

Figure 17–1. This photograph illustrates rheumatoid nodules in the soft tissues of the fingers.

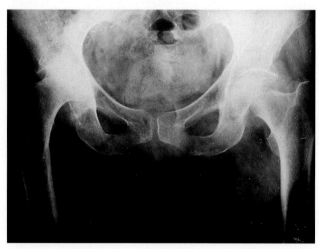

Figure 17–2. This radiograph shows rheumatoid disease with marked degenerative change.

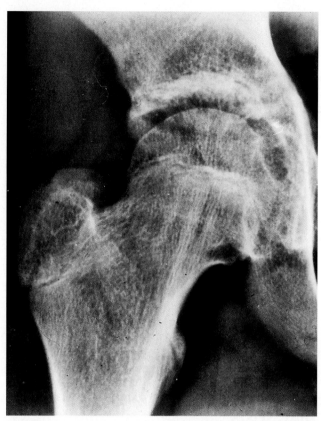

Figure 17–3. This radiograph illustrates juvenile rheumatoid arthritis involving the hip. Patients with juvenile rheumatoid arthritis may have systemic symptoms.

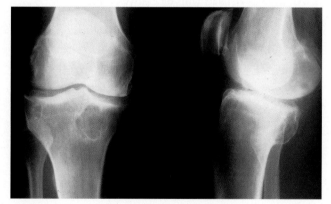

Figure 17–4. This radiograph of the knee shows joint space narrowing related to rheumatoid arthritis. In addition, a degenerative cyst is present in the proximal tibia.

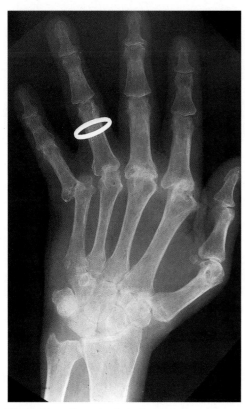

Figure 17–5. This radiograph of the hand shows subluxation of the metacarpophalangeal joints secondary to rheumatoid disease. Joint laxity related to the underlying process contributes to the subluxation. Joint space narrowing and osteopenia are also present.

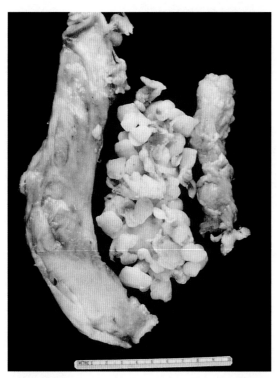

Figure 17–6. This photograph of a gross specimen illustrates the features of hyperplastic synovium and multiple "rice bodies" from the knee of a patient with rheumatoid arthritis.

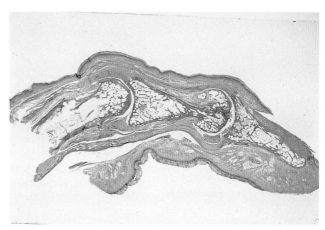

Figure 17–7. This photograph demonstrates the gross pathologic changes associated with rheumatoid arthritis of the finger. Periarticular bony erosion and ligamentous laxity are present. Ligamentous laxity leads to subluxation, as shown in Figure 17–5.

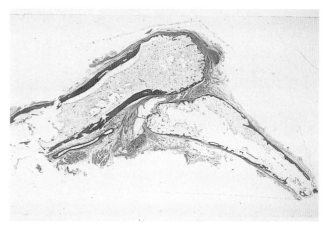

Figure 17–8. This photograph illustrates subluxation of the metacarpophalangeal joint in a patient with rheumatoid arthritis.

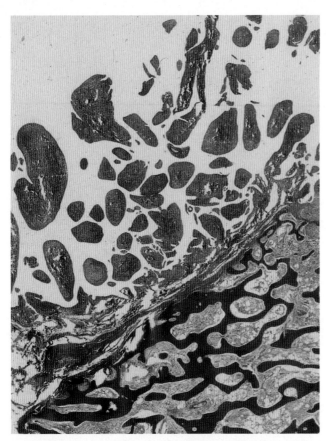

Figure 17–9. This photomicrograph illustrates the dramatic villous hyperplasia of the synovium present in rheumatoid arthritis. Lymphoid nodules are identifiable within the hyperplastic synovial villi.

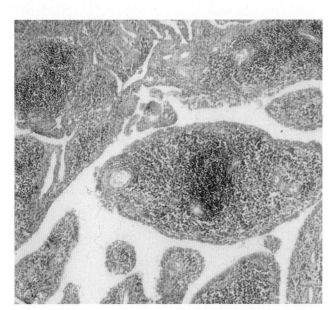

Figure 17–10. This photomicrograph reveals the lymphoid hyperplasia of rheumatoid disease at higher magnification. Plasma cells may form a significant proportion of the lymphoplasmacytic synovial infiltrate.

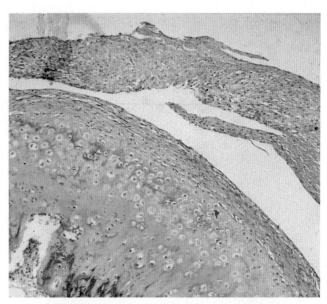

Figure 17–11. This photomicrograph illustrates hyperplastic synovial proliferation extending over the articular surface of the femoral head. Such pannus proliferation results in destruction of the articular cartilage.

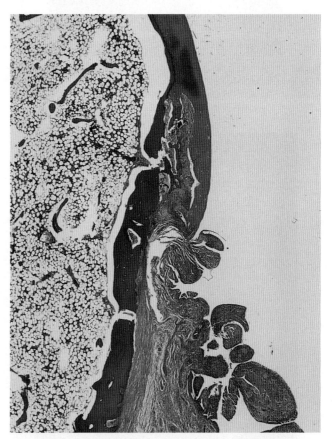

Figure 17–12. Further encroachment of the proliferative synovium onto the articular surface of the femoral head is illustrated in this photomicrograph. Erosion of the articular cartilage may result in eburnation of the underlying bone in longstanding rheumatoid disease.

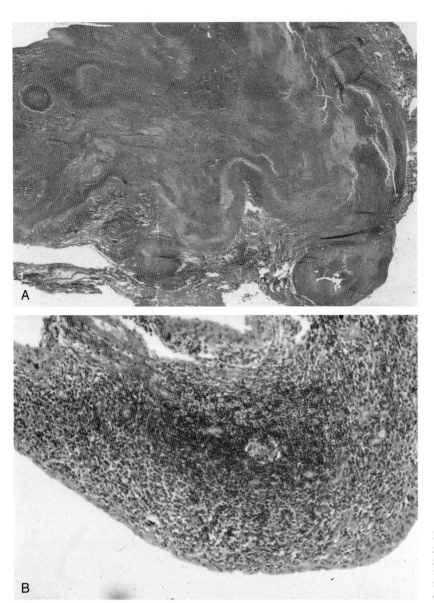

Figure 17–13. *A* and *B*, These two photomicrographs reveal the histologic features of rheumatoid granulomas. Such rheumatoid nodules may simulate infectious granulomas. Central necrosis and surrounding histiocytic and giant cell reaction are present in the necrotic region.

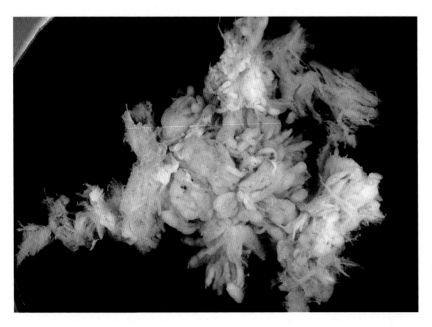

Figure 17–14. This photograph of a gross specimen illustrates villous hyperplasia of the synovium in rheumatoid arthritis. Similar features would be evident at arthroscopy.

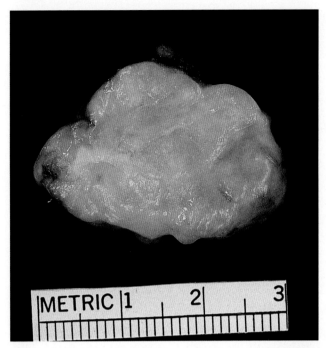

Figure 17–15. This photograph of a nodule specimen from the index finger exemplifies the appearance of a rheumatoid nodule. Rheumatoid nodules are variable in color and may show foci of necrosis grossly.

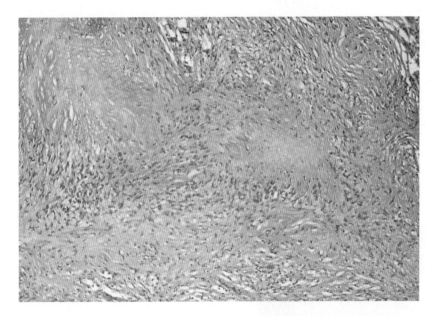

Figure 17–16. The histologic features of a rheumatoid nodule are shown in this photomicrograph. The central necrosis with peripheral histiocytic palisading may mimic the appearance of an infectious granuloma. Special stains for fungi and mycobacteria are negative in such rheumatoid nodules.

CHAPTER 18

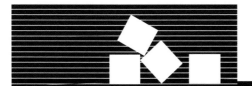

Ochronosis—Disorder of Tyrosine and Phenylalanine Catabolism Secondary to Homogentisic Acid and Related Compounds

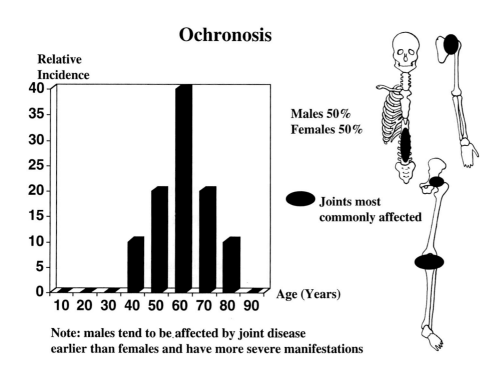

Ochronosis

Males 50%
Females 50%

Joints most commonly affected

Note: males tend to be affected by joint disease earlier than females and have more severe manifestations

INHERITANCE

Inheritance is autosomal recessive (related to deficiency of homogentisic acid oxidase).

CLINICAL SIGNS

1. Alkaptonuria (homogentisic acid in the urine) is present.

2. Sclerae may be darkened (due to deposition of homogentisic acid in collagen in this tissue).
3. The ear lobes may be discolored (due to deposition of homogentisic acid in collagen in this tissue).
4. Black discoloration of other tissues related to the accumulation of homogentisic acid (e.g., cardiovascular, genitourinary, and respiratory tissues, as well as sclerae and skin) may be exhibited.

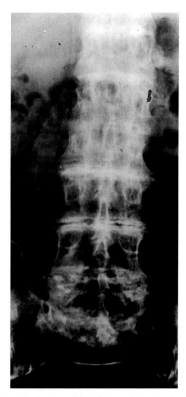

Figure 18–1. This radiograph of the vertebrae illustrates the changes in ochronosis. There is narrowing of the disc spaces and deposition of calcium in the degenerated disc material.

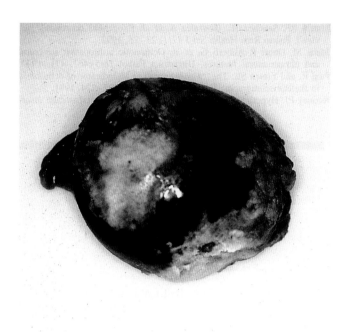

Figure 18–3. This gross specimen of the femoral head from a patient with ochronosis illustrates the black discoloration of the cartilage. In addition, there is degeneration of the articular cartilage and eburnation of the underlying bone.

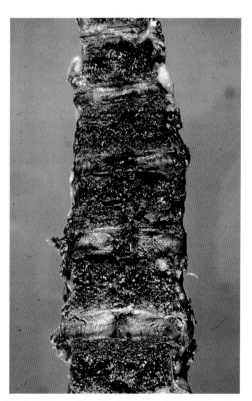

Figure 18–2. This gross specimen of the vertebrae shows the characteristic appearance of degenerated disc material in patients with ochronosis. The black discoloration is present in disc material and in cartilage.

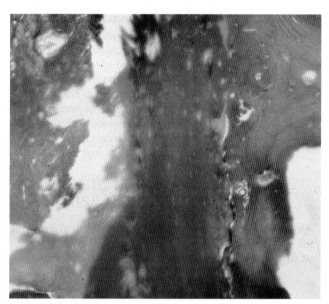

Figure 18–4. This photomicrograph illustrates the appearance of articular cartilage in a patient with ochronosis. Hematoxylin and eosin–stained sections are brown to black, depending upon the extent of homogentisic acid deposition in the tissue. The articular cartilage may be frayed.

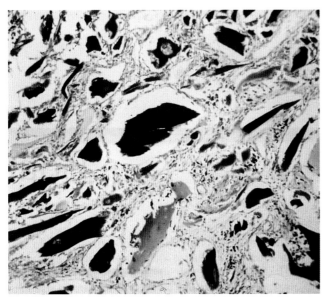

Figure 18–5. The deposition of homogentisic acid leads to altered mechanical properties and degeneration of the cartilage. Flaking of the cartilage into the synovium results in mild inflammatory changes and fibrosis as shown on this photomicrograph.

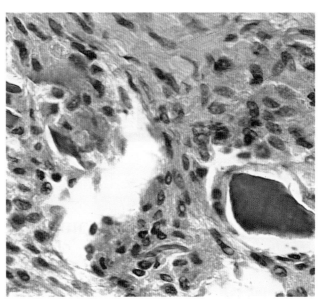

Figure 18–7. Fragments of ochronotic cartilage embedded in the synovium of the knee are illustrated in this photomicrograph. Histiocytic and giant cell reaction surrounds the brownish discolored cartilage.

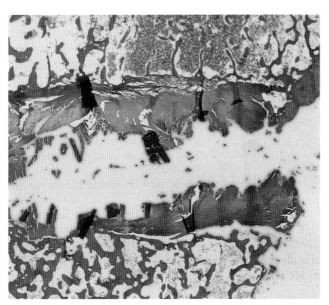

Figure 18–6. This low-power photomicrograph shows the discoloration of an intervertebral disc due to ochronosis. The mechanical properties of the disc tissue are altered and thus subject to degeneration.

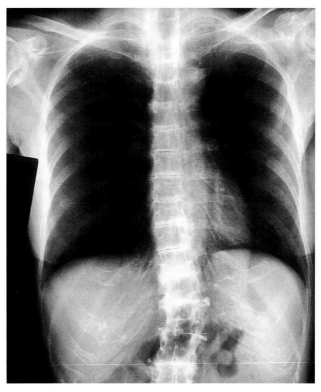

Figure 18–8. The chest radiograph of this 56-year-old woman shows mineralization of the intervertebral disc secondary to ochronosis.

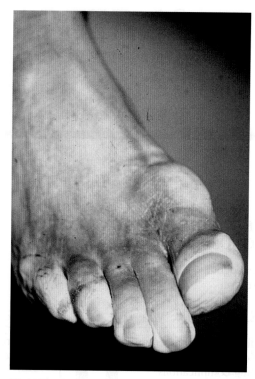

Figure 19–1. The first metatarsophalangeal joint of the foot is the most common location for an acute gouty attack. Such attacks are frequently associated with an extremely painful, red, and swollen joint. Aspiration of the joint yields synovial fluid containing negatively birefringent urate crystals.

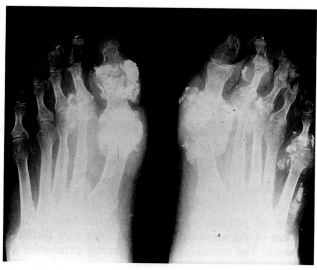

Figure 19–3. A later stage of the disease with associated tophaceous gouty deposits is shown in this radiograph. Destruction of multiple joints in a distribution atypical of rheumatoid disease is often evident at this late stage of the process.

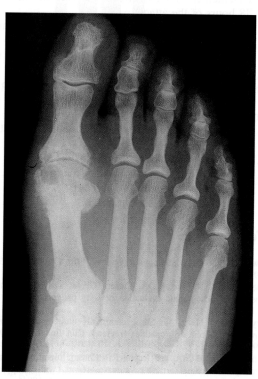

Figure 19–2. The radiographic features of gouty arthritis involving the first metatarsophalangeal joint are illustrated in this radiograph. Soft tissue swelling is seen early in the course of the disease. Later the characteristic punched-out bony erosion without adjacent bony reaction is evident, as shown in this radiograph.

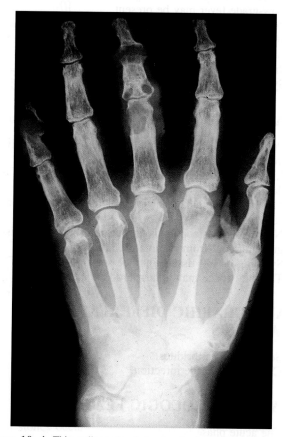

Figure 19–4. This radiograph of the hand of a patient with gouty arthropathy demonstrates periarticular punched-out lytic lesions similar to those commonly seen in the foot.

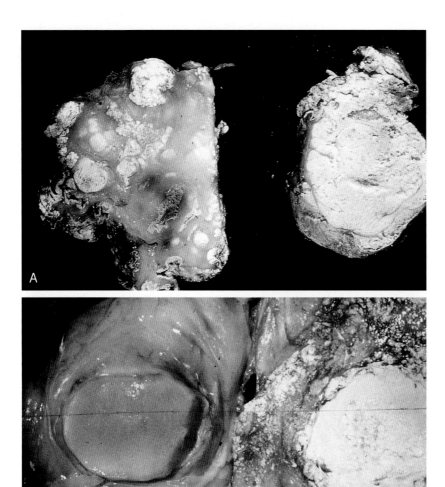

Figure 19–5. *A* and *B*, These gross photographs illustrate tophaceous deposits of urate crystals in the soft tissues about the knee. The white crystals can be spread on a slide and viewed under polarized light to confirm the diagnosis of gout.

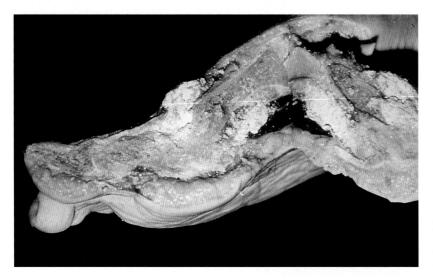

Figure 19–6. This photograph of a soft tissue gross specimen from the foot also shows the appearance of gouty tophi. Urate crystal deposition may occur in tendons, bone, and even articular cartilage.

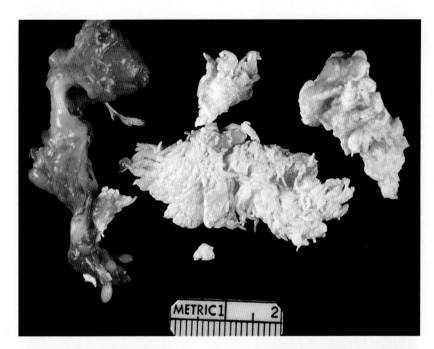

Figure 19–7. Crystalline material from other sources may mimic the gross appearance of gouty tophi. This gross specimen illustrates the appearance of crystalline debris in the soft tissues related to a steroid injection. Such crystalline debris does not show the characteristic birefringence of urates.

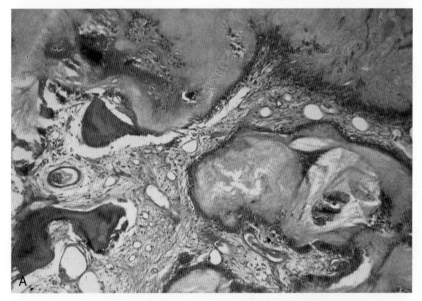

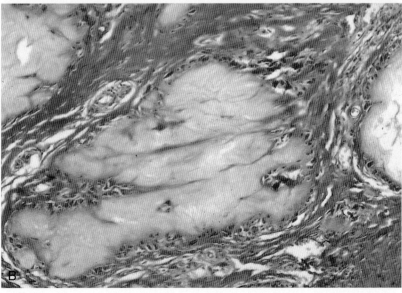

Figure 19–8. *A* and *B*, These two photomicrographs illustrate the histologic appearance of urate in tissue sections stained with hematoxylin and eosin. The urate crystals may be dissolved in processing through water-based solutions, but if present in significant quantities the crystals will frequently be found even after routine processing.

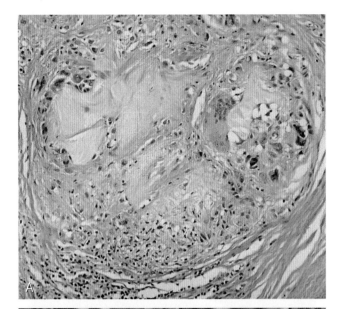

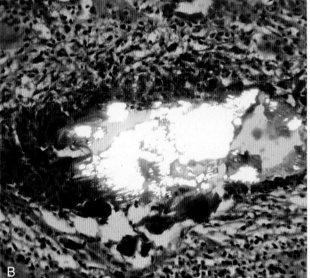

Figure 19–9. *A* and *B*, These two photomicrographs illustrate a histiocytic and giant cell reaction to urate deposits that is common in the soft tissues surrounding gouty tophi. Processing of tissue in alcohol and staining with the De Galantha technique may aid in the identification of these deposits.

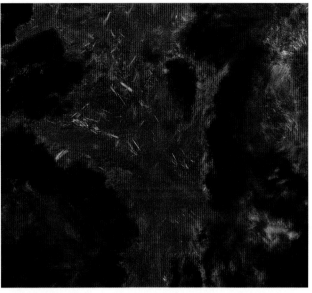

Figure 19–10. This photomicrograph demonstrates the appearance of urate crystals in a frozen section stained with toluidine blue. With this technique the crystals appear brown.

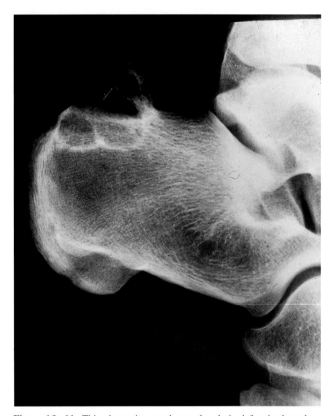

Figure 19–11. This photomicrograph reveals a lytic defect in the calcaneus of a 25-year-old female patient. The characteristic punched-out pattern of lytic bone destruction without the reaction of gout is present. This patient was asymptomatic (see Fig. 19–12).

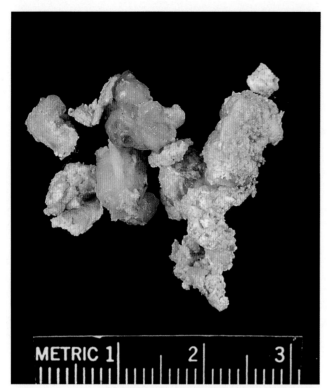

Figure 19–12. This photograph of a gross specimen illustrates the appearance of the curetted material from the calcaneal lytic lesion shown in Figure 19–11. Whitish urate crystalline islands are identifiable within reactive connective tissue.

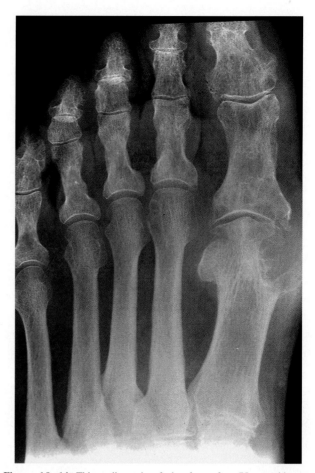

Figure 19–14. This radiograph of the foot of a 75-year-old man demonstrates the punched-out lytic lesions typical of gout involving the metacarpophalangeal joint of the great toe.

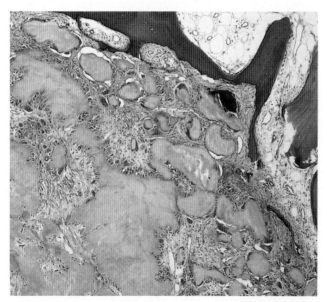

Figure 19–13. Histologically, urate crystals within the bony lytic defects of gout are frequently surrounded by a giant cell reaction. At low magnification, the pattern may mimic that of a caseating granulomatous infectious disease.

CHAPTER 20

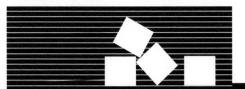

Chondrocalcinosis (Pseudogout, Calcium Pyrophosphate Dihydrate Crystal Deposition Disease)

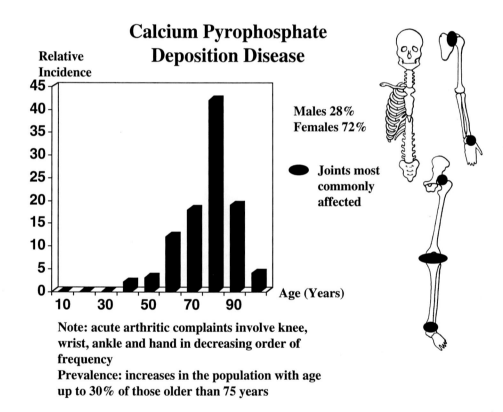

Calcium Pyrophosphate Deposition Disease

Males 28%
Females 72%

● Joints most commonly affected

Age (Years)

Note: acute arthritic complaints involve knee, wrist, ankle and hand in decreasing order of frequency
Prevalence: increases in the population with age up to 30% of those older than 75 years

CLINICAL SIGNS

1. The earliest signs are most commonly related to the knee joint. (Although the lower limb joints are most commonly involved in both men and women, the predilection is more marked in men.)

2. Multiple joints commonly affected, in order of frequency, are knees, ankles, wrists, elbows, hips, and shoulders.

115

3. Hyperuricemia may be present (gout must be ruled out).
4. Effusion of the knee joint is seen in patients with chronic disease.
5. Heberden's nodes may be seen.
6. Diseases associated with calcium pyrophosphate deposition disease include
   a. Hemochromatosis.
   b. Hypophosphatasia.
   c. Hypomagnesemia.
   d. Hyperparathyroidism.
   e. Hypothyroidism.

CLINICAL SYMPTOMS

1. Acute swelling (gout-like symptoms) can occur and may be associated with trauma, surgery, or other illness.
2. The majority of patients are asymptomatic.
3. Onset is in the sixth or seventh decade of life.
4. Multiple joints may be symmetrically affected, simulating rheumatoid disease.
5. Rapid joint destruction simulates Charcot's arthropathy.
6. Stiffening of the spine, usually familial, may occur.
7. Although patients may present with acute attacks, the mean duration of symptoms prior to diagnosis is approximately ten years.

MAJOR RADIOGRAPHIC FEATURES

1. Punctate or linear mineralization is evident in fibrocartilage and possibly in hyaline cartilage, usually bilaterally.
2. Fibrocartilage is most intensely mineralized in the knee menisci, triangular ligament of the wrist, and pubic symphysis.
3. Capsular mineralization involving the hips and shoulders, as well as the metacarpophalangeal and metatarsophalangeal joints, may be seen.
4. Subchondral linear mineralization parallel to the end plate may be evident.
5. The joint space may show narrowing.
6. Calcification of the interspinous and supraspinous ligaments as well as the ligamentum flavum may be seen.

7. Spinal canal narrowing may occur related to massive crystal deposition ("tophaceous pseudogout") and osteophyte formation.
8. Large, weight-bearing joints tend to show the greatest probability for progressive degenerative changes.

RADIOGRAPHIC DIFFERENTIAL DIAGNOSIS

1. Hemochromatosis.
2. Hyperparathyroidism.
3. Diabetes mellitus.
4. Rheumatoid arthritis.
5. Gout.

MAJOR PATHOLOGIC FEATURES

1. Grossly, deposits are chalky white and may be either crystalline or amorphous.
2. Deposits are usually surrounded by a cuff of histiocytes and multinucleated giant cells.
3. The crystals are more rhomboid than needle-like (as in gout) and are weakly positively birefringent.
4. The cartilaginous lacunae become enlarged and may coalesce.
5. The cartilage matrix adjacent to the lacunae undergoes a mucoid degenerative change.

PATHOLOGIC DIFFERENTIAL DIAGNOSIS

1. Gout.
2. Residual effect from prior steroid injection.

TREATMENT

1. Primary disease, if present (e.g., hemochromatosis, hyperparathyroidism, diabetes, ochronosis), must be identified and treated.
2. For acute attacks, the following may be used:
   a. Nonsteroidal anti-inflammatory agents (NSAIDs) (e.g., indomethacin, naproxen).
   b. Aspiration and intra-articular injection of steroids (e.g., triamcinolone, 10 to 40 mg).

3. Prophylaxis may be accomplished with colchicine (0.6 mg by mouth twice a day).

References

Agarwal AK: Gout and pseudogout [review]. Prim Care 20(4):839–855, 1993.

Doherty M: Calcium pyrophosphate in joint disease [review]. Hosp Pract (Off Ed) 29(11):93–96, 99–100, 103–104, 1994.

Elborn JS, Kelly J, and Roberts SD: Pseudogout, chondrocalcinosis and the early recognition of haemochromatosis. Ulster Med J 61(1):119–123, 1992.

Keen CE, Crocker PR, Brady K, et al: Calcium pyrophosphate dihydrate deposition disease: morphological and microanalytical features. Histopathology 19(6):529–536, 1991.

Masuda I, Ishikawa K, and Usuku G: A histologic and immunohisto-chemical study of calcium pyrophosphate dihydrate crystal deposition disease. Clin Orthop Rel Res (263):272–287, 1991.

Pritzker KP: Calcium pyrophosphate dihydrate crystal deposition and other crystal deposition diseases [review]. Curr Opin Rheumatol 6(4):442–447, 1994.

Ryan LM: Calcium pyrophosphate dihydrate crystal deposition and other crystal deposition diseases [review]. Curr Opin Rheumatol 5(4):517–521, 1993.

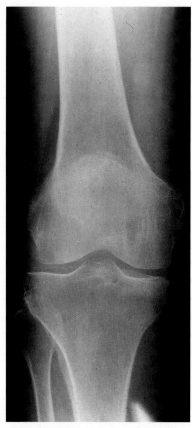

Figure 20–1. This radiograph illustrates the features of chondrocalcinosis of the knee in a 94-year-old woman. Calcification of the menisci and articular cartilage is common in this condition.

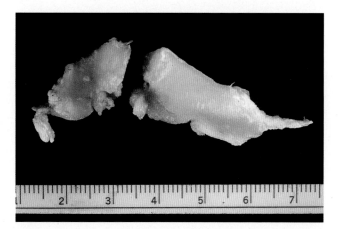

Figure 20–2. The gross appearance of chondrocalcinosis is demonstrated in this specimen from a meniscus. Grossly, the whitish crystalline deposition of calcium pyrophosphate can mimic the appearance of urate tophi.

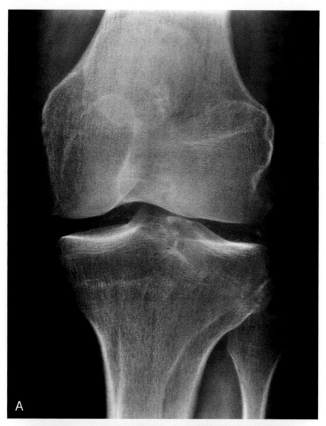

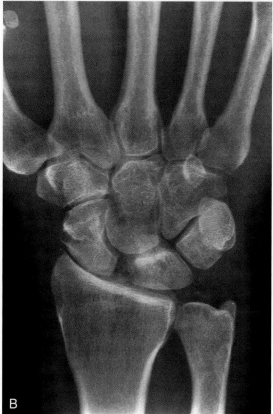

Figure 20–3. Radiographs of the knee (*A*) and wrist (*B*) illustrate chondrocalcinosis involving the joints of a 64-year-old female patient.

CHAPTER 21

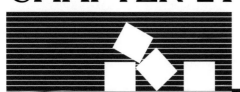

Amyloidosis

CLINICAL SIGNS

1. Clinically evident masses of amyloid are uncommon.
2. Generally, amyloidosis involves multiple joints bilaterally, as it is a systemic process.
3. Patients with hemodialysis-related amyloidosis may present with trigger finger, flexor tendon contracture, spontaneous tendon rupture, or pathologic fracture.
4. Carpal tunnel syndrome, most often bilateral, may be seen.
5. Findings related to other organ malfunction—e.g., chronic renal failure or cardiomyopathy—may be present.

CLINICAL SYMPTOMS

1. The patient may be asymptomatic.
2. Symptoms of carpal tunnel syndrome may be present.
3. Pain secondary to compression fracture may be experienced.
4. Joint pain is the most common presenting complaint of patients with hemodialysis–related amyloidosis.
5. Joint stiffness may be present.

MAJOR RADIOGRAPHIC FEATURES

1. Juxta-articular osteoporosis may be seen.
2. Soft tissue swelling may be present.
3. Subchondral bone cysts may be evident.
4. The joint spaces appear relatively preserved.
5. Vertebral compression fractures may be seen.
6. The localized lytic form of the disease tends to affect the long bones, skull, and ribs, resulting in well-marginated lytic lesions.
7. Pathologic fracture may be present.

8. Dialysis-associated amyloid bone disease may also be associated with changes resulting from secondary hyperparathyroidism (due to renal failure) as well as aluminum-induced osteomalacia.

RADIOGRAPHIC DIFFERENTIAL DIAGNOSIS

1. Metastases.
2. Lymphoma.
3. Myeloma.

MAJOR PATHOLOGIC FEATURES

1. Deposits of eosinophilic amorphous material may be seen in soft tissues or bone.
2. Congo red stains reveal apple green birefringent masses when viewed with polarized light.
3. Deposits tend to occur in vessel walls.
4. When turnefactive deposits are present, histiocytic and giant cell reactions are commonly seen.
5. Dialysis-associated amyloid bone disease likely shows the histologic changes associated with chronic renal failure, as patients who develop amyloid bone disease in this setting have almost invariably been on dialysis for longer than ten years.

PATHOLOGIC DIFFERENTIAL DIAGNOSIS

1. Dense fibrosis.
2. Amyloid deposition associated with plasma cellular proliferative disorders.

119

TREATMENT
Medical

1. The predisposing disease must be treated. Most cases at this time are related to an underlying plasma cell dyscrasia, which may require chemotherapy.

Surgical

1. Localized amyloid deposits (amyloidomas) may be excised.
2. Symptoms due to carpal tunnel syndrome may be treated with carpal tunnel decompression.

References

Boccalatte M, Pratesi G, Calabrese G, et al: Amyloid bone disease and highly permeable synthetic membranes. Int J Artif Organs 17(4):203–208, 1994.
Gravallese EM, Baker N, Lester S, et al: Musculoskeletal manifestations in beta 2-microglobulin amyloidosis. Case discussion [clinical conference]. Arthritis Rheum 35(5):592–602, 1992.
Kurer MH, Baillod RA, and Madgwick JC: Musculoskeletal manifestations of amyloidosis. A review of 83 patients on haemodialysis for at least 10 years. J Bone Joint Surg (Br) 73(2):271–276, 1991.
Ross LV, Ross GJ, Mesgarzadeh M, et al: Hemodialysis-related amyloidomas of bone. Radiology 178(1):263–265, 1991.

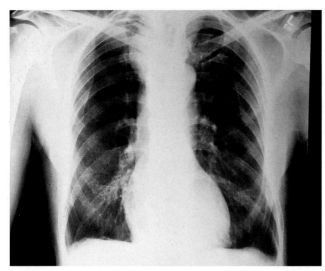

Figure 21–1. This radiograph of the chest of a 78-year-old man demonstrates a lytic lesion in the fourth thoracic vertebra.

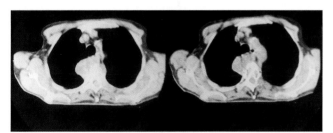

Figure 21–2. The lesion of Figure 21–1 is better seen in this computed tomographic (CT) scan. The patient had an amyloid tumor destroying the vertebra and had no evidence of myeloma at the time of diagnosis.

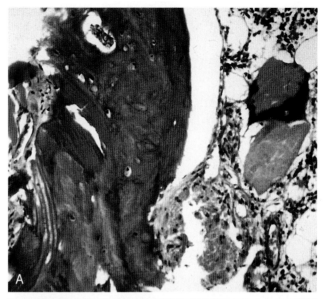

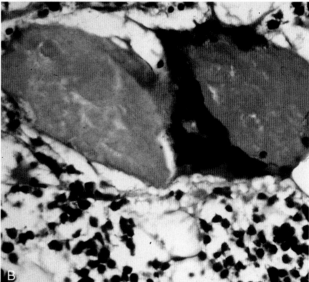

Figure 21–3. *A* and *B*, A region of calcified amyloid is identified adjacent to a bony trabecula in this biopsy specimen from a 55-year-old woman. The surrounding marrow does not show evidence of a plasmacytosis.

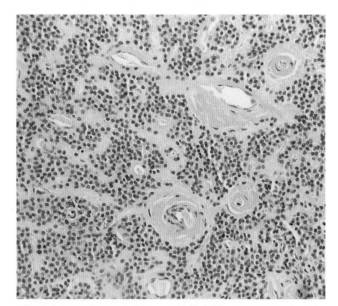

Figure 21–4. This photomicrograph illustrates amyloid deposition in the region of a plasmacellular proliferation from the 12th thoracic vertebra of a 51-year-old man. This was a solitary lesion at the time of diagnosis. The condition is best diagnosed as a solitary plasmacytoma rather than an amyloid tumor because of the presence of a plasmacellular proliferation in the region of the amyloid.

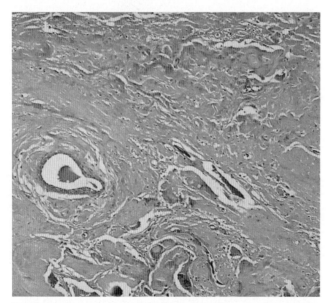

Figure 21–5. At times the amyloid deposited in regions of myeloma may be so dense as to almost totally replace any plasmacellular proliferation, as shown in this example of myeloma involving the scapula. Any plasmacellular proliferation associated with amyloid deposition should raise doubts about a diagnosis of any amyloid tumor.

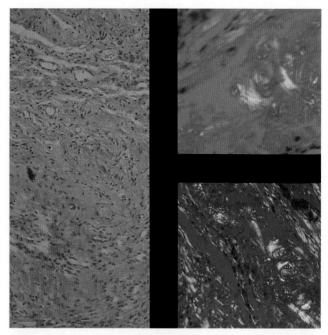

Figure 21–6. This set of photomicrographs shows specimens from the carpal tunnel of an elderly patient who presented with signs of carpal tunnel syndrome. A dense eosinophilic amorphous deposit of amyloid is visible in the tissue from the carpal ligament. When the specimen is viewed under polarized light, Congo red stains show the congophilic material to have the apple green birefringent characteristic of amyloid.

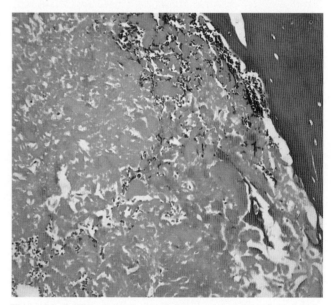

Figure 21–7. This photomicrograph illustrates a nodule of amyloid in the femur. Only when there are no identifiable plasma cells in the region of the amyloid, as in this case, is it reasonable to make a diagnosis of an amyloid tumor of bone. The majority of such lesions are associated with myeloma.

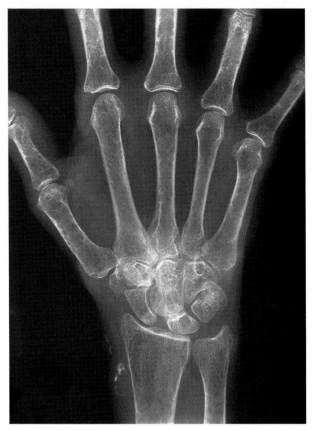

Figure 21–8. Amyloid deposition associated with long-term renal dialysis complicates the changes seen in the small bones of the hand in this 50-year-old dialysis patient.

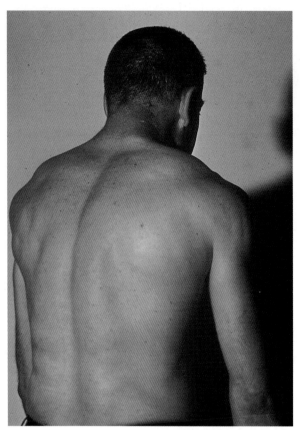

Figure 21–9. Amyloid deposition in skeletal muscle may result in striking changes, as illustrated in this clinical photograph. There is a great disparity between the clinical appearance of well-formed muscle masses and the deterioration of strength associated with amyloid deposition.

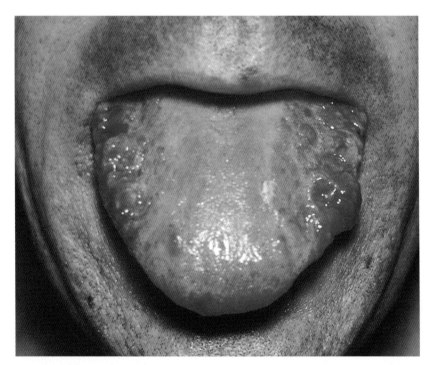

Figure 21–10. Masses of amyloid involve the tongue in this patient. Macroglossia may be associated with amyloidosis.

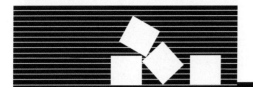

CHAPTER 22

Xanthomatosis

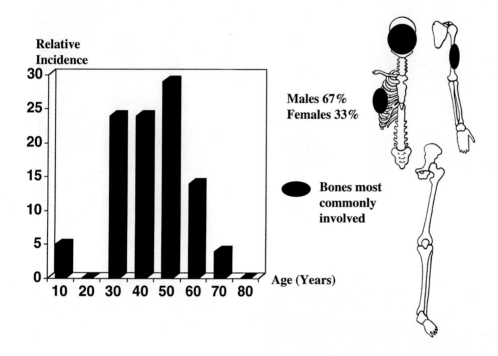

Males 67%
Females 33%

⬤ Bones most
commonly
involved

CLINICAL SIGNS

1. Lipid may accumulate in histiocytes, forming skin nodules (particularly over the extensor tendons of the fingers and the Achilles tendon).
2. Hypercholesterolemia may be present.

CLINICAL SYMPTOMS

1. Pain may be experienced.
2. There may be incidental skeletal findings.
3. Involvement of the orbital bones may result in proptosis or diplopia or both.

MAJOR RADIOGRAPHIC FEATURES

1. Xanthomatosis rarely results in skeletal abnormalities; but when it does, patchy sclerosis and focal lytic destruction can be seen.
2. Cortical bone may be thinned secondary to endosteal erosion.
3. Lesions tend to be round to oval and less than 4 cm.
4. Lesions are sharply marginated, with a rim of surrounding sclerosis.
5. Cortical expansion may be present.
6. Periosteal new bone formation is rarely present.

124

RADIOGRAPHIC DIFFERENTIAL DIAGNOSIS

1. Giant cell tumor.
2. Sinus histiocytosis with massive lymphadenopathy.
3. Fibrous dysplasia.
4. Metaphyseal fibrous defect.
5. Unicameral bone cyst.
6. Osteoblastoma.
7. Langerhans' cell histiocytosis.

MAJOR PATHOLOGIC FEATURES

1. Grossly, the lesional tissue is yellowish.
2. Histologically, the marrow is replaced by foamy histiocytes and shows varying degrees of fibrosis and inflammation.
3. Cleft-like spaces are present amid the lipid-laden histiocytes, and these spaces represent cholesterol crystals that have been dissolved during tissue processing.
4. Multinucleated giant cells are commonly present.
5. Hemosiderin pigment is present in approximately 60 per cent of lesions.
6. Fibrosis is commonly seen.
7. Scattered foci of calcification may be evident.

PATHOLOGIC DIFFERENTIAL DIAGNOSIS

1. Erdheim-Chester disease.
2. Langerhans' cell histiocytosis.
3. Sinus histiocytosis with massive lymphadenopathy (Rosai-Dorfman disease).

4. Osteomyelitis.
5. Metastatic clear cell carcinoma (particularly if the biopsy is a needle biopsy or aspiration cytology).
6. Benign fibrous histiocytoma.

TREATMENT

Medical

1. Underlying hyperlipoproteinemias must be recognized and treated.
2. Articular, tendinous, and periarticular manifestations are treated symptomatically (e.g., nonsteroidal anti-inflammatory drugs [NSAIDs]).

Surgical

1. Symptomatic xanthomas are excised.

References

Bertoni F, Capanna R, Calderoni P, Bacchini P: Case report 223. Benign fibrous histiocytoma. Skeletal Radiol 9:215–217, 1983.

Eble JN, Rosenberg AE, and Young RH: Retroperitoneal xanthogranuloma in a patient with Erdheim-Chester disease [review]. Am J Surg Pathol 18(8):843–848, 1994.

Fink MG, Levinson DJ, Brown NL, et al: Erdheim-Chester disease. Case report with autopsy findings. Arch Pathol Lab Med 115(6):619–623, 1991.

Hamilton WC, Ramsey PL, Hanson SM, and Schiff DC: Osseous xanthoma and multiple hand tumors as a complication of hyperlipidemia. Report of a case. J. Bone Joint Surg (Am) 57:551–553, 1975.

Yaghmai I: Intra- and extraosseous xanthomata associated with hyperlipidemia. Radiology 128:49–54, 1978.

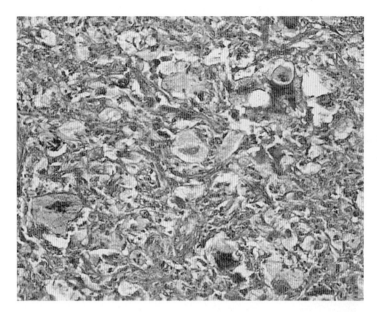

Figure 22–1. This photomicrograph illustrates numerous lipid-laden histiocytes and scattered giant cells in a xanthoma. Many benign bone tumors may undergo degenerative changes and show a similar xanthomatous morphology.

Figure 22–2. Numerous cholesterol clefts, the result of cholesterol crystal formation that is subsequently removed by tissue processing, are present in this lesion from the ilium. If no residual identifiable benign tumor is present in such a lesion, then xanthoma may be used as a descriptive diagnosis.

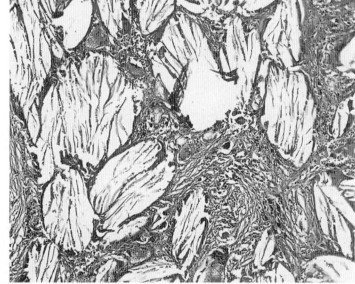

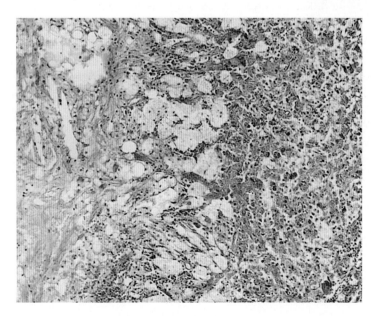

Figure 22–3. This photomicrograph illustrates xanthomatous degenerative changes in a giant cell tumor of the proximal tibia. Hemorrhage and necrosis frequently precede the xanthomatous degeneration in giant cell tumors. If the lesion involves the epiphysis of a long bone in a patient older than 20 years of age, then such histologic features most likely represent degenerative change in a pre-existing giant cell tumor.

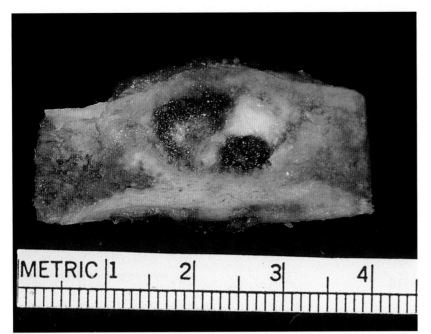

Figure 22–4. This photograph of a gross specimen shows a portion of resected rib with a well-circumscribed defect. The yellow portion of the lesion represents a region of lipid-laden histiocytes, which microscopically have a xanthomatous appearance. Such xanthomatous degeneration of fibrous dysplasia, a lesion commonly found in the ribs, may be mistaken for other tumors when sampled with fine-needle aspiration.

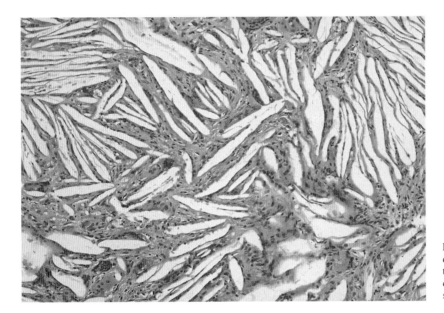

Figure 22–5. This photomicrograph illustrates the degenerative pattern that can be seen in giant cell tumors. Cholesterol clefts and multinucleated giant cells are present. This pattern may simulate that seen in a xanthoma of bone.

CHAPTER 23

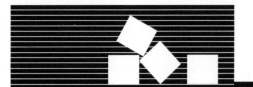

Fibrous Dysplasia

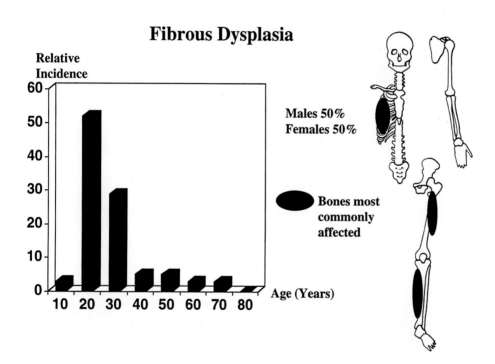

Fibrous Dysplasia

Males 50%
Females 50%

Bones most commonly affected

CLINICAL SYMPTOMS

1. Most patients are asymptomatic.
2. Abnormal bone growth may result in deformity.
3. Pain may be present.
4. Swelling may be noted; when the process involves the skull bones, the patient may present with exophthalmos.
5. Involvement of the femoral neck may result in weakening and resultant pathologic fracture.

CLINICAL SIGNS

1. A localized swelling may be found.
2. Exophthalmos may be present if skull bones are involved.

3. Cutaneous pigmentation may be seen in association with polyostotic disease (Albright's syndrome).
4. Precocious puberty in girls may be associated with polyostotic disease (Albright's syndrome).
5. Soft tissue myxomas have been reported in association with fibrous dysplasia (Mazabraud's syndrome).

MAJOR RADIOGRAPHIC FEATURES

1. The location of the lesion is metaphyseal or diaphyseal.
2. The lesion is usually lytic or ground glass–like in density.
3. The affected bone shows expansion and sharp margination of the lesion.
4. Bowing and pathologic fracture may be seen.

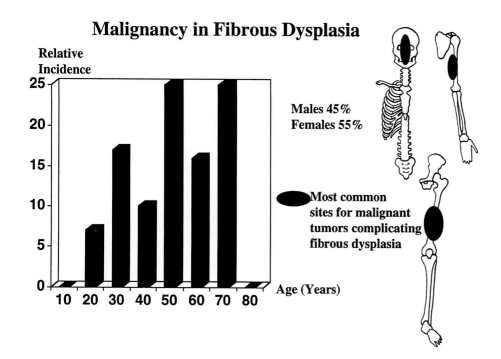

Malignancy in Fibrous Dysplasia

Males 45%
Females 55%

Most common sites for malignant tumors complicating fibrous dysplasia

5. The lesion may be surrounded by a thick rind of sclerotic bone.
6. Multiple bones may be affected (polyostotic).

RADIOGRAPHIC DIFFERENTIAL DIAGNOSIS

1. Fibroma (metaphyseal fibrous defect, nonossifying fibroma).
2. Unicameral bone cyst (simple cyst).
3. Chondromyxoid fibroma.
4. Aneurysmal bone cyst.

MAJOR PATHOLOGIC FEATURES

Gross

1. Lesional tissue is usually dense and fibrous.
2. Osteoid trabeculae within the fibrous tissue impart a gritty quality to the lesion when it is cut.
3. Prominent cyst formation may be present; such cysts are most commonly filled with a clear, yellowish fluid.
4. Dense ossification may also occur within the lesional tissue.

Microscopic

1. At low magnification, the lesion is composed of proliferating fibroblasts that produce a dense collagenous matrix.
2. Osteoid trabeculae course irregularly through the connective tissue.
3. The trabeculae are arranged in a haphazard, nonfunctional manner, and they may contain reversal lines mimicking the appearance of Paget's disease.
4. A metaplastic chondroid component may be present and rarely is so prominent as to raise the question of whether the lesion represents a hyaline cartilage neoplasm.
5. Cystic degeneration may be identified. These regions of degeneration may also show numerous lipophages and benign multinucleated giant cells. Rarely, the lesion shows marked myxoid change.
6. At higher magnification, no cytologic atypia is seen.

PATHOLOGIC DIFFERENTIAL DIAGNOSIS

Benign lesions:

1. Paget's disease.
2. Giant cell reparative granuloma.

Malignant lesions:

1. Low-grade central osteosarcoma.
2. Parosteal osteosarcoma (if the location is not known).

TREATMENT

Primary Modality: observation if the lesion is asymptomatic.

Other Possible Approaches: curettage and grafting or resection.

References

Campanacci M, and Laus M: Osteofibrous dysplasia of the tibia and fibula. J Bone Joint Surg (Am) *63*:367–375, 1981.

Huvos AG, Higginbotham NL, and Miller TR: Bone sarcoma arising in fibrous dysplasia. J Bone Joint Surg (Am) *54*:1047–1056, 1972.

Nager GT, Kennedy DW, and Kopstein E: Fibrous dysplasia: a review of the disease and its manifestations in the temporal bone. Ann Otol Rhinol Laryngol (Suppl) *92*:1–52, 1982.

Nakashima Y, Yamamuro T, Fumiwara Y, et al: Osteofibrous dysplasia (ossifying fibroma of long bones): a study of 12 cases. Cancer *52*:909–914, 1983.

Ruggieri P, Sim FH, Bond JR, Unni KK: Malignancies in fibrous dysplasia. Cancer *73*:1411–1424, 1994.

Weatherby RP, Dahlin DC, and Ivins JC: Postradiation sarcoma of bone: review of 78 Mayo Clinic cases. Mayo Clin Proc *56*:294–306, 1981.

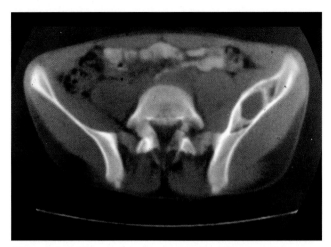

Figure 23–1. This computed tomographic (CT) scan illustrates a sharply marginated lesion of fibrous dysplasia expanding the left iliac bone.

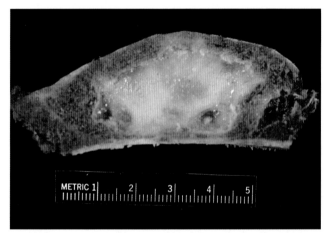

Figure 23–2. The gross pathologic features of the case shown in Figure 23–1 are seen in this photograph. The lesional tissue is whitish. Cystic degeneration is common in old fibrous dysplasia; such degeneration may be accompanied by the presence of numerous lipid-laden histiocytes seen on histologic examination.

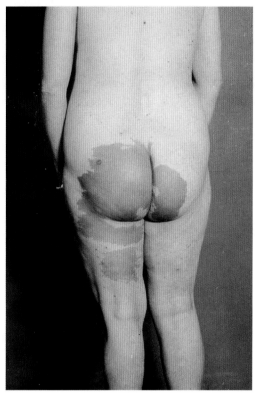

Figure 23–3. Pigmentation, as shown in this photograph, may be seen in cases of Albright's syndrome (polyostotic fibrous dysplasia).

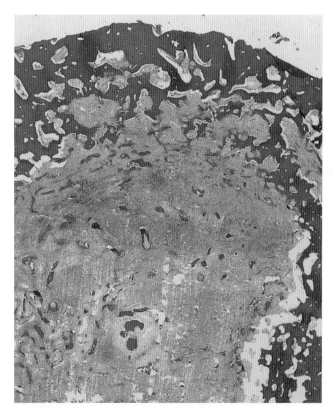

Figure 23–4. At low magnification, fibrous dysplasia is relatively hypocellular and composed of a spindle cell stroma, within which numerous irregular trabeculae of osteoid are present.

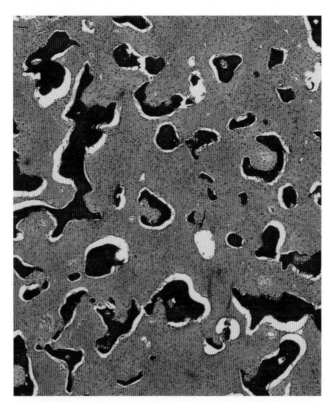

Figure 23–5. At higher magnification, the osteoid is seen to be arranged in a nonfunctional manner. The shape of the osteoid may be irregular or round to oval, as in this case of fibrous dysplasia involving the rib.

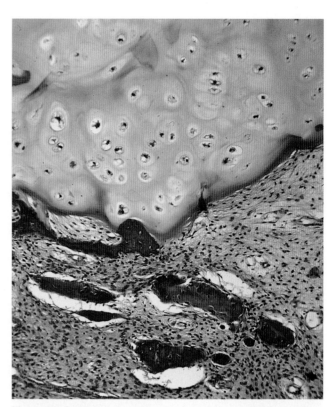

Figure 23–7. Fibrous dysplasia may also have a cartilaginous component; in such cases, the designation of "fibrocartilaginous dysplasia" is appropriate. This example of such a lesion was taken from the femur of a patient with Albright's syndrome.

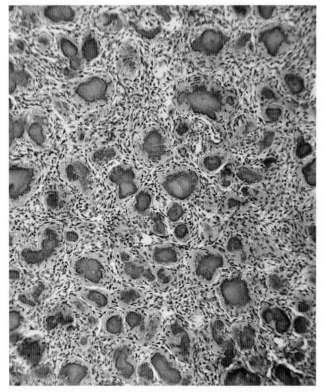

Figure 23–6. Occasionally, the osteoid produced in fibrous dysplasia may mimic the appearance of cementum or even psammomatous calcification, as seen in a meningioma. Such is the case in this lesion of the ilium.

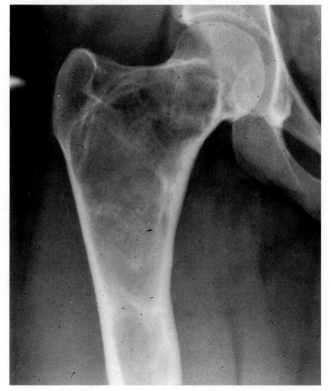

Figure 23–8. The proximal femur is a common location for fibrous dysplasia. This lesion, which has resulted in extensive expansion of the proximal femur, shows the sharp margination and sclerotic rim associated with a benign process.

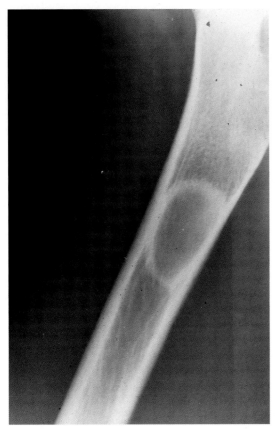

Figure 23–9. The "ground glass" density of fibrous dysplasia is evident in this radiograph of a lesion involving the medulla of the femur. Note the thick rind of surrounding sclerosis.

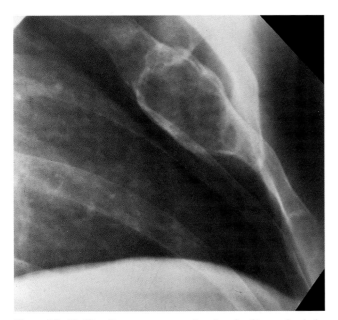

Figure 23–10. The ribs are a common location for fibrous dysplasia. This example shows expansion of the affected rib, frequently seen in such cases, and sclerosis of the surrounding bone.

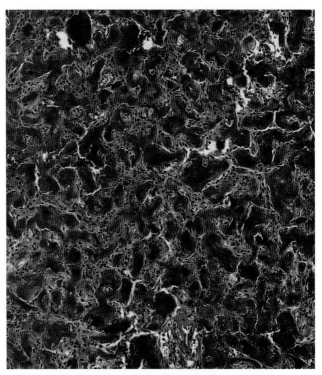

Figure 23–11. Fibrous dysplasia may involve the flat bones of the skull, as in this case. In such cases, the irregular psammoma body–like ossification of the lesion may result in a pattern simulating that of a meningioma secondarily involving the affected bone.

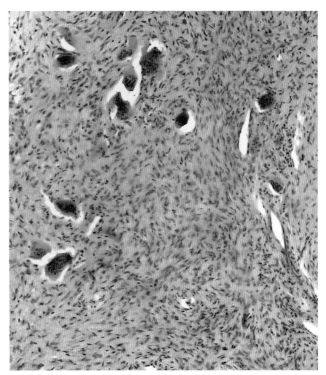

Figure 23–12. Benign multinucleated giant cells may be seen in fibrous dysplasia, as in this case involving the humerus. Like other lesions that contain numerous giant cells, this lesion may be confused with giant cell tumor and other giant cell–containing bone lesions.

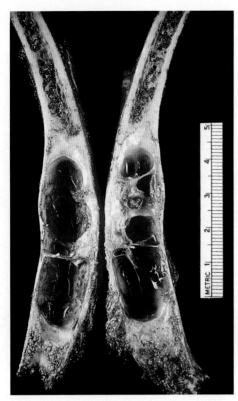

Figure 23–13. Cystic degeneration is most commonly associated with fibrous dysplasia of the rib, as in this case.

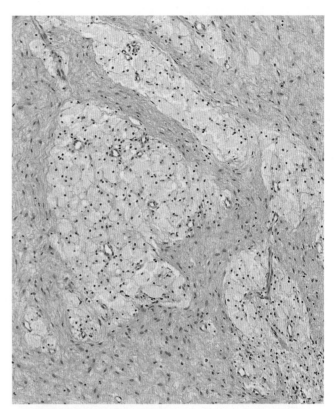

Figure 23–14. Foam cells, or lipid-laden macrophages, also indicate a degenerative process. Such foci are evident in this example of fibrous dysplasia involving the proximal femur.

CHAPTER 24

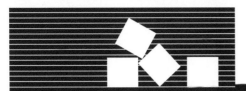

Osteofibrous Dysplasia

CLINICAL SIGNS

1. Bowing of the lower extremity may be seen.
2. Abnormal gait (limp) may be present.
3. Leg length discrepancy may be seen.
4. Pathologic fracture may occur through the lesion.

CLINICAL SYMPTOMS

1. A painless or, less commonly, painful mass is usually associated with minor trauma.
2. An enlarging mass may be present.
3. Bowing of the lower extremity may be seen.

MAJOR RADIOGRAPHIC FEATURES

1. Osteofibrous dysplasia almost exclusively involves the tibia. (The adjacent fibula may be involved in up to 20 per cent of cases.)
2. Multiple eccentric lytic defects may be seen, most commonly affecting the cortex anteriorly.
3. A diaphyseal location is most common, but the dysplasia may extend to involve the metaphysis.
4. Some cases show a "ground glass" appearance similar to that of fibrous dysplasia.
5. The cortex is thinned or, rarely, absent in areas of involvement. (Generally, a thin rim of cortex separates the lesion from the medullary bone.)
6. The tibia may be bowed anteriorly.
7. The lesion may have a multiloculated appearance.
8. The periosteum is preserved.
9. Calcifications may be identified within the lesion.
10. Computed tomographic (CT) scans demonstrate cortical involvement without extension to involve the medullary bone.
11. Increased signal on both T1- and T2-weighted magnetic resonance (MR) images may be seen.
12. Isotopic bone scan shows increased uptake by the lesional tissue.

RADIOGRAPHIC DIFFERENTIAL DIAGNOSIS

1. Adamantinoma.
2. Fibrous dysplasia.
3. Infection.

MAJOR PATHOLOGIC FEATURES

Gross

1. Lesional tissue is gray-white and firm.
2. Bony sclerosis may surround the lesional tissue.
3. Lesional tissue is identified within the cortex, which is commonly expanded.

Microscopic

1. Lesional tissue is composed of irregularly shaped trabecular bone lying in fibrous connective tissue.
2. In contrast to typical fibrous dysplasia, the trabecular bone is characteristically surrounded by prominent osteoblastic "rimming."
3. Foci of hemorrhage may be present.
4. Foamy macrophages, presumably degenerative in origin, may be present.

5. In contrast to adamantinoma, epithelial islands are absent.
6. Isolated, scattered individual keratin-positive cells may be identified immunohistochemically within the fibrous connective tissue.

PATHOLOGIC DIFFERENTIAL DIAGNOSIS

1. Adamantinoma.
2. Fibrous dysplasia.
3. Paget's disease.

TREATMENT

1. Observation is essential, as the process "involutes" with skeletal maturity.
2. Biopsy should be performed if the diagnosis is in question.
3. Resection may be necessary.

References

Campanacci M, and Laus M: Osteofibrous dysplasia of the tibia and fibula. J Bone Joint Surg (Am) 63:367–375, 1981.

Castellote A, Garcia-Pena P, Lucaya J, and Lorenzo J: Osteofibrous dysplasia. Skeletal Radiol 17:483–486, 1988.

Park YK, Unni KK, McLeod RA, and Pritchard DJ: Osteofibrous dysplasia: clinicopathologic study of 80 cases. Hum Pathol 24:1339–1347, 1993.

Wang JW, Shih CH, and Chen WJ: Osteofibrous dysplasia (ossifying fibroma of long bones). Clin Orthop 278:235–243, 1992.

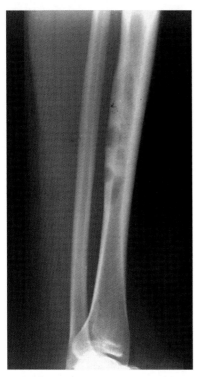

Figure 24–1. This radiograph illustrates the typical appearance of osteofibrous dysplasia involving the tibial cortex. Multiple areas of lucency are surrounded by bony sclerosis. The corresponding gross pathologic appearance of the lesion is shown in Figure 24–2.

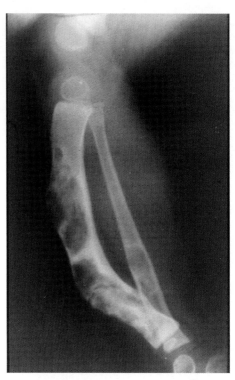

Figure 24–3. This radiograph of the tibia from a three-year-old girl shows marked bowing of the tibia due to its involvement by osteofibrous dysplasia. Although osteofibrous dysplasia is likely a "developmental" condition, congenital cases have only rarely been documented.

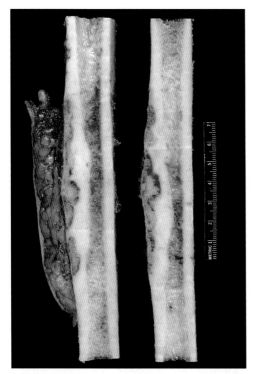

Figure 24–2. This gross specimen is from a case of osteofibrous dysplasia treated with resection. The gray-white lesional tissue involving the cortex is clearly distinct from the surrounding sclerotic reactive bone. Note that the process docs not involve the underlying medullary bone.

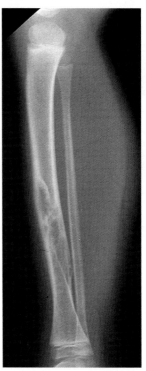

Figure 24–4. Figures 24–4 and 24–5 show the radiographic and computed tomographic (CT) appearance, respectively, of osteofibrous dysplasia in a five-year-old male patient. Note the bony sclerosis surrounding the regions of osteolysis and the lack of periosteal reaction.

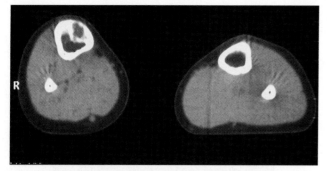

Figure 24–5. This CT scan of the patient in Figure 24–4 shows that the cortex is expanded and deformed by the process of osteofibrous dysplasia and the underlying medullary bone is uninvolved.

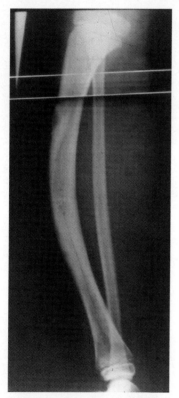

Figure 24–6. This radiograph illustrates osteofibrous dysplasia involving the tibia. Significant bowing is present. This case of a ten-year-old girl had been followed since birth, and the process appeared to be resolving radiographically. Osteofibrous dysplasia generally "involutes" with skeletal maturity.

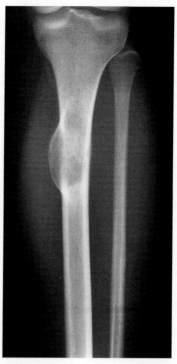

Figure 24–7. This 17-year-old girl presented with a mass lesion involving the anterior aspect of her lower extremity. The radiograph illustrates a more "aneurysmal" expansion of the tibia than is commonly seen in osteofibrous dysplasia. No significant periosteal reaction is evident. Aneurysmal bone cyst change can be seen in a wide variety of bone lesions.

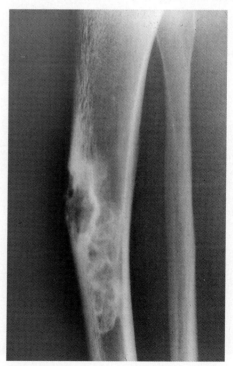

Figure 24–8. This 15-year-old boy has osteofibrous dysplasia of the tibia. The cortex is partially absent, but no significant periosteal reaction is evident. The differential diagnosis for such a lesion most commonly includes adamantinoma.

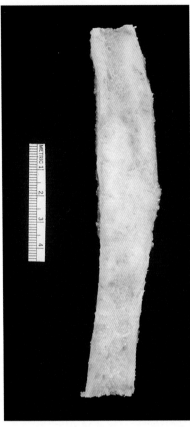

Figure 24–9. This photograph of a gross specimen illustrates osteofibrous dysplasia involving the tibia in a nine-year-old female patient. Longstanding cases of osteofibrous dysplasia have been reported to occasionally extend to involve the medullary bone.

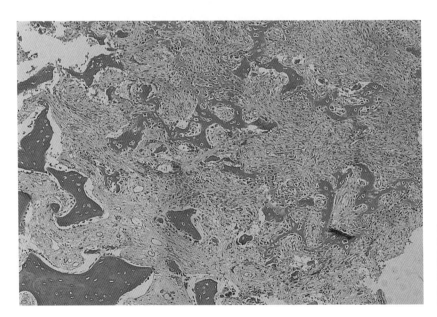

Figure 24–10. The low-power histologic appearance of osteofibrous dysplasia is illustrated in this photomicrograph. The irregularly arranged bony trabeculae lying within a relatively hypocellular fibroblastic proliferation is typical of the lesion and suggests the pathologic differential diagnosis of fibrous dysplasia.

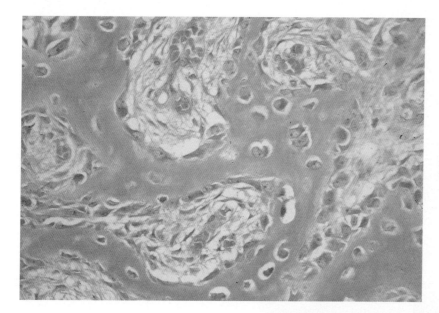

Figure 24–11. This high-power photomicrograph illustrates the prominent osteoblastic rimming of bony trabeculae, which helps distinguish osteofibrous dysplasia from fibrous dysplasia.

Figure 24–12. The bone produced by osteofibrous dysplasia may be relatively thin, as shown in this photomicrograph. Given this appearance, the pathologist may be concerned about the possible diagnosis of low-grade central osteosarcoma. Considering the histologic appearance in the context of the clinical and radiographic features helps to avoid this potential diagnostic problem.

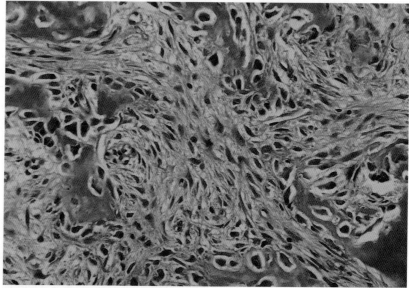

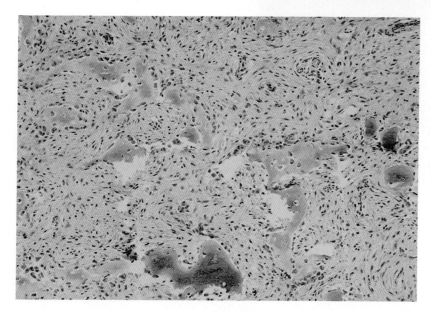

Figure 24–13. This low-power photomicrograph shows a portion of a tibial lesion of osteofibrous dysplasia that is relatively devoid of bony trabeculae. Such regions may raise concern regarding a diagnosis of adamantinoma. Although immunohistochemical stains for keratin can be helpful in such cases, it should be remembered that individual cells may be keratin-positive in osteofibrous dysplasia.

CHAPTER 25

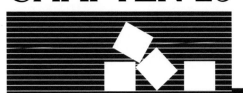

Ankylosing Spondylitis

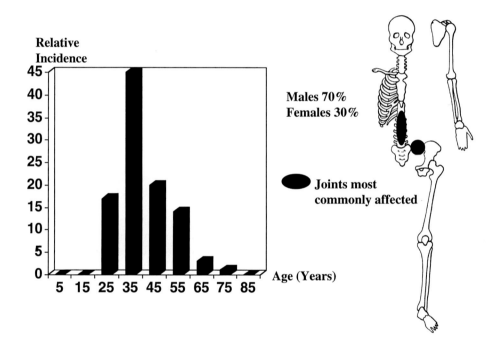

Males 70%
Females 30%

● **Joints most commonly affected**

INCIDENCE

The incidence of ankylosing spondylitis is approximately 6.6 per 100,000 population, with a peak incidence in the third and fourth decades. An association exists between the presence of HLA-B27 and a high incidence of ankylosing spondylitis.

PREVALENCE

The prevalence of ankylosing spondylitis is approximately 400 per 100,000 population. The peak prevalence is in the fifth and sixth decades.

CLINICAL SIGNS

1. Males are affected more commonly than females.
2. Movement of the spine is restricted in all three planes (anterior flexion, lateral flexion, and extension).
3. Approximately 90 per cent of patients have HLA-B27. (*Note:* HLA-B27 is associated with the other spondyloarthropathies as well.)
4. Expansion of the chest is limited, as measured at the level of the fourth intercostal space.
5. Morning stiffness may be present.
6. Symptoms may improve with exercise.
7. A family history of similar disease may be present.

8. Diagnostic criteria for ankylosing spondylitis include
   a. Low back pain and stiffness of greater than three months' duration.
   b. Thoracic pain and stiffness.
   c. Limitation of motion of the lumbar vertebrae.
   d. Limitation of chest expansion.
   e. History of iritis or its sequelae.
   f. Bilateral sacroiliac changes on radiography that are characteristic of ankylosing spondylitis.

CLINICAL SYMPTOMS

1. Low back pain may be present.
2. Stiffness of the back is greater in the early morning.
3. Involvement of the peripheral joints with arthritic symptoms generally occurs late in the course of the disease.
4. Fatigue, weight loss, and low-grade fever may be present during periods of active disease.

MAJOR RADIOGRAPHIC FEATURES

1. Squaring of the margins of the vertebral bodies may be seen.
2. A "bamboo spine" appearance may be evident.
3. Sclerosis may be present on both sides of the sacroiliac joint.
4. The sacroiliac joint may show fusion.

RADIOGRAPHIC DIFFERENTIAL DIAGNOSIS

1. Psoriatic arthritis.
2. Reiter's syndrome.
3. Enteropathic spondylitis.
4. Diffuse idiopathic skeletal hyperostosis (DISH).

MAJOR PATHOLOGIC FEATURES

1. Active endochondral ossification across the intervertebral disc or articular cartilage may be apparent.
2. Inflammatory changes in the synovium are similar but less intense than those seen in rheumatoid arthritis.

PATHOLOGIC DIFFERENTIAL DIAGNOSIS

1. Rheumatoid arthritis.
2. Psoriatic arthritis.
3. Reiter's syndrome
4. Enteropathic spondylitis.

TREATMENT

Medical

1. Supportive care, education, and proper nutrition are mainstays of treatment.
2. Physical therapy, exercise to maintain motion, and prevention of spinal deformity are important.
3. Nonsteroidal anti-inflammatory drugs (NSAIDs) may be used. (Aspirin is not as effective as other agents.)
4. Common spine fractures must be recognized and subsequently braced.

Surgical

1. Vertebral wedge osteotomy may be used to correct severe kyphosis.
2. Total joint replacement may be performed in advanced disease.

References

Barozzi L, Olivieri I, De Matteis M, et al: Seronegative spondylarthropathies: imaging of spondylitis, enthesitis and dactylitis. Eur J Radiol *27 (Suppl 1)*:S12–S17, 1998.

Braun J, Bollow M, and Sieper J: Radiologic diagnosis and pathology of the spondyloarthropathies. Rheum Dis Clin North Am *24(4)*:697–735, 1998.

Calin A: Differentiating the seronegative spondyloarthropathies: how to characterize and manage ankylosing spondylitis. J Musculoskel Med *3*:14, 1986.

Gran JT, and Husby G: Clinical, epidemiologic, and therapeutic aspects of ankylosing spondylitis. Curr Opin Rheumatol *10(4)*:292–298, 1998.

Olivieri I, Barozzi L, Padula A, et al: Clinical manifestations of seronegative spondylarthropathies. Eur J Radiol *27 (Suppl 1)*:S3–S6, 1998.

Van der Linden S, van der Heijde D: Ankylosing spondylitis. Clinical features. Rheum Dis Clin North Am *24(4)*:663–766, 1998.

Wordsworth P: Genes in the spondyloarthropathies. Rheum Dis Clin North Am *24(4)*:845–863, 1998.

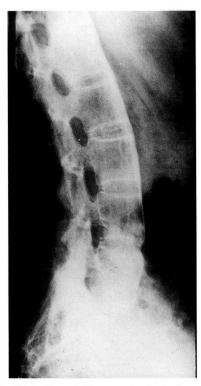

Figure 25–1. This radiograph illustrates the classic features of ankylosing spondylitis, including squaring of the vertebrae, ossification of the anterior ligament, and fusion of the facets.

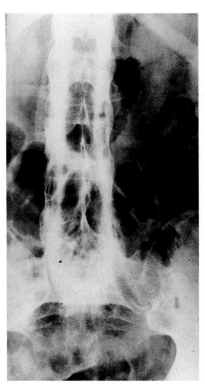

Figure 25–3. This radiograph illustrates the "bamboo spine" appearance of well-developed ankylosing spondylitis.

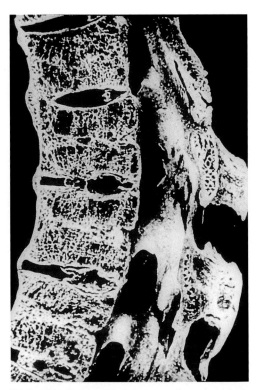

Figure 25–2. This photograph of a macerated specimen is from a patient with ankylosing spondylitis. Some squaring of the vertebrae is evident, but the major feature illustrated is ossification of the anterior ligament and fusion of the vertebral facets.

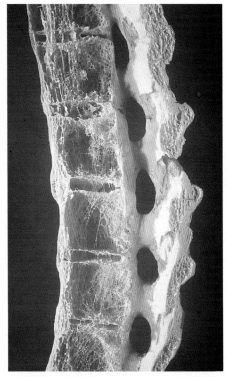

Figure 25–4. This photograph of a macerated specimen from a 71-year-old man who suffered from ankylosing spondylitis demonstrates squaring of the vertebrae as well as bony ankylosis.

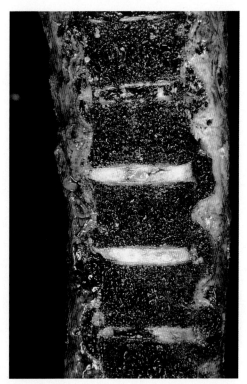

Figure 25–5. This photograph of a gross specimen shows a coronal cross-section of vertebrae in a patient who had well-developed ankylosing spondylitis. Bony ankylosis is evident, and hematopoietic marrow occupies the medullary space of the ankylosed bone.

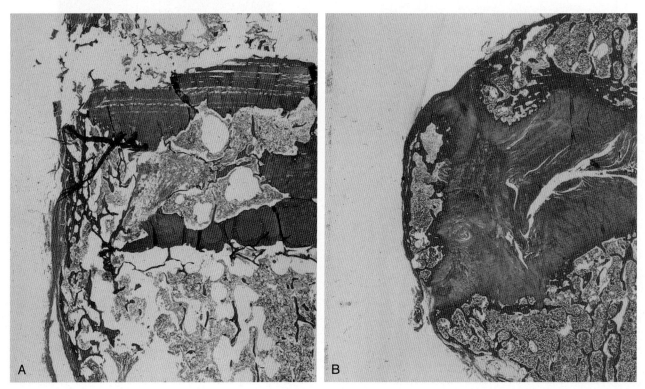

Figure 25–6. *A* and *B*, These two photomicrographs illustrate the histologic appearance of bony ankylosis of the vertebrae. Active endochondral ossification may be seen.

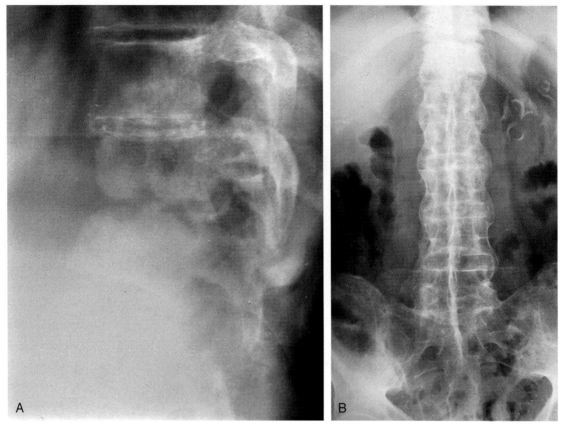

Figure 25–7. Ankylosing spondylitis is shown in these lateral (*A*) and anteroposterior (AP) (*B*) radiographs from a 71-year-old male patient. Bony ankylosis is particularly evident in the AP radiograph.

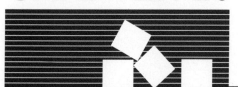

CHAPTER 26

Synovial Chondromatosis

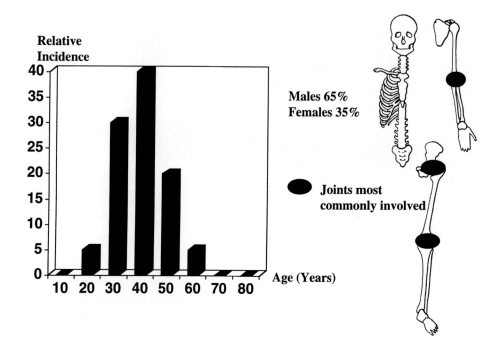

Relative Incidence

Males 65%
Females 35%

● **Joints most commonly involved**

Age (Years)

CLINICAL SIGNS

1. A monoarticular process is noted.
2. The knee, hip, and elbow are most commonly involved.
3. Joint effusion may be present.
4. Joint aspiration may reveal hemorrhagic fluid, but no crystals are identified.
5. Palpable loose bodies may be present.
6. Progressive arthropathy may occur.

CLINICAL SYMPTOMS

1. Pain may be experienced in the affected joint. (An insidious course is common.)
2. The affected joint may show swelling.
3. Palpable loose bodies may be present.
4. The affected joint may exhibit loss of motion.
5. "Locking" of the joint may be seen.
6. The affected joint may show instability.

MAJOR RADIOGRAPHIC FEATURES

1. There are soft tissue masses with varying amounts of calcification in the region of the affected joint.
2. Bony erosion may be seen (particularly in joints with tight capsules).
3. Calcific bodies may be present in the soft tissues adjacent to the joint.
4. Joint effusion may be evident.
5. Secondary arthropathy may be present in advanced cases.
6. Arthrogram outlines space-occupying masses in the joint.
7. Bone scan is generally unremarkable.

8. The appearance on magnetic resonance imaging (MRI) is characterized by
   a. Lobulated, homogeneous intra-articular signal isointense to slightly hyperintense to muscle on T1-weighted images and hyperintense on T2-weighted images.
   b. Pattern a with foci of signal void on all pulse sequences (the majority).
   c. Patterns a and b with foci of peripheral low signal surrounding a central fat-like signal.

RADIOGRAPHIC DIFFERENTIAL DIAGNOSIS

1. Osteoarthritis.
2. Pigmented villonodular synovitis.
3. Lipoma arborescens.
4. Chondrosarcoma.
5. Xanthoma (localized nodular synovitis).
6. Popliteal cyst.
7. Gout.

MAJOR PATHOLOGIC FEATURES

Gross

1. The synovium is hyperplastic.
2. Nodular projections are present on the synovial surface.
3. Pedunculated masses may be present.
4. Loose bodies may be found in the joint.
5. Masses of cartilage with osseous metaplasia may "invade" the adjacent soft tissue.
6. Secondary osteoarthritic changes may occur, with bony erosion and extension of cartilaginous masses into the eroded bone.

Microscopic

1. Masses of hyaline cartilage are arranged in a nodular pattern.
2. The hyaline cartilage is relatively hypercellular.
3. Mild cytologic atypia may be present.
4. Osseous metaplasia may be seen (particularly at the periphery of the hyaline cartilage masses).
5. Myxoid stromal change of the chondroid matrix is generally absent.

Note: The histologic features resemble those of intramedullary low-grade chondrosarcoma.

PATHOLOGIC DIFFERENTIAL DIAGNOSIS

1. Chondrosarcoma.
2. Osteoarthritis.

TREATMENT

1. Total synovectomy (open or arthroscopic) with removal of loose bodies may be performed in patients with active disease.
2. Partial synovectomy (open or arthroscopic) with removal of loose bodies may be performed in patients with localized disease.
3. Loose bodies may be removed in the late phase of the disease.
4. Reconstructive surgery, i.e., total joint arthroplasty, may be performed in patients with advanced arthropathy.

References

Hamilton A, Davis RI, and Nixon JE: Synovial chondrosarcoma complicating synovial chondromatosis: report of a case and review of the literature. J Bone Joint Surg (Am) 69:1084–1088, 1987.

Kramer J, Recht M, Deely DM, et al: MR appearance of idiopathic synovial osteochondromatosis. J Comput Assist Tomogr 17:772–776, 1993.

Maurice H, Crone M, and Watt I: Synovial chondromatosis. J Bone Joint Surg (Br) 70:807–811, 1988.

Milgram JW: Synovial osteochondromatosis: a histological study of thirty cases. J Bone Joint Surg (Am) 59:792–801, 1977.

Murphy FP, Dahlin DC, and Sullivan CR: Articular synovial chondromatosis. J Bone Joint Surg (Am) 44:77, 1962.

Ogilvie-Harris DJ, and Saleh K: Generalized synovial chondromatosis of the knee: a comparison of removal of the loose bodies alone with arthroscopic synovectomy. Arthroscopy 10:166–170, 1994.

Shpitzer T, Ganel A, and Engelberg S: Surgery for synovial chondromatosis: 26 cases followed up for 6 years. Acta Orthop Scand 61:567–569, 1990.

Sim FH: Synovial proliferative disorders: role of synovectomy. Arthroscopy 1:198–204, 1985.

Sim FH, Dahlin DC, and Ivins JC: Extra-articular synovial chondromatosis. J Bone Joint Surg (Am) 59:492–495, 1977.

Sundaram M, McGuire MH, Fletcher J, et al: Magnetic resonance imaging of lesions of synovial origin. Skeletal Radiol 15:110–116, 1986.

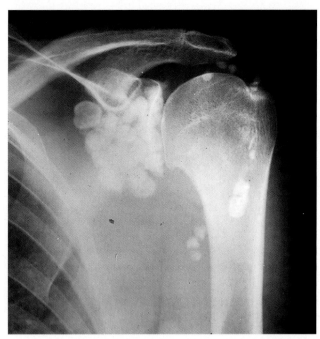

Figure 26–1. This radiograph illustrates synovial chondromatosis involving the shoulder joint. Multiple well-circumscribed calcific densities are noted. Extension into the soft tissues surrounding the joint can occur.

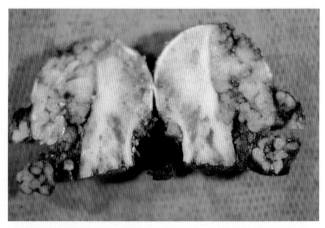

Figure 26–3. This photograph of a gross specimen shows recurrent synovial chondromatosis involving the hip joint. The recurrent lesion has eroded into the head and neck of the femur.

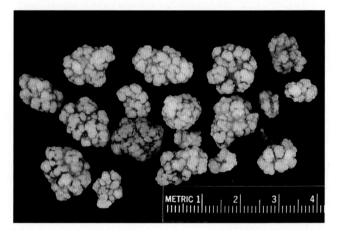

Figure 26–4. This photograph of a gross specimen illustrates the multilobulated nature of loose bodies in synovial chondromatosis. Such loose bodies may be large or small and may mimic the "rice bodies" of osteoarthritis.

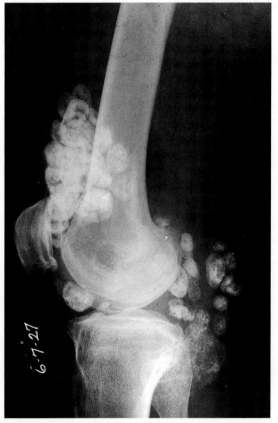

Figure 26–2. This radiograph illustrates synovial chondromatosis involving the knee. Well-circumscribed calcific densities are present both anteriorly and posteriorly. Bony destruction on either side of the joint may occur in such cases.

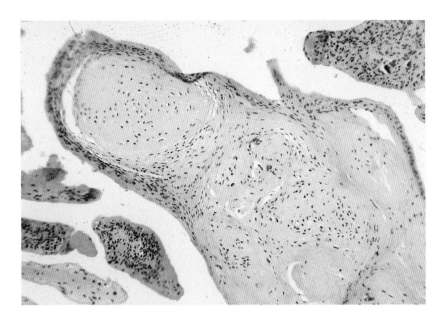

Figure 26–5. This photomicrograph demonstrates the pattern of synovial chondromatosis as seen at low magnification. The synovial lining is identified as overlying the cartilage.

Figure 26–6. This photomicrograph illustrates the histologic features of synovial chondromatosis as seen at high magnification. The cartilage is characteristically relatively hypercellular and may show some nuclear enlargement. These features may mimic a low-grade chondrosarcoma. The lesion is usually lobulated, as shown in this example.

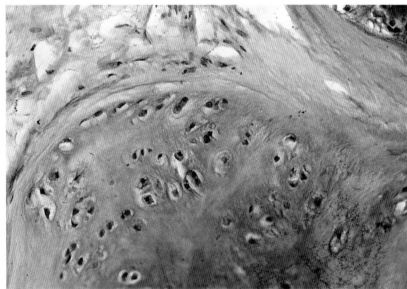

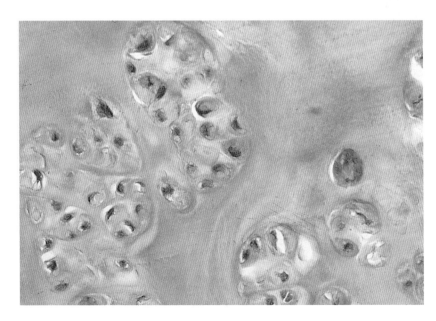

Figure 26–7. This photomicrograph shows the degree of nuclear pleomorphism that can be seen in synovial chondromatosis. The histologic criteria used to differentiate benign from malignant intraosseous cartilage tumors do not apply to cartilaginous lesions of the synovium.

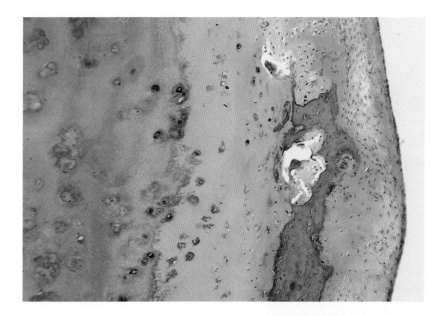

Figure 26–8. This photomicrograph illustrates the osseous metaplasia that often accompanies the chondroid metaplasia of synovial chondromatosis. The bone in such cases most frequently is at the periphery of the cartilage islands.

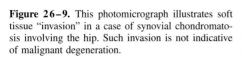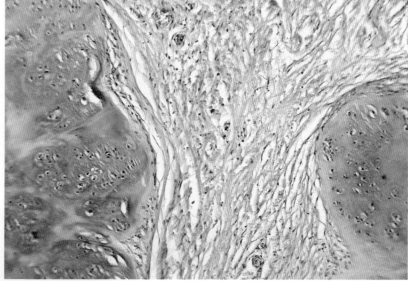

Figure 26–9. This photomicrograph illustrates soft tissue "invasion" in a case of synovial chondromatosis involving the hip. Such invasion is not indicative of malignant degeneration.

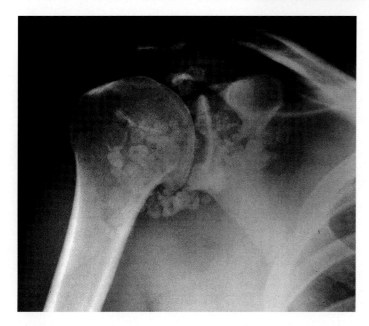

Figure 26–10. This radiograph reveals synovial chondromatosis in the shoulder of a 24-year-old man.

CHAPTER 27

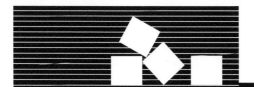

Pigmented Villonodular Synovitis

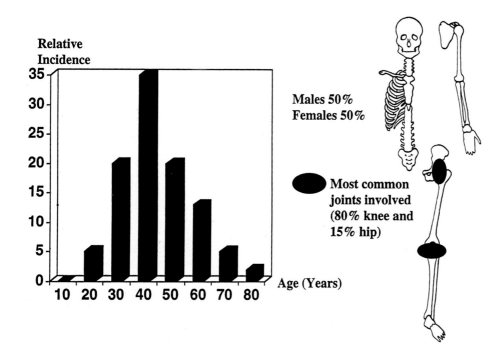

Males 50%
Females 50%

Most common joints involved (80% knee and 15% hip)

CLINICAL SIGNS

1. Joint mobility is limited (up to 90 per cent of cases).
2. A palpable mass may be present (approximately 10 per cent of cases).
3. Skin temperature is increased.
4. The clinical examination is often nonspecific.
5. Laboratory tests are generally within normal limits.
6. Synovial fluid is variable in color (yellow to brown or bloody).
7. Recurrent bloody effusions may occur.

CLINICAL SYMPTOMS

1. The process is monoarticular.
2. Pain may be experienced with motion of the affected joint.
3. Painful swelling of the affected joint may occur.
4. The motion of the affected joint may be limited. ("Locking" of the joint may be described.)
5. Symptoms are generally present for months (average, approximately four years).
6. A sudden exacerbation of pain is due to torsion of nodules that result from the pathologic process.

MAJOR RADIOGRAPHIC FEATURES

1. Plain radiograph shows the following characteristics:
   a. Lucencies on either side of the affected joint. When present, these are generally multiple and have a thin, sclerotic margin.
   b. Joint space narrowing, particularly if the disease involves the hip.
   c. Associated osteoporosis.
   d. Associated osteosclerosis.
   e. Osteophytes, which are uncommonly present.
   f. Soft tissue swelling.
2. Magnetic resonance imaging (MRI) shows the following characteristics:
   a. Low signal on both T1- and T2-weighted images (due to hemosiderin deposition and fibrous connective tissue in the lesion).
   b. Presence of "fat" signal within the mass lesion.
   c. Erosion of bone (most common in the hips, tibiofibular joint, and lumbar facet joints and detected in approximately 60 per cent of cases on MRI).
   d. Preservation of the joint space.
   e. Grape-like mass with a signal density approximately equal to that of muscle.
   f. Effusion, which is present in the majority of patients with knee involvement.

RADIOGRAPHIC DIFFERENTIAL DIAGNOSIS

1. Synovial chondromatosis.
2. Rheumatoid arthritis.
3. Synovial hemangioma.
4. Lipoma arborescens.
5. Osteoarthritis.
6. Hemophilia.

MAJOR PATHOLOGIC FEATURES

Gross

1. The synovium is characterized as the following:
   a. Nodular.
   b. Villous.
   c. Diffuse.
   d. Combination of the above.
2. The cut surface of the synovium is red-brown to yellow-brown, depending upon whether regions rich in hemosiderin-laden macrophages or lipid-laden macrophages predominate.

Microscopic

1. There is proliferation of round to polygonal cells, with scant cytoplasm forming villous finger-like or rounded masses underlying the synovial lining.
2. Nuclei are small and round to oval.
3. Nuclear grooves may be identifiable.
4. Variable amounts of fibrous connective tissue are present.
5. Mitoses are generally inconspicuous.
6. Lipid-laden histiocytes are scattered throughout the lesion or gathered in clusters.
7. Multinucleated giant cells are scattered throughout the lesion.
8. Hemosiderin-laden macrophages are variable in number but may be present in large numbers, giving the synovium a dark brown appearance.

PATHOLOGIC DIFFERENTIAL DIAGNOSIS

1. Metaphyseal fibrous defect (if location is not known).
2. Benign fibrous histiocytoma (if location is not known).
3. Giant cell tumor of tendon sheath (if location is not known).
4. Malignant fibrous histiocytoma.

Note: The histologic features of pigmented villonodular synovitis, metaphyseal fibrous defect (nonossifying fibroma), giant cell tumor of tendon sheath type, and benign fibrous histiocytoma overlap entirely. The location of the lesion is the differentiating feature of these conditions.

TREATMENT

1. Total synovectomy by open or arthroscopic techniques is necessary in the diffuse type of disease. Usually anterior and posterior synovectomy of the knee is re-

quired, and the recurrence rate is approximately 20 to 40 per cent.

2. Intra-articular yttrium-90 radiation synovectomy is experimental.
3. Surgical excision (arthroscopic or open) is curative in patients with localized disease.
4. Reconstructive surgery is indicated for patients with extensive joint destruction, i.e., arthrodesis or joint replacement.

References

Bertoni F, Unni KK, Beabout JW, and Sim FH: Malignant giant cell tumor of the tendon sheaths and joints (malignant pigmented villonodular synovitis). Am J Surg Pathol *21*:153–163, 1997.

Cotten A, Flipo RM, Chastanet P, et al.: Pigmented villonodular synovitis of the hip: review of radiographic features in 58 patients. Skeletal Radiol *24*:1–6, 1995.

Dorwart RH, Genant HK, Johnston WH, and Morris JM: Pigmented villonodular synovitis of synovial joints: clinical, pathologic and radiologic features. AJR Am J Radiol *143*:886–888, 1984.

Flandry F, and Hughston JC: Current Concepts Review. Pigmented villonodular synovitis. J Bone Joint Surg (Am) *69*:942–949, 1987.

Giannini C, Scheithauer BW, Wenger, DE, and Unni KK: Pigmented villonodular synovitis of the spine: a clinical, radiological and morphological study of 12 cases. J Neurosurg *84*:592–597, 1996.

Gitelis S, Heligman D, and Morton T: The treatment of pigmented villonodular synovitis of the hip. Clin Orthop *239*:154–160, 1989.

Goldman AB, and DiCarlo EF: Pigmented villonodular synovitis. Diagnosis and differential diagnosis. Radiol Clin North Am *26*:1327–1347, 1988.

Hughes TH, Sartoris DJ, Schweitzer ME, and Resnick DL: Pigmented villonodular synovitis: MRI characteristics. Skeletal Radiol *24*:7–12, 1995.

Ogilvie-Harris DJ, McLean J, and Zarnett ME: Pigmented villonodular synovitis of the knee. The results of total arthroscopic synovectomy, partial, arthroscopic synovectomy, and arthroscopic local excision. J Bone Joint Surg (Am) *74*:119–123, 1992.

Schwartz HS, Unni KK, and Pritchard DJ: Pigmented villonodular synovitis. A retrospective review of affected large joints. Clin Orthop *247*:243–255, 1989.

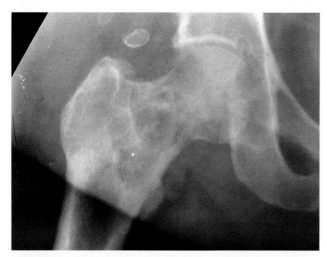

Figure 27–1. This radiograph illustrates bony destruction on either side of the hip joint in a 66-year-old woman with pigmented villonodular synovitis. Well-defined lytic defects with some adjacent sclerosis are identified.

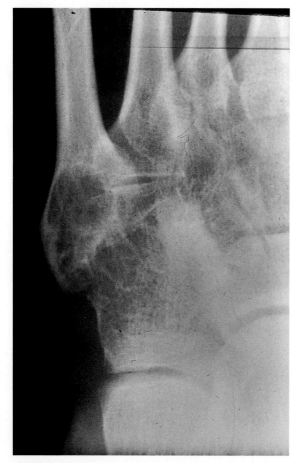

Figure 27–2. This radiograph illustrates the bony destruction associated with pigmented villonodular synovitis of the foot in a 50-year-old woman. Peripheral sclerosis adjacent to the bony lytic defects is well illustrated. Soft tissue masses may also be appreciated in such cases.

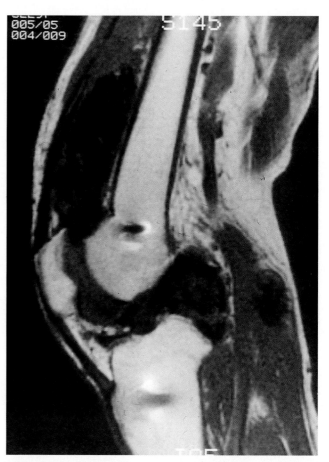

Figure 27–3. The magnetic resonance imaging (MRI) appearance of pigmented villonodular synovitis involving the knee is illustrated in this figure. The low-signal-intensity lesion extends posteriorly into the popliteal fossa as well as into the distal femur and proximal tibia.

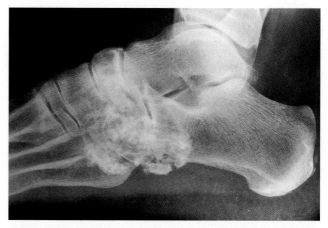

Figure 27–4. Calcification within masses of pigmented villonodular synovitis is uncommon. This example from a 64-year-old male patient with pigmented villonodular synovitis of the foot shows calcification (see Figure 27–5).

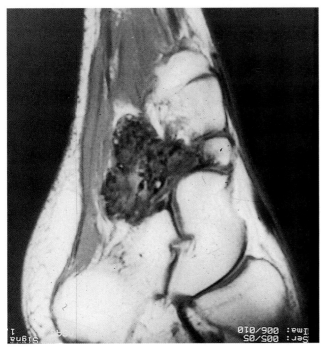

Figure 27–5. This MRI scan corresponds to the case illustrated in Figure 27–4. Foci of high signal intensity within the low-signal mass correspond to regions with numerous lipid-laden histiocytes. Regions of proliferation with abundant hemosiderin show low signal on T1- and T2-weighted images.

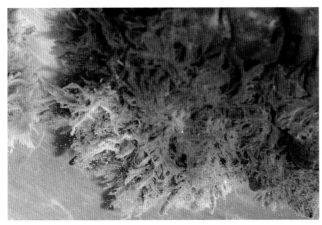

Figure 27–6. This photograph of a gross specimen of resected synovium placed in water illustrates the characteristic villous proliferation of the synovium in pigmented villonodular synovitis. Arthroscopically this same pattern may be seen.

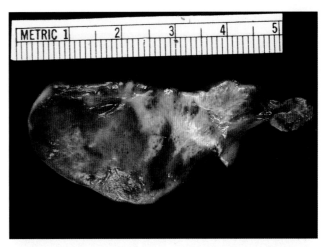

Figure 27–7. Pigmented villonodular synovitis may present grossly in a localized nodular pattern, as seen in this case.

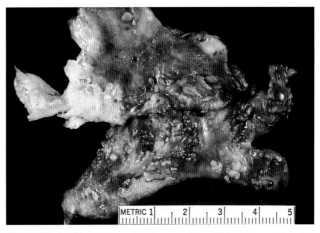

Figure 27–8. Other causes for pigmentation within the synovium include synovial hemorrhage, ochronosis, and metallic synovitis after total joint arthroplasty. This photograph illustrates the appearance of metallic synovitis.

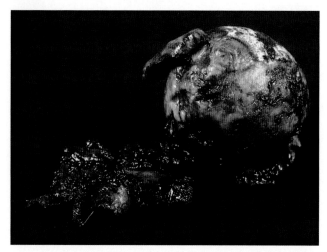

Figure 27–9. This femoral head was resected at the time of placement of a total hip prosthesis in a patient with pigmented villonodular synovitis. Bony erosion by the synovial proliferation is evident. The color of lesional tissue grossly varies, depending upon the relative numbers of hemosiderin-laden and lipid-laden macrophages in the specimen.

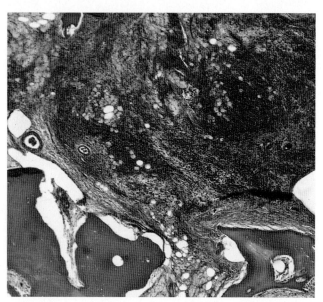

Figure 27–10. This photomicrograph shows the low-magnification pattern of pigmented villonodular synovitis invading the acetabulum. The defect is well circumscribed, mirroring the radiographic appearance.

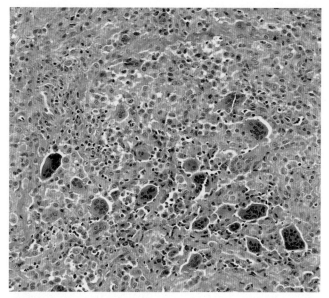

Figure 27–11. At low magnification, pigmented villonodular synovitis shows scattered multinucleated giant cells lying within a mononuclear cell background with varying degrees of fibrosis, as illustrated in this photomicrograph.

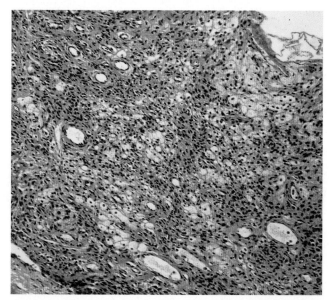

Figure 27–12. Regions of lipid-laden macrophages often form small clusters within the proliferation, as illustrated in this photomicrograph. Adjacent hemosiderin-laden macrophages show brownish discoloration of the cytoplasm.

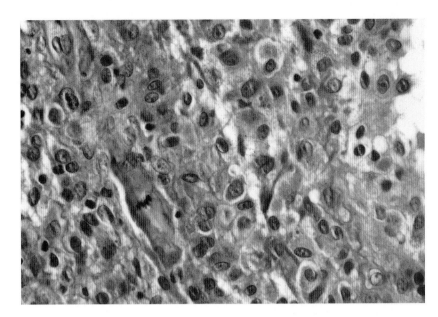

Figure 27–13. At high magnification, pigmented villonodular synovitis shows mononuclear cells with abundant cytoplasm as well as multinucleated giant cells. The mononuclear cells are eosinophilic, with clear or brown-staining cytoplasm.

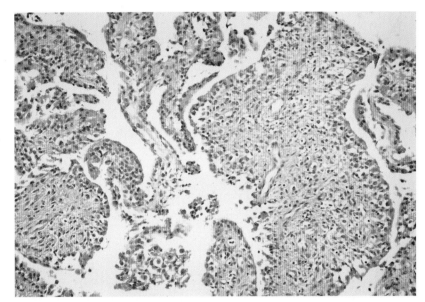

Figure 27–14. This photomicrograph shows a residual synovial cell layer overlying hemosiderin-laden macrophages in pigmented villonodular synovitis.

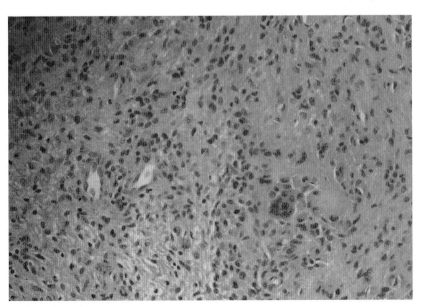

Figure 27–15. This photomicrograph illustrates the microscopic features of giant cell tumor of tendon sheath type. Histologically this entity is indistinguishable from pigmented villonodular synovitis. Giant cell tumors of tendon sheath type are well-circumscribed soft tissue masses, as illustrated in this photomicrograph.

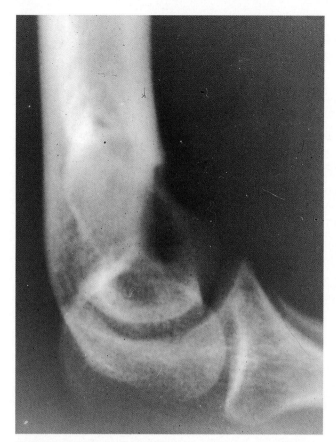

Figure 27–16. This radiograph illustrates pigmented villonodular synovitis of the elbow in a 13-year-old girl.

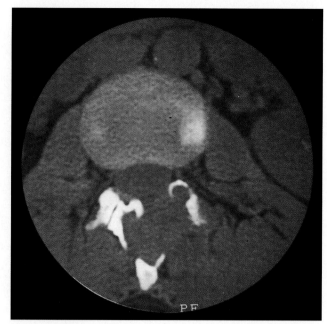

Figure 27–18. CT scan showing pigmented villonodular synovitis of the lumbar spine in a 47-year-old man.

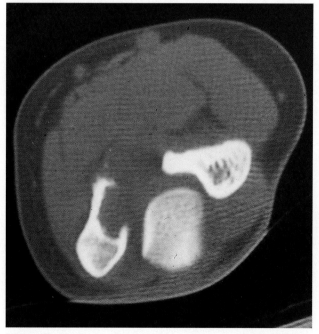

Figure 27–17. Computed tomographic (CT) scan of the patient in Figure 27–16.

CHAPTER 28

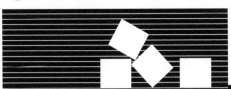

Arthroplasty Effect

CLINICAL SIGNS

1. Most patients are asymptomatic if the implant remains well fixed.

CLINICAL SYMPTOMS

1. Pain is the most common symptom related to implant loosening.
2. Joint dysfunction is related to implant loosening.

MAJOR RADIOGRAPHIC FEATURES

1. Nonseptic periprosthetic osteolysis has two patterns:
   a. Diffuse benign pattern:
      i. Radiolucency surrounds the bone-prosthesis interface.
      ii. The affected area may be surrounded by radiodense lines.
   b. Focal aggressive pattern:
      i. Isolated lytic lesions, 0.5 to 2.0 cm, may be seen.
      ii. Little reactive bone is present.
      iii. The lesions may coalesce to form contiguous lytic zones of destruction.
2. With loosening, cement or implant fractures result in a position change of components.

RADIOGRAPHIC DIFFERENTIAL DIAGNOSIS

1. Sepsis.
2. Stress shielding resorption.
3. Osteoporosis.

MAJOR PATHOLOGIC FEATURES

1. There may be a foreign body granulomatous reaction to particulate implant materials, e.g., polyethylene, methacrylate, or metal.

2. Fibrovascular, villous membrane infiltrated with sheets of foamy macrophages and giant cells may be seen.
3. Patients with prostheses in which metal articulates on metal may show gray-black discoloration of the synovium due to metallic debris.
4. Polyethylene may engender a host reaction producing a pseudotumor.

PATHOLOGIC DIFFERENTIAL DIAGNOSIS

1. Sepsis.
2. Granulomatous infection.
3. Pigmented villonodular synovitis.

TREATMENT

1. Improvement in implant design and techniques should prevent this condition.
2. Medical treatment includes symptomatic measures and close follow-up for cases in which there is mild osteolysis.
3. Surgical treatment consists of revision arthroplasty for patients with
   a. Symptomatic loosening and osteolysis.
   b. Significant osteolysis compromising bone stock even in asymptomatic patients.

References

Fehring TK, and McAlister JA Jr: Frozen histologic section as a guide to sepsis in revision joint arthroplasty. Clin Orthop (304):229–237, 1994.

Mauerhan DR, Nelson CL, Smith DL, et al: Prophylaxis against infection in total joint arthroplasty. One day of cefuroxime compared with three days of cefazolin. J Bone Joint Surg (Am) 76:39–45, 1994.

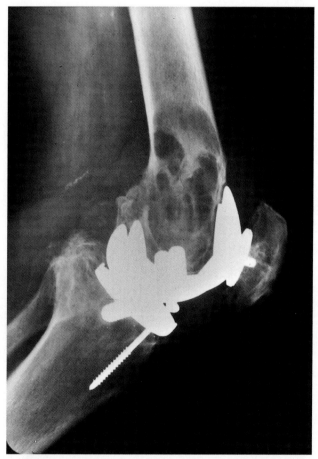

Figure 28–1. Radiograph of the knee in a 77-year-old man who presented with knee pain after total knee arthroplasty. Although infection was thought to be the most likely cause of the bony destruction adjacent to the prosthesis, cultures and histologic evaluation yielded negative findings, and the changes were thus ascribed to periprosthetic osteolysis.

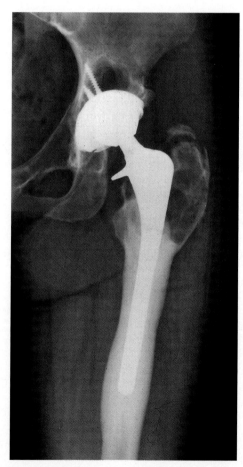

Figure 28–2. Radiograph of the hip in a 40-year-old woman who had previously had a total hip arthroplasty after suffering avascular necrosis of the femoral head. She presented with a three-month history of pain. Pathologic evaluation, including cultures, confirmed a diagnosis of aseptic periprosthetic osteolysis.

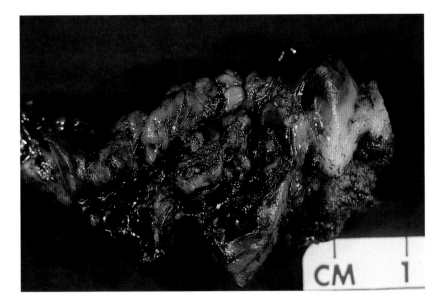

Figure 28–3. This photograph of a gross specimen illustrates the deeply stained appearance of synovium that can be seen in "metallic synovitis." Similar changes may be seen in the synovium in patients who suffer from aseptic periprosthetic osteolysis.

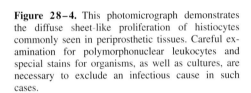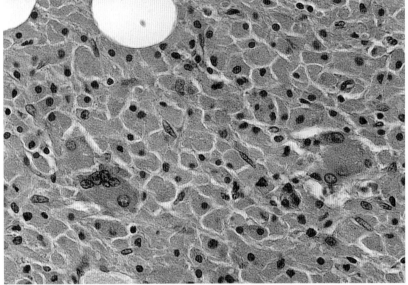

Figure 28–4. This photomicrograph demonstrates the diffuse sheet-like proliferation of histiocytes commonly seen in periprosthetic tissues. Careful examination for polymorphonuclear leukocytes and special stains for organisms, as well as cultures, are necessary to exclude an infectious cause in such cases.

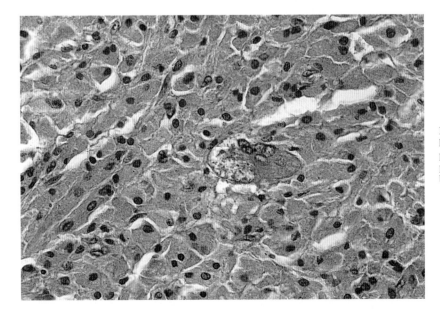

Figure 28–5. This photomicrograph illustrates the histiocytic proliferation associated with aseptic periprosthetic osteolysis. Immediately adjacent to the prosthesis, a zone of dense collagenous tissue may be present.

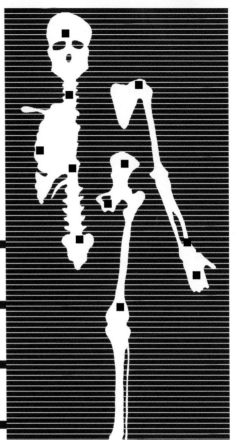

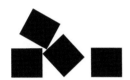

SECTION ■ 2

BONE TUMORS AND TUMOR-LIKE CONDITIONS

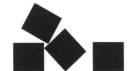

BONE-FORMING
TUMORS

CHAPTER 29

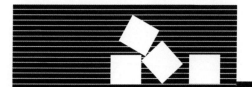

Osteoid Osteoma

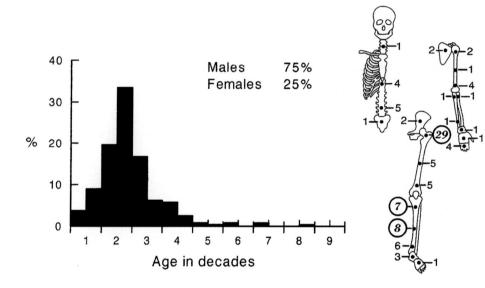

Males 75%
Females 25%

CLINICAL SIGNS

1. Lower extremity lesions often cause dysfunction manifested as a limp.
2. Muscle atrophy may be present in the affected extremity.
3. Neurologic disorder may be suspected in some cases owing to the combination of pain, decreased muscle stretch reflexes, and muscular atrophy. Approximately 3 per cent of patients have symptoms clinically suggestive of lumbar disc disease.

CLINICAL SYMPTOMS

1. The patient's complaints can be virtually diagnostic. The most important complaint is pain of increasing severity. The pain is frequently noted to be worse at night and is relieved with aspirin.
2. The pain may be referred to an adjacent joint.
3. If the involved bone is superficial, a painful local swelling may be noted.
4. If the tumor involves the vertebra, the patient may present with scoliosis.
5. Arthritic symptoms may be produced by tumors near a joint.

MAJOR RADIOGRAPHIC FEATURES

1. A small round lucency, usually lying in the cortex, is identified on plane radiography.
2. Surrounding the lucency are sclerosis and cortical reaction.

3. At the center of the lucency or nidus, there may be central ossification.
4. Twenty-five per cent of tumors are not demonstrated on plain radiography and therefore require isotope bone scan, tomography, or computed tomography (CT) for identification.
5. Tumors in cancellous bone, subperiosteal tumors, and intracapsular tumors provoke little or no sclerosis.

RADIOGRAPHIC DIFFERENTIAL DIAGNOSIS

1. Brodie's abscess.
2. Stress fracture.
3. Osteoblastoma.

MAJOR PATHOLOGIC FEATURES

Gross

1. The lesional tissue is red.
2. The tumor is granular but may be soft or densely sclerotic.
3. The nidus is generally distinct from the surrounding sclerotic bone.
4. The lesional tissue is generally less than 1 cm in its greatest dimension.
5. The nidus may be difficult to identify grossly. In such cases, preoperative tetracycline labeling may be of help because the nidus tends to stand out when viewed under ultraviolet light.

Microscopic

1. At low magnification, the nidus consists of an interlacing network of osteoid trabeculae.
2. The trabeculae are usually thin and arranged in a haphazard manner.
3. Mineralization of the osteoid is variable, but the greatest degree of mineralization generally occurs at the center of the nidus.

4. Between the osteoid trabeculae there is a loose fibrovascular connective tissue.
5. Multinucleated giant cells may be identified within the fibrovascular connective tissue.
6. At higher magnification, the osteoblasts surrounding the osteoid trabeculae are uniform in their cytologic characteristics, having round, regular nuclei and abundant cytoplasm.
7. Cartilage is not present.
8. The nidus is well demarcated from the surrounding bone, which generally has undergone sclerotic changes.

PATHOLOGIC DIFFERENTIAL DIAGNOSIS

Benign lesions:

1. Osteoblastoma.

Malignant lesions:

1. Osteosarcoma.

TREATMENT

Primary Modality: radiofrequency ablation of the nidus via a percutaneous approach.

Other Possible Approaches: complete resection of the nidus with bone grafting as indicated, depending upon the size of the defect.

References

McLeod RA, Dahlin DC, and Beabout, JW: The spectrum of osteoblastoma. Am J Roentgenol 26:321–335, 1976.
Sim FH, Dahlin DC, and Beabout JW: Osteoid-osteoma: diagnostic problems. J Bone Joint Surg (Am) 57:154–159, 1975.
Sim FH, Dahlin DC, Stauffer RN, and Laws ER Jr: Primary bone tumors simulating lumbar disc syndrome. Spine 2:65–74, 1977.
Swee RG, McLeod RA, and Beabout JW: Osteoid osteoma: detection, diagnosis and localization. Radiology 130:117–123, 1979.
Vigorita VJ, and Ghelman B: Localization of osteoid osteomas—use of radionuclide scanning and autoimaging in identifying the nidus. Am J Clin Pathol 79:223–225, 1983.

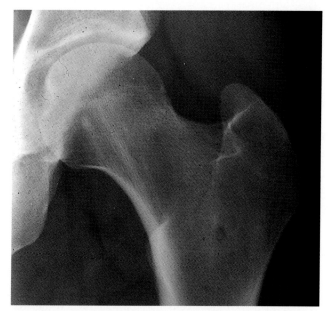

Figure 29–1. This radiograph illustrates a small oval lucent lesion in the intertrochanteric region of the femur. The radiographic features are compatible with the diagnosis of osteoid osteoma.

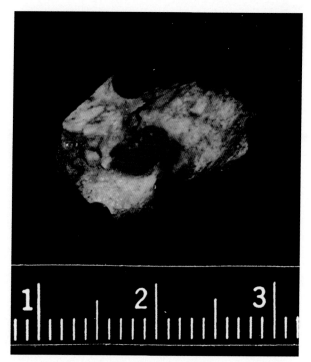

Figure 29–3. Grossly, the nidus of osteoid osteoma is reddish and appears hemorrhagic, as shown in this photograph. The nidus tends to stand out from the surrounding sclerotic bone.

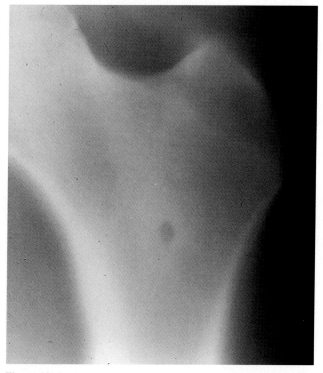

Figure 29–2. Tomograms may be helpful in evaluating such lesions. The surrounding sclerosis is identifiable.

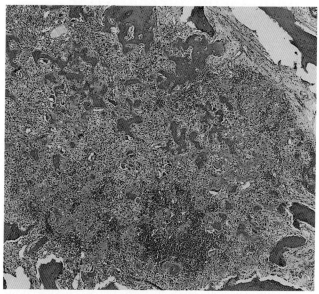

Figure 29–4. At low magnification, the nidus of osteoid osteoma is well circumscribed. The surrounding bone is sclerotic, a reactive change that may extend for a considerable distance from the nidus.

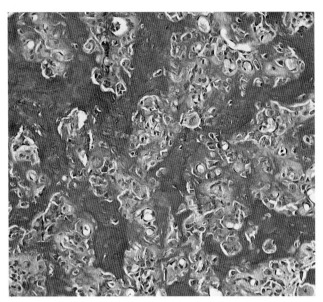

Figure 29–5. At the center of the nidus, the lesion is composed of irregular trabeculae of bone, which lie in a hypocellular, fibrovascular connective tissue. These features are identical with those of osteoblastoma.

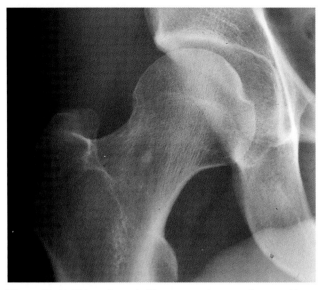

Figure 29–7. This radiograph illustrates an intracapsular osteoid osteoma of the femoral neck. The central ossification is typical of this lesion; however, the tumor has not provoked any surrounding sclerosis.

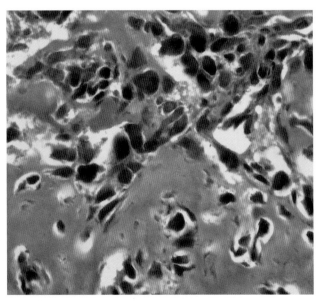

Figure 29–6. At high magnification, the irregularity of the osteoid and the cellular proliferation may be misinterpreted as representing an osteosarcoma. Using low power and paying attention to the radiographic features help the pathologist avoid this mistake.

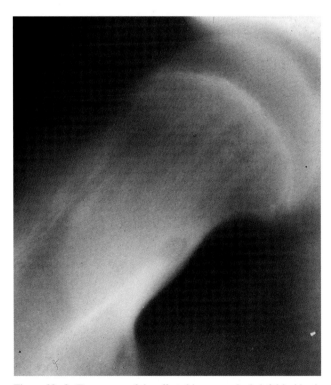

Figure 29–8. Tomograms of the affected bone may be helpful in identifying the nidus when the plain radiograph is unrevealing. Sclerosis is seen to surround the nidus in this tomogram of the proximal femur.

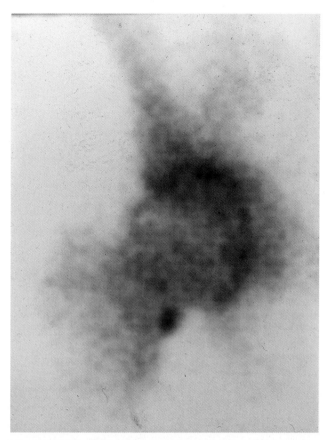

Figure 29–9. An isotope bone scan is also extremely useful in identifying small osteoid osteomas that are radiographically inapparent, as this bone scan illustrates.

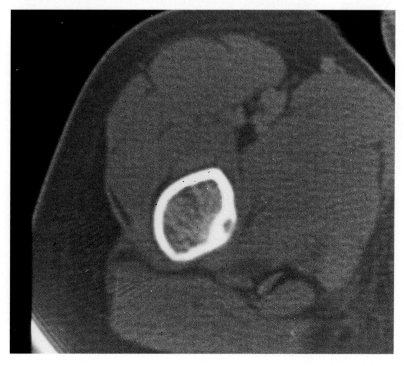

Figure 29–10. A computed tomographic (CT) scan may also be helpful in some instances. In this case, a cortical subtrochanteric osteoid osteoma of the femur was identified on a CT scan.

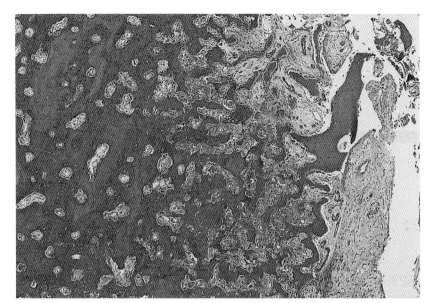

Figure 29–11. Some osteoid osteomas show extensive ossification of the nidus, as illustrated in this photomicrograph. Note the marked circumscription, which results in the lesion's appearing to "break away" from the surrounding bone.

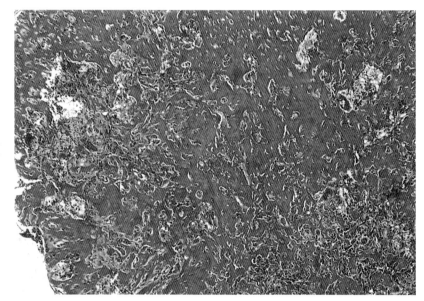

Figure 29–12. In cases with extensive ossification of the nidus, cytologic evaluation of the lesion is difficult.

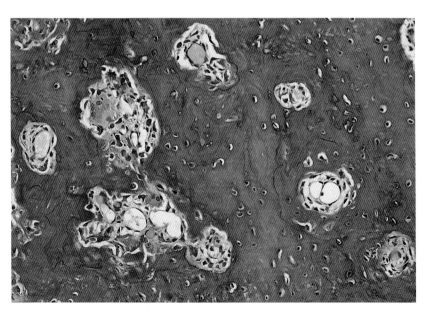

Figure 29–13. At higher magnification, the histologic features may resemble those of pagetoid bone. Attention to the radiographic features helps to avoid a misdiagnosis in such cases.

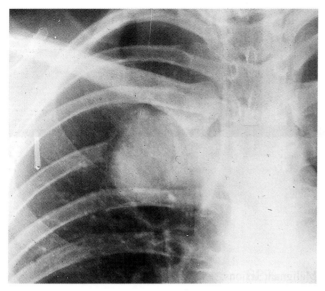

Figure 30–1. This radiograph illustrates a partially ossified mass lesion involving a rib posteriorly. There is associated bone destruction and a soft tissue mass indicative of an aggressive lesion.

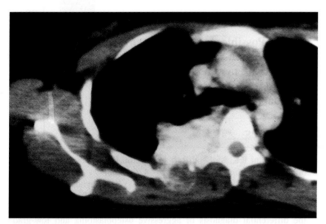

Figure 30–2. The computed tomographic (CT) scan in this case shows the same features that are evident in the plain radiograph.

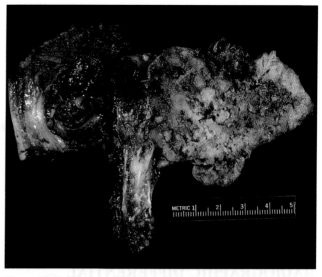

Figure 30–3. The gross pathologic features in this case correlate well with the plain radiographic and CT appearance of this lesion. The tumor was confirmed histologically to be an osteoblastoma.

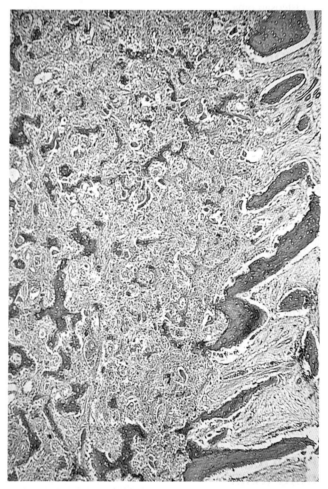

Figure 30–4. At low magnification, the periphery of an osteoblastoma is well circumscribed, as illustrated in this photomicrograph.

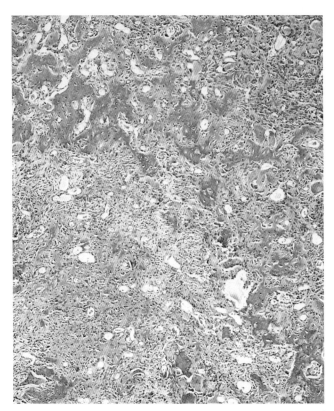

Figure 30–5. The tumor is composed of numerous irregularly shaped bony trabeculae between which there is hypocellular fibrovascular connective tissue.

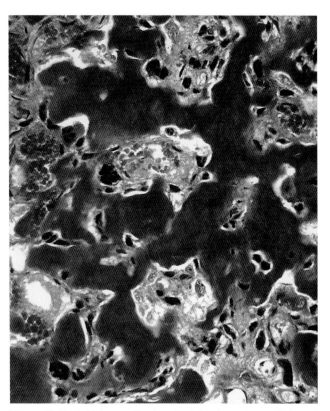

Figure 30–7. At high magnification, the lesion is not hypercellular and nuclear pleomorphism is generally not marked. However, some lesions can show cytologic changes that may simulate osteosarcoma, as demonstrated in this photomicrograph.

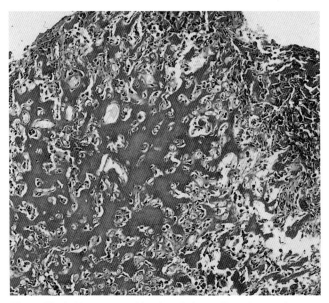

Figure 30–6. Numerous multinucleated giant cells and a prominent osteoblastic rimming of the bony trabeculae are evident. Vascular spaces are generally prominent.

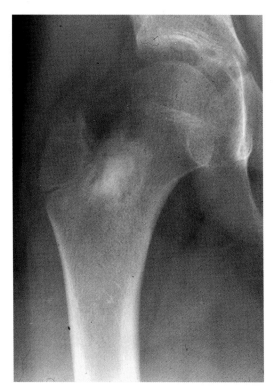

Figure 30–8. This radiograph of the proximal femur shows a heavily ossified oval osteoblastoma. A lucent halo surrounds the ossified lesion and is itself surrounded by a zone of sclerosis—features that support a benign diagnosis.

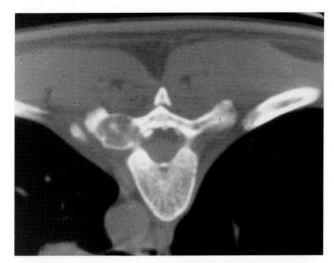

Figure 30–9. Osteoblastomas commonly involve the vertebrae; the dorsal elements are usually the location of such lesions, as illustrated in this case. The central ossification is also characteristic of this tumor.

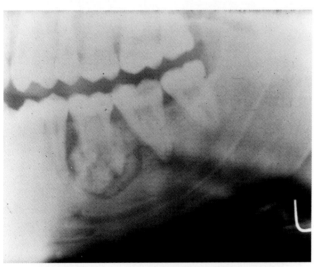

Figure 30–10. Lesions histologically indistinguishable from osteoblastoma also involve the maxilla and mandible, as shown here. Such lesions have been termed "cementoblastomas." Note the ossified tumor surrounding the tooth root with a lucent halo.

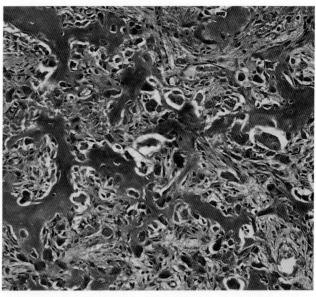

Figure 30–11. Although the irregular bony trabeculae of osteoblastoma may simulate the osteoid produced by osteosarcomas, the hypocellular nature of the fibrovascular connective tissue seen between such trabeculae supports a diagnosis of osteoblastoma.

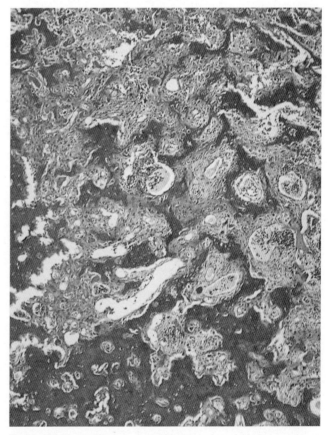

Figure 30–12. Ossification of osteoblastomas is variable from region to region in the tumor. This photomicrograph illustrates the transition from a more heavily ossified area to a less ossified region.

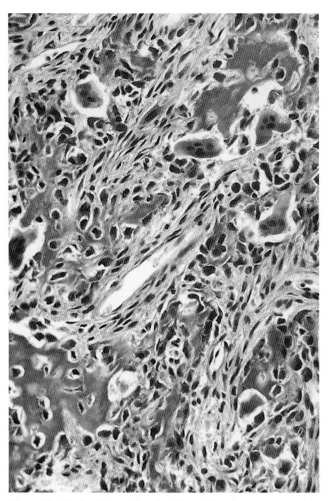

Figure 30–13. Careful attention should be paid to the appearance of the lesion at low magnification and to the radiographic features, as overemphasis on the high-power appearance of a lesion may lead to a mistaken diagnosis of malignancy.

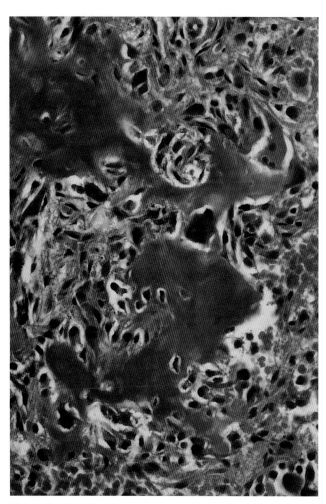

Figure 30–14. Although the nuclei in an osteoblastoma may be somewhat hyperchromatic, the cells do not lie "shoulder to shoulder" as in an osteosarcoma. Thus, the osteoblastoma has a looser appearance, as illustrated in this photomicrograph.

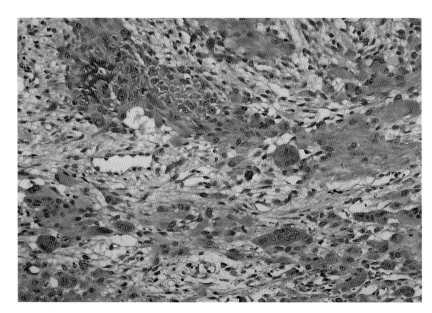

Figure 30–15. This photomicrograph of a femoral osteoblastoma shows the characteristic loose hypocellular fibrovascular connective tissue that helps differentiate osteoblastoma from osteoblastoma-like osteosarcomas.

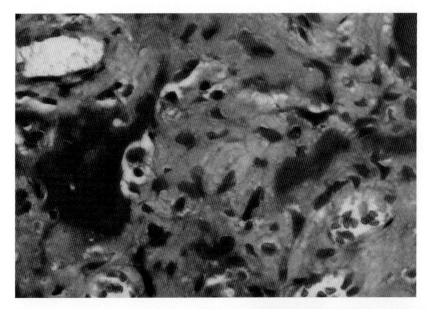

Figure 30–16. Cells showing degenerative cytologic atypia, resulting in irregularly shaped hyperchromatic nuclei, as seen in this photomicrograph, can be mistaken for malignant osteoblastomas. This photomicrograph of a femoral osteoblastoma shows these cytologic features.

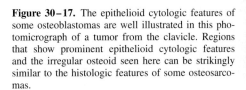

Figure 30–17. The epithelioid cytologic features of some osteoblastomas are well illustrated in this photomicrograph of a tumor from the clavicle. Regions that show prominent epithelioid cytologic features and the irregular osteoid seen here can be strikingly similar to the histologic features of some osteosarcomas.

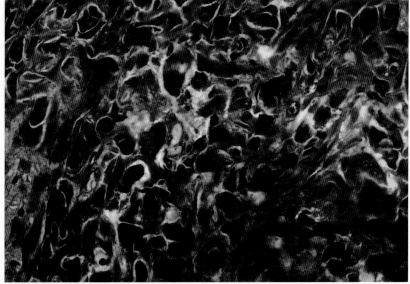

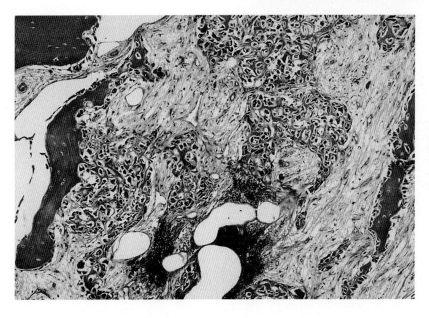

Figure 30–18. Although osteoblastomas form a solitary lesion radiographically, microscopically they may appear multicentric, as illustrated in this photomicrograph. Presumably, such "dangling lobules" of tumor may result in recurrence if the osteoblastoma is not thoroughly curetted.

CHAPTER 31

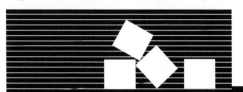

Osteosarcoma (Conventional)

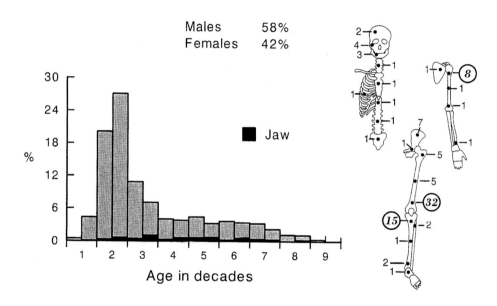

Males 58%
Females 42%

■ Jaw

%

30
24
18
12
6
0

1 2 3 4 5 6 7 8 9

Age in decades

CLINICAL SIGNS

1. A tender mass generally is palpable on physical examination, because soft tissue extension is common.
2. When the mass is very large, dilated, and engorged, veins may be seen overlying it.
3. Edema distal to the lesion due to blockage of lymphatics or venous compression occurs uncommonly.
4. Elevation of serum alkaline phosphatase concentrations occurs in about 50 per cent of patients.

CLINICAL SYMPTOMS

1. Pain, which may be intermittent initially, is universally present.
2. A swelling in the region of the affected bone is also a cardinal, although nonspecific, symptom.
3. Pathologic fracture is uncommon as the presenting complaint.

4. The duration of symptoms is generally short, varying from weeks to several months.

MAJOR RADIOGRAPHIC FEATURES

1. The favored site is the metaphysis of a long bone, especially the knee.
2. There may be lytic, blastic, or mixed bone destruction and production.
3. Trabecular and cortical destruction is usually geographic and poorly marginated.
4. Periosteal new bone is frequent and often takes the form of spiculation or Codman's triangles.
5. Soft tissue extension is the rule in larger lesions.
6. Magnetic resonance imaging (MRI) and computed tomography (CT) are essential for pretreatment staging.

RADIOGRAPHIC DIFFERENTIAL DIAGNOSIS

1. Ewing's sarcoma.
2. Fibrosarcoma or malignant fibrous histiocytoma.
3. Chondrosarcoma.
4. Osteomyelitis.
5. Osteoblastoma.
6. Giant cell tumor.

MAJOR PATHOLOGIC FEATURES

Gross

1. The tumors generally have violated the cortex of the affected bone at the time of diagnosis.
2. An associated soft tissue mass is commonly found.
3. The tumor may extend within the medullary cavity beyond the abnormality defined by plane radiography. (MRI is particularly helpful in defining the extent of intramedullary disease.)
4. The tumor is variable in consistency and may be distinctly sclerotic; in general, however, soft areas are identifiable as well.
5. The tumor varies from yellow-brown to whitish, depending upon whether the predominant differentiation is fibroblastic, chondroblastic, or osteoblastic.
6. Necrosis, cyst formation, and hemorrhage are most commonly seen in the softer portions of the tumor.

Microscopic

1. At low magnification, the tumor may show great variability. However, all tumors classified as osteosarcoma must show a frankly sarcomatous stroma that produces osteoid. (Frequently, the osteoid shows a fine, lace-like pattern.)
2. The tumor is hypercellular, and generally the stromal cells are spindled.
3. Zones of chrondroid matrix may be identified.
4. Sclerotic zones of extensive ossification may appear hypocellular, having undergone degeneration.
5. The spindle cells may be arranged in a "herring bone" or storiform pattern.
6. At higher magnification, the spindle cells show marked pleomorphism. The nuclei are extremely variable in size and shape and are hyperchromic.
7. Mitotic figures are generally abundant.
8. The degree to which osteoid is produced is greatly variable, and a careful search may be needed to identify the eosinophilic matrix surrounding atypical cells.

9. Variable numbers of benign multinucleated giant cells are seen; when abundant, they may focally mimic the appearance of a giant cell tumor.

PATHOLOGIC DIFFERENTIAL DIAGNOSIS

Benign lesions:

1. Osteoblastoma.
2. Osteoid osteoma.
3. Giant cell tumor.
4. Fracture callus.

Malignant lesions:

1. Fibrosarcoma.
2. Chondrosarcoma.
3. Malignant fibrous histiocytoma.

TREATMENT

Primary Modality: surgical ablation by amputation or limb-saving resection with a wide margin. If preoperative staging indicates that a successful limb-salvage procedure can be performed, the extremity can be reconstructed with a custom joint prosthesis, an osteochondral allograft, or a resection arthrodesis. The reconstructive procedure should be tailored to the needs of the individual. Protocols employing preoperative (neoadjuvant) chemotherapy use the extent of tumor "necrosis" at the time of definitive operation as a measure of effectiveness. Current advances in chemotherapy are making an important contribution to the improved survival of patients with osteosarcoma. An aggressive approach with thoracotomy is saving approximately one third of the patients who develop pulmonary metastases.

Other Possible Approaches: radiation therapy, possibly combined with neutron beam radiation for lesions of inaccessible sites such as the spine and sacrum.

References

Campanacci M, Bacci G, Bertoni F, et al: The treatment of osteosarcoma of the extremities: twenty years experience at the Istituto Ortopedico Rizzoli. Cancer 48:1569–1581, 1981.

Harvei S, and Solheim O: The prognosis in osteosarcoma: Norwegian national data. Cancer 48:1719–1723, 1981.

Marcove RC, and Rosen G: En bloc resection for osteogenic sarcoma. Cancer 45:3040–3044, 1980.

Martin SE, Dwyer A, Kissane JM, and Cost J: Small-cell osteosarcoma. Cancer 50:990–996, 1982.

Sanerkin NG: Definitions of osteosarcoma, chondrosarcoma and fibrosarcoma of bone. Cancer 46:178–185, 1980.

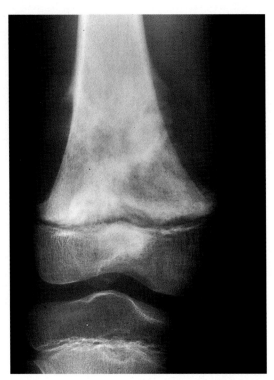

Figure 31–1. This anteroposterior (AP) radiograph demonstrates a mixed lytic and sclerotic lesion in the distal femur of a skeletally immature patient. Codman's triangle is present superiorly. The radiographic features are those of an osteosarcoma.

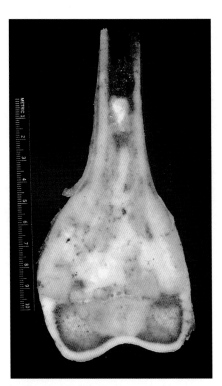

Figure 31–2. The gross pathologic features in this case correspond well to the plain x-ray film appearance shown in Figure 31–1. The tumor crosses the open physis, which often acts as a relative barrier to the intraosseous extension of osteosarcomas. The tumor is firm and gritty; however, soft areas are nearly always present.

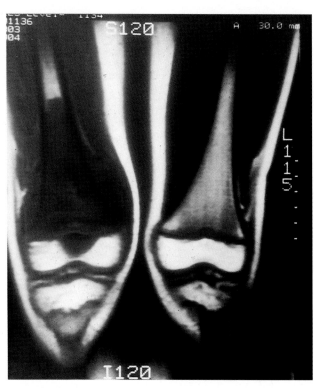

Figure 31–3. This coronal magnetic resonance imaging (MRI) scan of the same patient's distal femur demonstrates the extent of the low-signal tumor seen in contrast to the high-signal normal marrow. The extension of the tumor across the physis into the epiphysis is also readily demonstrated.

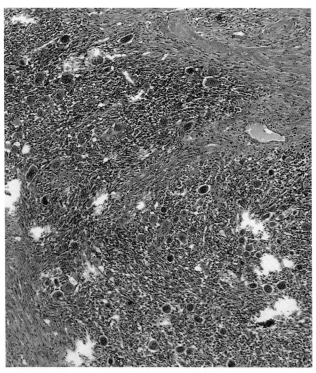

Figure 31–4. At low magnification, osteosarcomas show a variety of histologic patterns. This photomicrograph illustrates a tumor that is predominantly composed of spindle cells (fibroblastic) in which numerous benign multinucleated giant cells are present.

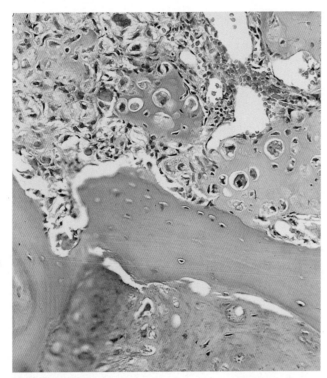

Figure 31–5. This photomicrograph illustrates the permeative growth of a chondroblastic osteosarcoma of the distal femur. Residual bony trabeculae are present. The chondroid portion of such a tumor may not show as significant a cytologic atypia as the spindle cell components of the lesion and thus, if taken out of context, may suggest the diagnosis of chondrosarcoma.

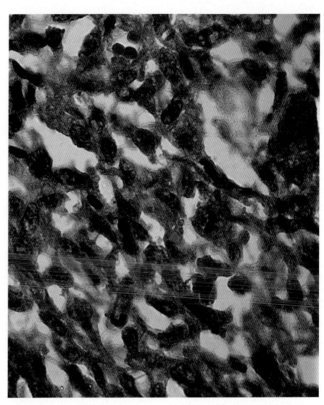

Figure 31–7. At high magnification, ordinary osteosarcomas are poorly differentiated or high-grade tumors. They show nuclear pleomorphism and anaplasia, and mitotic activity is generally brisk.

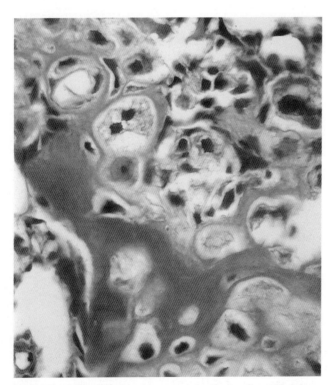

Figure 31–6. Osteoblastic osteosarcomas may be heavily ossified; however, the cytologic atypia of the proliferating cells is generally obvious in such cases, as is shown in this photomicrograph.

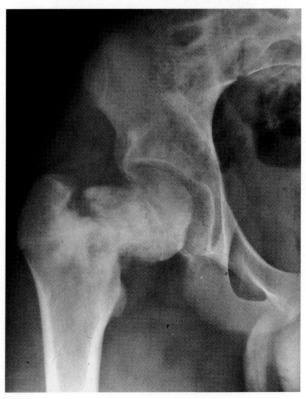

Figure 31–8. This radiograph of the proximal femur shows a sclerotic osteosarcoma that has resulted in a pathologic fracture.

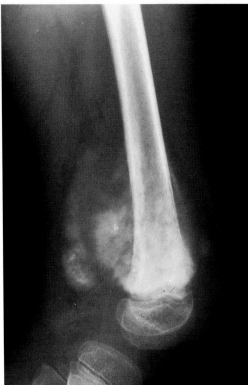

Figure 31–9. This radiograph illustrates a large, heavily ossified osteosarcoma of the lower femoral metaphysis, with a large soft tissue component.

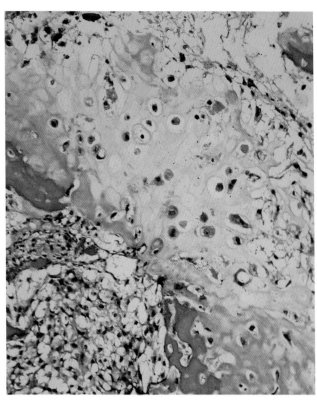

Figure 31–11. Ossification within a chondroblastic osteosarcoma may occur at the periphery of the cartilaginous masses, as illustrated in this photomicrograph, or within a spindle cell component of the lesion.

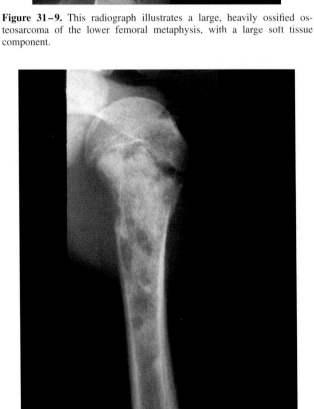

Figure 31–10. A mixed lytic and sclerotic radiographic appearance is common in osteosarcoma, as in this case involving the upper diametaphyseal region of the humerus.

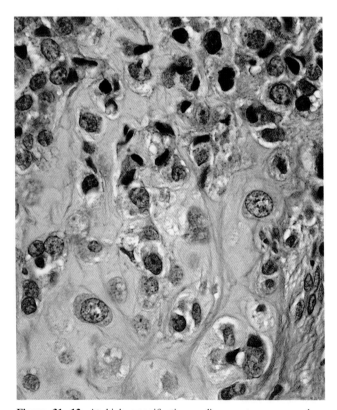

Figure 31–12. At high magnification, ordinary osteosarcomas show marked cytologic atypia. The "lace-like" osteoid that identifies the tumor as an osteosarcoma may be only focally present.

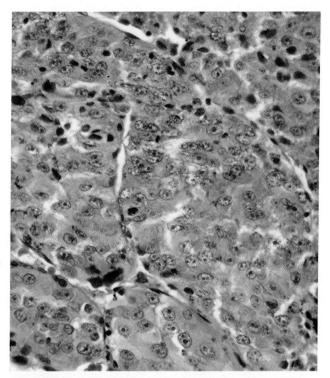

Figure 31–13. Some osteosarcomas show a distinctly epithelioid histologic pattern of growth, as illustrated in this photomicrograph of a tumor from the radius. Given the young age of most patients with osteosarcoma, such a pattern generally does not result in misdiagnosis.

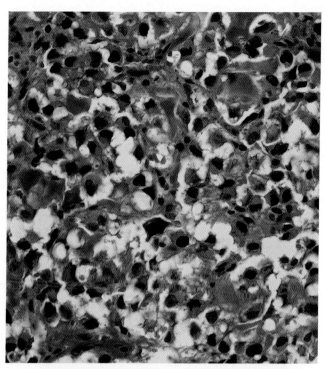

Figure 31–15. Conventional osteosarcomas may show epithelioid cytologic characteristics, as in this tumor from the distal femur. In elderly patients, such epithelioid differentiation may be sufficiently prominent to cause confusion with metastatic carcinoma.

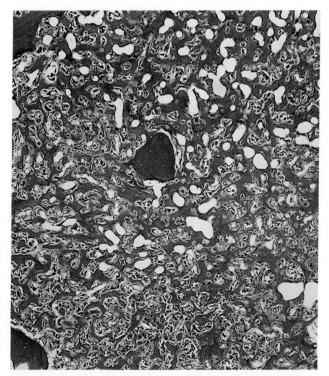

Figure 31–14. This photomicrograph illustrates the infiltrative pattern commonly seen in malignant bone tumors. Residual pre-existing bony trabeculae are surrounded by the osteoblastic osteosarcoma.

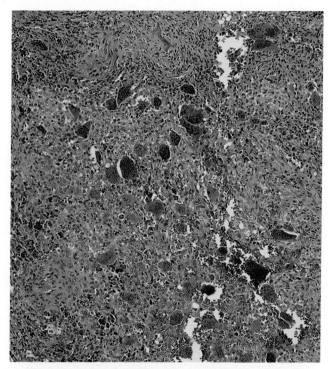

Figure 31–16. Another histologic pattern that may be seen in conventional osteosarcoma is a "giant cell–rich pattern," as illustrated in this photomicrograph. Such tumors may be easily confused with giant cell tumors of bone. This problem is further complicated by the fact that giant cell tumors may show a malignant appearance radiographically.

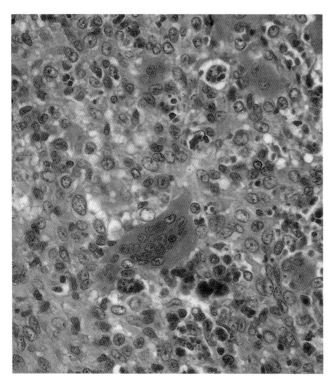

Figure 31–17. This photomicrograph illustrates the cytologic appearance of the giant cell–rich osteosarcoma depicted in Figure 31–16. The cytologic atypia of the mononuclear cells in such tumors is greater than that seen in benign giant cell tumors of bone.

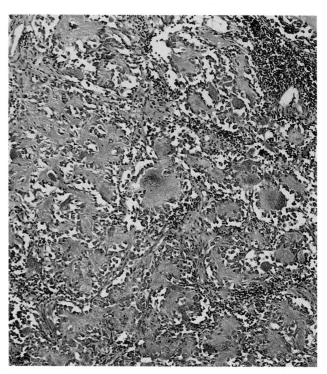

Figure 31–19. This photomicrograph demonstrates the histologic pattern seen in an osteoblastoma-like osteosarcoma. Such tumors are difficult to distinguish from osteoblastoma. The presence of cartilage in such a lesion favors the diagnosis of osteosarcoma.

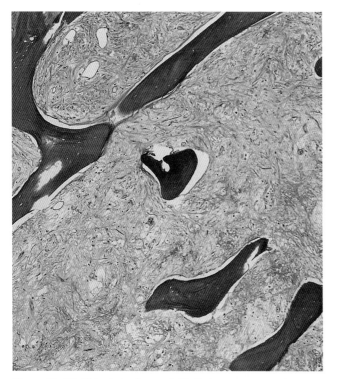

Figure 31–18. This photomicrograph illustrates a common pattern seen in postchemotherapy osteosarcoma. Regions such as this may be totally replaced by collagenized stroma devoid of malignant cells.

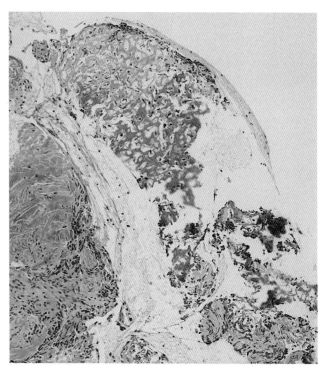

Figure 31–20. Needle biopsy is increasingly used to diagnose primary bone tumors. This photomicrograph illustrates the pattern seen in an osteosarcoma of the tibia. Careful correlation with the radiographic appearance of the lesion is even more critical when the amount of tissue sampled is limited, as in needle biopsy specimens.

CHAPTER 32

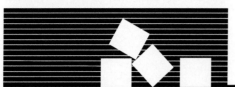

Parosteal Osteosarcoma

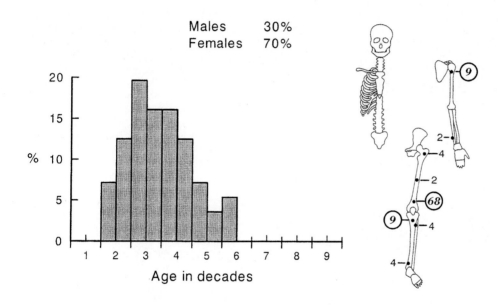

Males   30%
Females   70%

% — 20, 15, 10, 5, 0

Age in decades

CLINICAL SIGNS

1. A large mass lesion involves the affected bone.
2. The tumor may be tender to palpation.

CLINICAL SYMPTOMS

1. A painless mass is present in the posterior distal thigh.
2. The mass is generally of long duration (up to several years).
3. If the mass is sufficiently large, some patients complain of an inability to bend the knee.
4. Pain is uncommon.

MAJOR RADIOGRAPHIC FEATURES

1. A lobulated and ossified mass arises on the metaphyseal surface of a long bone.
2. The posterior lower femur is a preferred site.
3. There is broad attachment to the adjacent cortex.
4. The cortex is thickened and deformed.
5. Larger tumors encircle the bone.

RADIOGRAPHIC DIFFERENTIAL DIAGNOSIS

1. Myositis ossificans.
2. Periosteal osteosarcoma.

3. Periosteal chondrosarcoma.
4. High-grade surface osteosarcoma.
5. Ordinary (conventional) osteosarcoma.
6. Osteochondroma.

MAJOR PATHOLOGIC FEATURES

Gross

1. The tumor seems to be applied to the surface of the affected bone.
2. Medullary extension is absent unless the tumor is recurrent or has been present for many years.
3. The tumor is ossified and rock hard; if soft areas exist, they should be sampled because the tumor may have a higher-grade component in it.
4. Cartilaginous foci may be grossly evident and may form a "cap" over the tumor similar to an osteochondroma.

Microscopic

1. At low magnification, the pattern is that of a low-grade tumor. Osteoid trabeculae lie parallel to one another in a hypocellular fibroblastic stroma.
2. The fibroblastic component of the tumor shows minimal cytologic atypia, and only rarely are mitoses present.
3. At the surface of the tumor, a cartilaginous cap may be present, giving the tumor the appearance of an osteochondroma. However, between the bony trabeculae of an osteochondroma there is fatty or hematopoietic marrow, in contrast with the fibrous stroma of a parosteal osteosarcoma. In addition, the chondrocytes show mild cytologic atypia and do not exhibit the columnar arrangement seen in an osteochondroma.

PATHOLOGIC DIFFERENTIAL DIAGNOSIS

Benign lesions:

1. Osteochondroma.
2. Myositis ossificans (heterotopic ossification).

Malignant lesions:

1. High-grade surface osteosarcoma.
2. Periosteal osteosarcoma.

TREATMENT

Primary Modality: en bloc resection with a marginal margin and grafting, depending upon location.

Other Possible Approaches: amputation if the tumor involves neurovascular structures and is not resectable.

References

Ahuja SC, Villacin AB, Smith J, et al: Juxtacortical (parosteal) osteogenic sarcoma: histological grading and prognosis. J Bone Joint Surg (Am) 59:632–647, 1977.
Chang CP, Chu YK, Chu LS, et al: Scintigraphic appearance of parosteal osteosarcoma. Clin Nucl Med 22(1):54–56, 1997.
Edeiken J, Farrell C, Ackerman LV, and Spjut HJ: Parosteal sarcoma. Am J Roentgenol 111:579–583, 1971.
Lin J, Yao L, Mirra JM, and Bahk WJ: Osteochondroma-like parosteal osteosarcoma: a report of six cases of a new entity. Am J Roentgenol 170(6):1571–1577, 1998.
Unni KK, Dahlin DC, and Beabout JW: Periosteal osteogenic sarcoma. Cancer 3:2476–2485, 1976.
Unni KK, Dahlin DC, Beabout JW, and Ivins JC: Parosteal osteogenic sarcoma. Cancer 37:2466–2475, 1976.
Wold LE, Unni KK, Beabout JW, et al: Dedifferentiated parosteal osteosarcoma. J Bone Joint Surg (Am) 66:53–59, 1984.

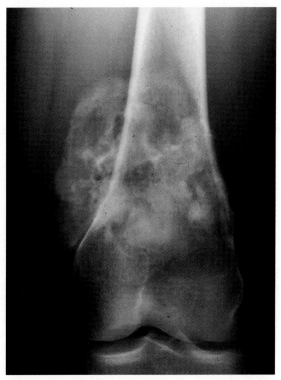

Figure 32–1. This anteroposterior (AP) radiograph illustrates the typical features of a parosteal osteosarcoma. The tumor is heavily ossified and broadly attached to the surface of the bone.

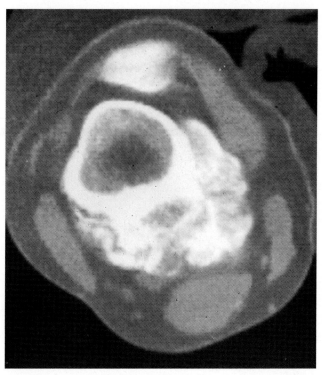

Figure 32–3. A computed tomographic (CT) scan of the tumor may be helpful in excluding medullary involvement. This scan shows the broad surface attachment of a parosteal osteosarcoma and the absence of medullary neoplasm.

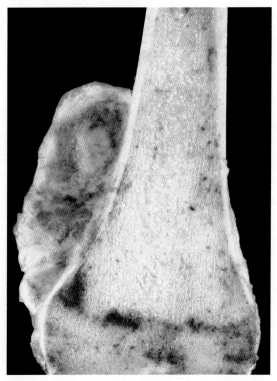

Figure 32–2. The gross pathologic features of the resected specimen correlate well with its radiographic appearance (see Fig. 32–1). The tumor is densely ossified, and no medullary involvement is present. Any soft areas of the tumor should be sampled, as they may represent "transformation" of the tumor.

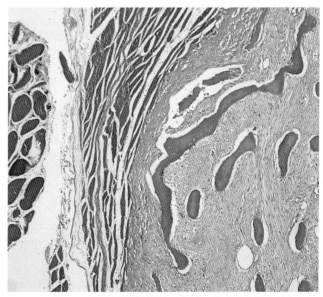

Figure 32–4. At low magnification, parosteal osteosarcoma shows an orderly appearance, with a hypocellular spindle cell component merging with mature-appearing, "normalized" bony trabeculae. The periphery of the lesion is generally well circumscribed, as shown in this photomicrograph.

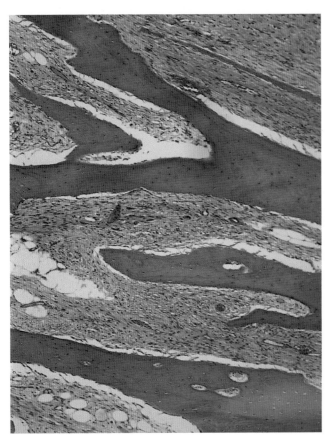

Figure 32–5. At higher magnification, the cytologic features of the spindle cell component of the tumor are more apparent. The juxtaposition of hypocellular spindle cells and mature bone may simulate the histologic features of fibrous dysplasia.

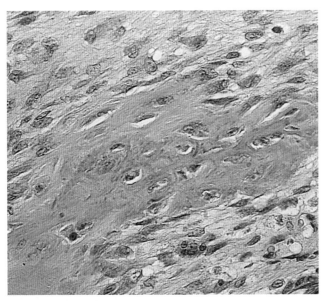

Figure 32–6. At high magnification, minimal cytologic atypia is apparent in the spindle cell component of the tumor.

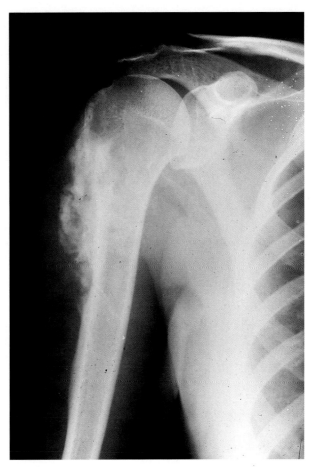

Figure 32–7. The proximal humerus is the second most common location for parosteal osteosarcoma. This tumor shows the characteristic broad-based bony attachment.

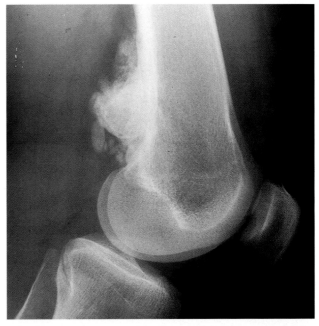

Figure 32–8. The distal posterior femur is the most common location for parosteal osteosarcoma. Medullary involvement is not identified in this lateral radiograph.

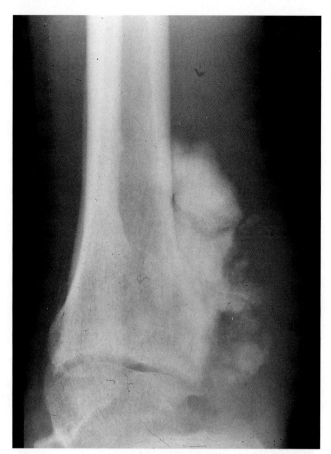

Figure 32–9. The radiographic features of this distal tibial parosteal osteosarcoma are identical with those of tumors in the more common location.

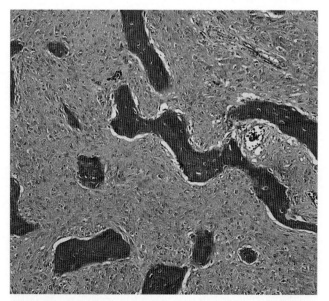

Figure 32–10. Irregular "matured" bony trabeculae of parosteal osteosarcoma may simulate the low-power pattern of fibrous dysplasia. However, the surface location of the lesion excludes the diagnosis of fibrous dysplasia.

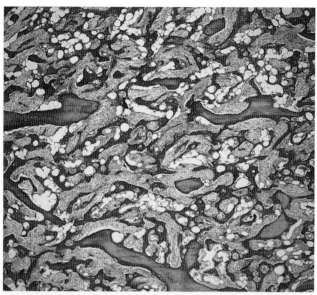

Figure 32–11. In recurrent or longstanding cases of parosteal osteosarcoma, the medullary cavity may be involved, as shown in this photomicrograph. The well-differentiated neoplasm is seen permeating the pre-existing medullary bony trabeculae.

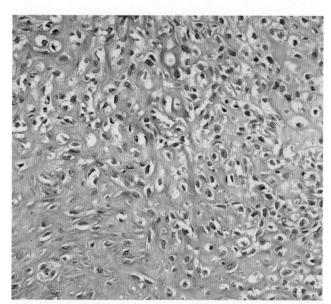

Figure 32–12. Any soft areas in a lesion that otherwise has the features of parosteal osteosarcoma should be histologically examined. This photomicrograph illustrates such a region in a recurrent tumor. The spindle cell proliferation shows much greater cytologic atypia than is seen in parosteal osteosarcoma. Such tumors have been termed "dedifferentiated parosteal osteosarcoma."

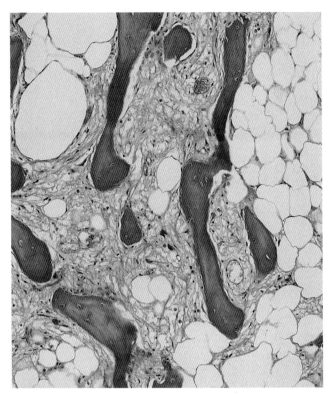

Figure 32–13. Minimal medullary invasion by low-grade parosteal osteosarcomas may be seen, as in this photomicrograph of a proximal humeral tumor. Such medullary invasion does not affect the patient's prognosis.

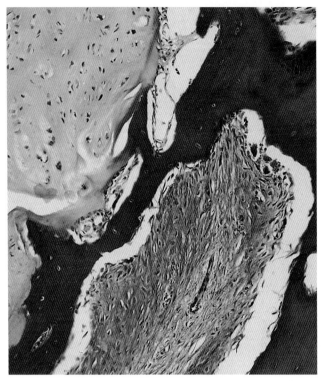

Figure 32–15. Parosteal osteosarcomas are generally composed of a bland fibroblastic proliferation lying between orderly trabecula-like bone. Occasionally, foci of cartilage differentiation may be present, as shown in this photomicrograph of a tumor from the distal posterior femur.

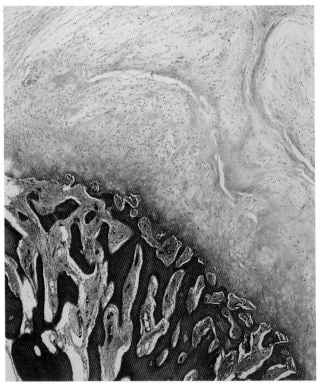

Figure 32–14. This photomicrograph illustrates the similarity between parosteal osteosarcoma and osteochondroma. Occasionally, as in this case, parosteal osteosarcomas have a well-developed cartilage cap.

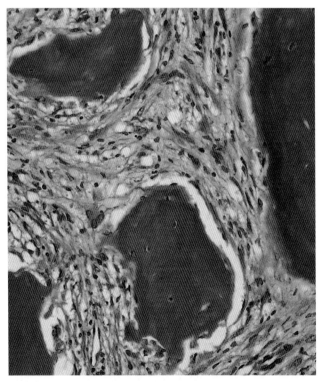

Figure 32–16. Parosteal osteosarcomas are low-grade tumors. The fibroblastic spindle cell portion of the neoplasm may show slight nuclear pleomorphism, as illustrated in this photomicrograph of a tumor from the distal posterior femur.

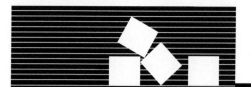

CHAPTER 33

Periosteal Osteosarcoma

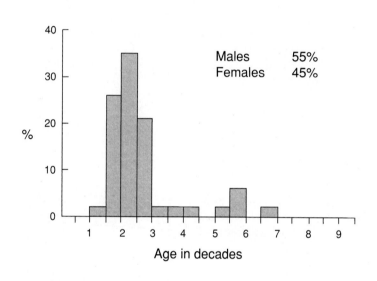

Males 55%
Females 45%

% (y-axis)
Age in decades (x-axis)

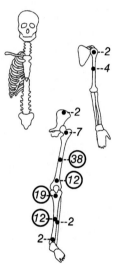

2
4
2
7
38
12
19
12
2
2

CLINICAL SIGNS

1. A mass may be palpable on physical examination.
2. The lesion may be tender to palpation.

CLINICAL SYMPTOMS

1. Pain is the most common presenting complaint.
2. A swelling may be noticed by the patient.

MAJOR RADIOGRAPHIC FEATURES

1. The lesion is diaphyseal in location, particularly in the tibia.
2. The lesion is located on the surface of the bone; the medullary canal is uninvolved.
3. Partial matrix mineralization may be seen.
4. The periphery of the soft tissue mass is free of mineral.

5. The adjacent cortex is thickened.
6. Periosteal reaction and Codman's triangle are common.

RADIOGRAPHIC DIFFERENTIAL DIAGNOSIS

1. Parosteal osteosarcoma.
2. High-grade surface osteosarcoma.
3. Periosteal chondrosarcoma.
4. Myositis ossificans (heterotopic ossification).

MAJOR PATHOLOGIC FEATURES

Gross

1. The tumor is lobulated, is situated on the surface of the bone, and may appear like a piece of putty applied to the periosteum.

2. The blue-gray color of a hyaline cartilage tumor is apparent.
3. Whitish spicules of bone may be seen to radiate through the tumor at right angles to the long axis of the underlying bone.
4. The medullary cavity is uninvolved.

Microscopic

1. At low magnification, the tumor exhibits abundant chondroid matrix production.
2. Traversing the chondroid matrix are spicules of osteoid.
3. The periphery is generally well circumscribed, and the tumor shows lobulation in these regions.
4. At the periphery of the lesion, the tumor exhibits a "condensation" of spindle-shaped cells.
5. At higher magnification, the cells lying within the chondroid matrix show mild cytologic atypia.
6. The spindled cells at the periphery also show cytologic atypia, and faint osteoid may be seen among them.
7. The cortical bone may be slightly eroded, but the medullary canal is free of tumor.
8. Mitotic activity is not brisk.

PATHOLOGIC DIFFERENTIAL DIAGNOSIS

Benign lesions:

1. Periosteal chondroma.

Malignant lesions:

1. Periosteal chondrosarcoma.
2. High-grade surface osteosarcoma.
3. Ordinary intramedullary osteosarcoma with a prominent surface component.

TREATMENT

Primary Modality: This lesion lends itself to surgical resection with a wide margin, and the bone can be reconstructed with use of an intercalary allograft or a vascularized fibular graft.

Other Possible Approaches: When an adequate margin cannot be achieved by en bloc resection, amputation is indicated. Preoperative chemotherapy may improve the low risk for local recurrence after local resection.

References

Bertoni FB, Boriani S, Laus M, and Campanacci M: Periosteal chondrosarcoma and periosteal osteosarcoma: two distinct entities. J Bone Joint Surg (Br) 64:370–376, 1982.
De Santos LA, Murray JA, Findlestein JB, et al: The radiographic spectrum of periosteal osteosarcoma. Radiology 127:123–129, 1978.
Ritts GD, Pritchard DJ, Unni KK, et al: Periosteal osteosarcoma. Clin Orthop 219:299–307, 1987.
Unni KK, Dahlin DC, and Beabout JW: Periosteal osteogenic sarcoma. Cancer 37:2476–2485, 1976.

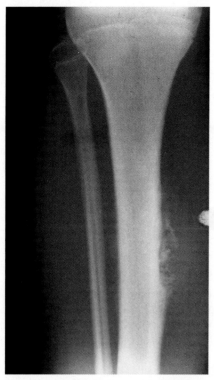

Figure 33–1. This radiograph illustrates the characteristic features of periosteal osteosarcoma. The tumor arises from the surface of the tibial diaphysis and is partially calcified.

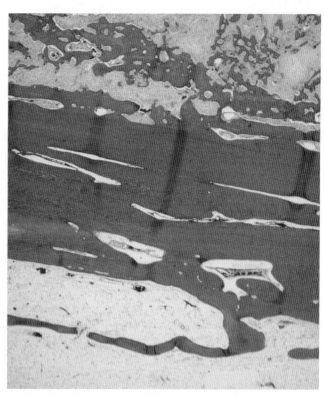

Figure 33–3. Periosteal osteosarcoma is a surface lesion of bone without medullary involvement. This photomicrograph at low magnification shows the uninvolved medullary region and the surface chondroblastic tumor.

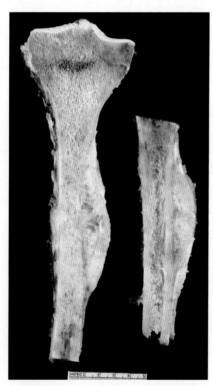

Figure 33–2. The bisected gross specimen of the tibial diaphysis shown in Figure 33–1 illustrates the surface nature of periosteal osteosarcoma as it affects the tibial diaphysis, the most commonly affected bone. Grossly, no visible tumor should be evident in the medullary portion of the affected bone.

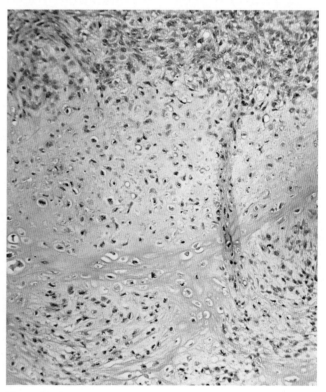

Figure 33–4. Periosteal osteosarcoma is characteristically chondroblastic, as shown in this photomicrograph. At the periphery of the chondroid islands a "condensation" of spindle cells is visible.

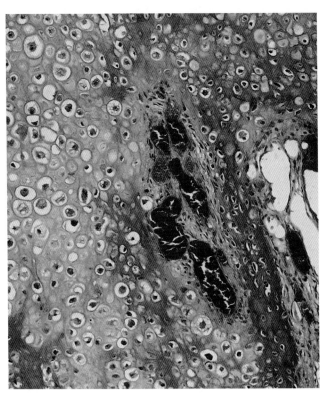

Figure 33–5. At higher magnification, osteoid is identified focally in the lesion. The focal nature of the osteoid production results in confusion of this tumor with periosteal chondrosarcoma and periosteal chondroma.

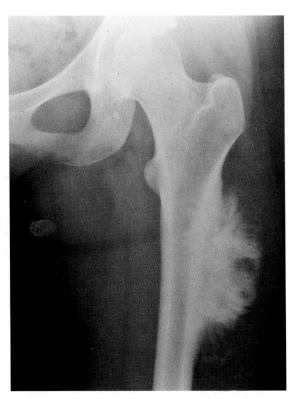

Figure 33–7. The femoral diaphysis is a common location for periosteal osteosarcoma, as shown in this radiograph. This tumor is large and shows the spiculated mineralization commonly identified in periosteal osteosarcoma.

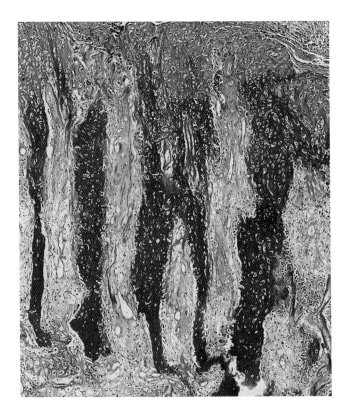

Figure 33–6. The radiating spicules of bone seen radiographically correspond to the bone seen at low magnification in the photomicrograph. Such osteoid frequently traverses the lesion perpendicularly to the underlying cortical bone.

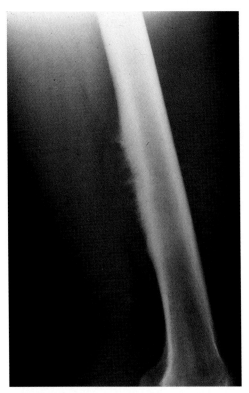

Figure 33–8. The radiating spicules of bone are seen centrally in this periosteal osteosarcoma of the lower femoral diaphysis. An unmineralized soft tissue mass is seen at the periphery of the tumor.

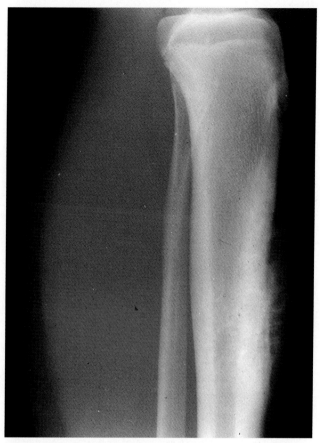

Figure 33–9. The most common location for periosteal osteosarcoma is the tibial diaphysis, as shown in this radiograph. The cortex in this case is thickened, but the underlying medulla is uninvolved.

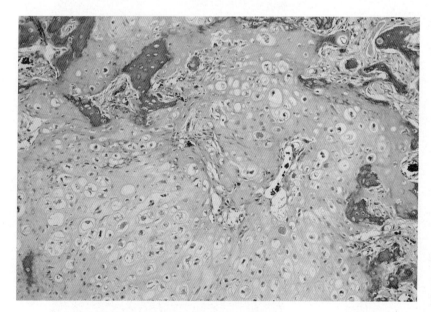

Figure 33–10. Chondroid matrix commonly predominates in periosteal osteosarcoma; however, osteoid is identifiable at the periphery of the chondroid zones in this photomicrograph.

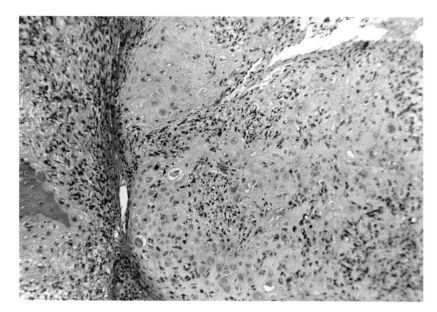

Figure 33–11. These tumors frequently show the lobulation that is commonly seen in cartilaginous tumors. However, at the periphery of the lobules, the tumor exhibits greater cellularity and atypia than is evident in chondrosarcomas.

Figure 33–12. Some periosteal osteosarcomas show greater regions of spindle cell proliferation, as in this photomicrograph. With such lesions, the differential diagnosis is between high-grade surface osteosarcoma and periosteal osteosarcoma.

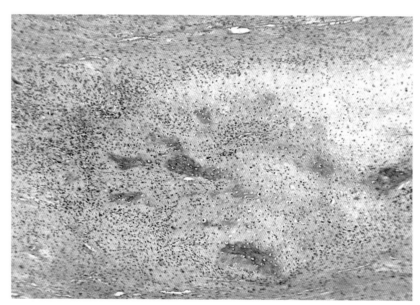

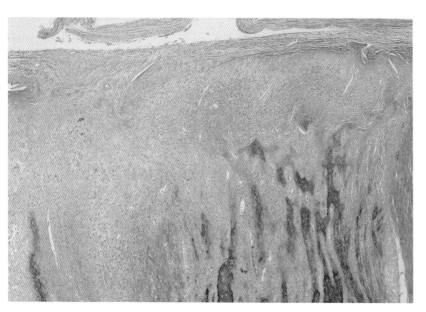

Figure 33–13. This low-power photomicrograph illustrates the classic histologic features of periosteal osteosarcoma. The chondroblastic tumor is transgressed by spiculated tumor osteoid that is arranged in a relatively orderly manner.

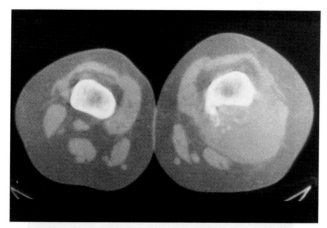

Figure 34–9. The computed tomographic (CT) scan of the same osteosarcoma shown in Figure 34–8 verifies the surface location of the tumor, delineating the soft tissue mass and confirming the absence of a medullary component of the lesion.

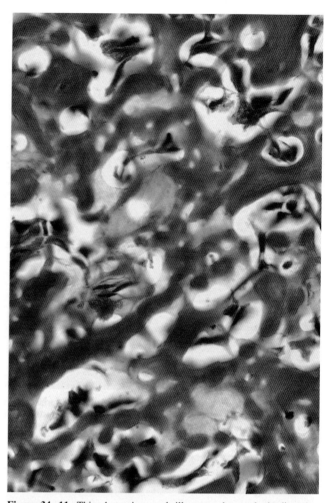

Figure 34–11. This photomicrograph illustrates the cytologic distortion that is commonly present in osteosclerotic osteosarcomas. This pattern may be seen in high-grade surface osteosarcomas or conventional high-grade intramedullary osteosarcomas.

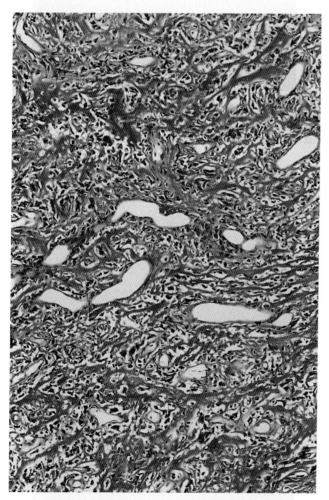

Figure 34–10. Abundant tumor osteoid arranged in a lace-like pattern is evident in this high-grade surface osteosarcoma of the femur.

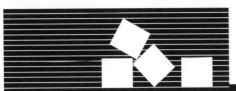

CHAPTER 35

Telangiectatic Osteosarcoma

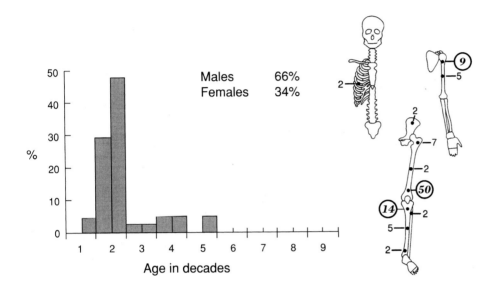

Males 66%
Females 34%

%

Age in decades

CLINICAL SIGNS

1. A tender mass lesion is noted.
2. Occasional pathologic fracture may be seen.

CLINICAL SYMPTOMS

1. Pain is present.
2. Swelling is noted in the region of the tumor.

MAJOR RADIOGRAPHIC FEATURES

1. The tumor is large and metaphyseal.
2. Medullary and cortical bone destruction is considerable.
3. The lesion is purely lytic and poorly marginated.
4. Periosteal new bone and soft tissue mass are common.

RADIOGRAPHIC DIFFERENTIAL DIAGNOSIS

1. Ordinary (conventional) osteosarcoma.
2. Fibrosarcoma.
3. Malignant fibrous histiocytoma.
4. Aneurysmal bone cyst.

MAJOR PATHOLOGIC FEATURES

Gross

1. Lesional tissue is hemorrhagic.
2. Firm, fleshy areas are not identifiable in tumor.
3. Lesional tissue is arranged in delicate strands coursing through the blood clot.

203

Microscopic

1. At low magnification, the features are similar to those of aneurysmal bone cyst.
2. Septa traverse and surround blood-filled spaces.
3. At higher magnification, the mononuclear cells are shown to be pleomorphic.
4. Benign multinucleated giant cells are almost uniformly present.
5. Osteoid production is generally focal and minimal.

PATHOLOGIC DIFFERENTIAL DIAGNOSIS

Benign lesions:

1. Aneurysmal bone cyst.

Malignant lesions:

1. Malignancy in giant cell tumor (malignant giant cell tumor).
2. Angiosarcoma.

TREATMENT

Primary Modality: as in conventional osteosarcoma, surgical ablation by amputation or limb-saving resection. Multidrug chemotherapy in a neoadjuvant setting is most commonly used.

Other Possible Approaches: radiation therapy for lesions in inaccessible sites.

References

Bertoni F, Pignatti G, Bacchini P, et al: Telangiectatic or hemorrhagic osteosarcoma of bone: a clinicopathologic study of 41 patients at the Rizzoli Institute. Prog Surg Pathol *10*:63–82, 1989.

Huvos AG, Rosen G, Bretsky SS, and Butler A: Telangiectatic osteogenic sarcoma: a clinicopathologic study of 124 patients. Cancer *49*:1679–1689, 1982.

Matsuno T, Unni KK, McLeod RA, and Dahlin DC: Telangiectatic osteogenic sarcoma. Cancer *38*:2538–2547, 1976.

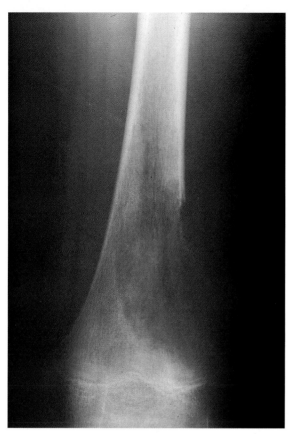

Figure 35–1. This radiograph illustrates a large, purely lytic, and poorly marginated tumor in the distal femoral metaphysis. Considerable destruction of the medullary and cortical bone is evident, with associated soft tissue extension. The purely lytic appearance is characteristic of telangiectatic osteosarcoma.

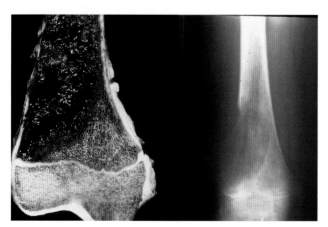

Figure 35–2. The gross pathologic features of telangiectatic osteosarcoma are illustrated in this photograph. The lesion is invariably hemorrhagic and may be quite cystic. Both grossly and microscopically, it may be mistaken for an aneurysmal bone cyst.

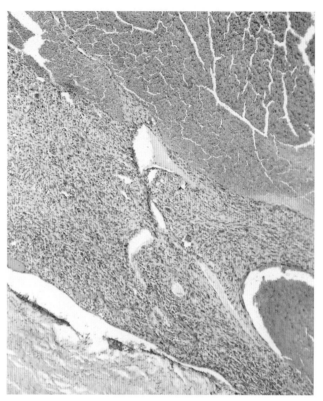

Figure 35–3. At low magnification, telangiectatic osteosarcoma contains large blood-filled spaces, similar to the pattern seen in an aneurysmal bone cyst.

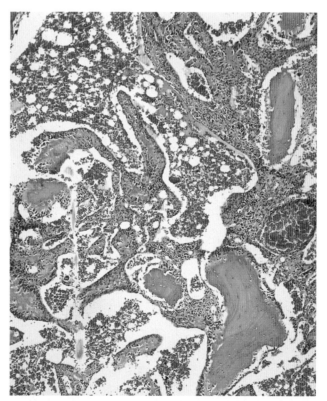

Figure 35–4. This photomicrograph shows the edge of a lesion demonstrating permeation of medullary bone. The bony trabeculae are normal and are not produced by the tumor.

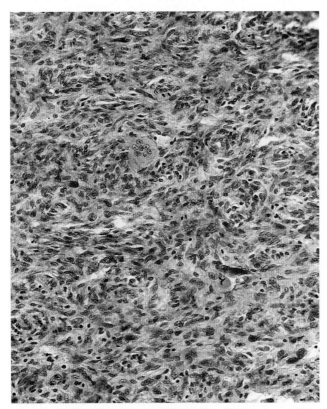

Figure 35–5. Solid areas of the tumor should be only a minor component of this tumor. Abnormal mitotic figures and benign giant cells are commonly found.

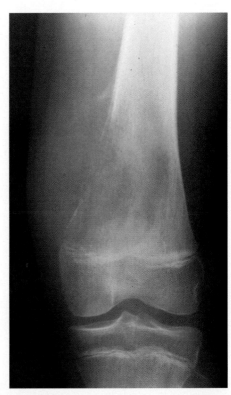

Figure 35–7. This lesion of the distal femur shows cortical destruction, Codman's triangle, and an associated soft tissue mass. These features support the diagnosis of a high-grade malignancy. The purely lytic nature of the lesion is compatible with the diagnosis of telangiectatic osteosarcoma, which it proved to be histologically.

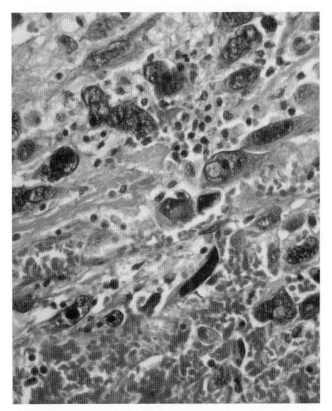

Figure 35–6. A rare telangiectatic osteosarcoma does not show septa and spaces but instead is composed of highly pleomorphic-appearing cells within a blood clot.

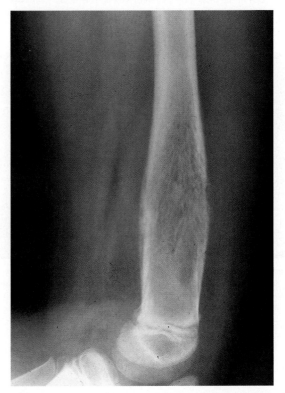

Figure 35–8. This diametaphyseal lytic lesion with poor margination and a permeative growth pattern also represents a telangiectatic osteosarcoma.

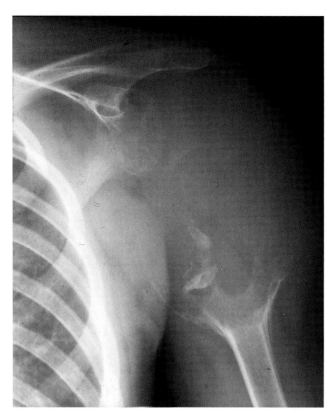

Figure 35–9. This proximal humeral lesion shows the "blown-out" appearance occasionally seen with an aneurysmal bone cyst. This lesion was confirmed histologically to be a telangiectatic osteosarcoma. The overlap of radiographic and histologic features of aneurysmal bone cyst and telangiectatic osteosarcoma presents particularly difficult diagnostic problems for the pathologist.

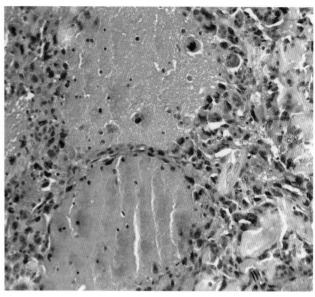

Figure 35–11. Careful examination of the septa is necessary in order to identify the cytologic atypia, shown in this photomicrograph, that distinguishes telangiectatic osteosarcoma from an aneurysmal bone cyst.

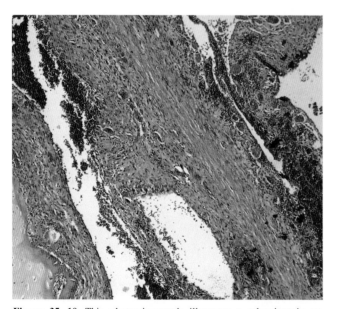

Figure 35–10. This photomicrograph illustrates a telangiectatic osteosarcoma that markedly simulates an aneurysmal bone cyst. Benign multinucleated giant cells are present, and some of the septa are fibrotic and hypocellular.

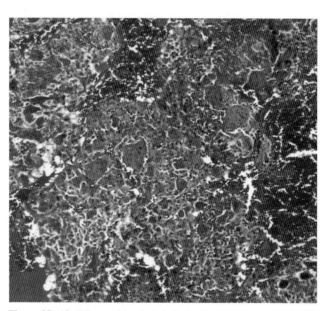

Figure 35–12. When multinucleated giant cells are numerous, as in this photomicrograph, a telangiectatic osteosarcoma may focally resemble a giant cell tumor.

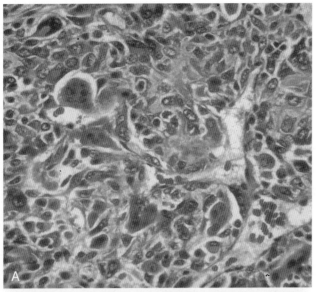

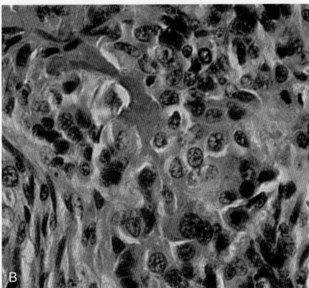

Figure 35–13. At high magnification, the cytologic atypia of the mononuclear cells illustrated in *A* and *B* distinguishes telangiectatic osteosarcoma from a giant cell tumor. Osteoid production (*B*) should be minimal.

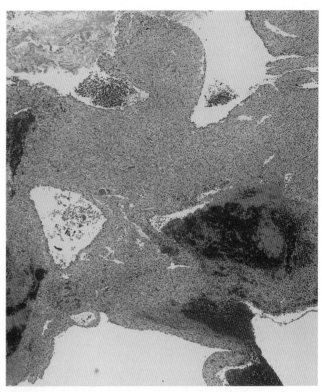

Figure 35–14. At low power, the histologic pattern of telangiectatic osteosarcoma, seen in this photomicrograph, mimics exactly the pattern of aneurysmal bone cyst.

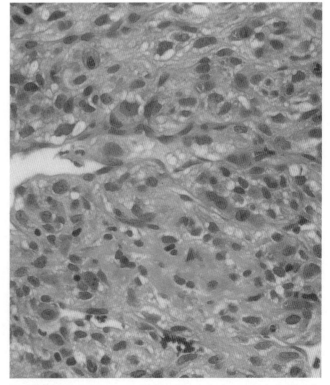

Figure 35–15. Moderate- to high-grade cytologic atypia is evident in the spindle cells of telangiectatic osteosarcoma. This photomicrograph shows the same tumor illustrated in Figure 35–14.

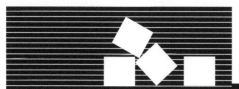

CHAPTER 36

Low-Grade Central Osteosarcoma

Males   50%
Females 50%

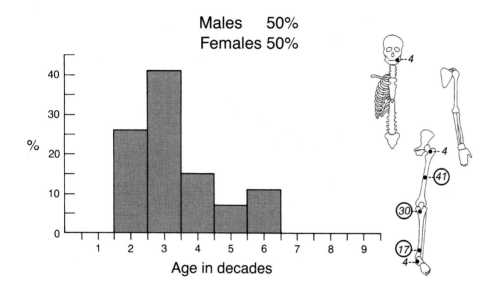

% — Age in decades

CLINICAL SIGNS

1. Usually, no specific signs are elicited on physical examination.

CLINICAL SYMPTOMS

1. Pain is a common presenting complaint.
2. A swelling is almost never noted.

MAJOR RADIOGRAPHIC FEATURES

1. Medullary lesions usually extend to the end of the bone.
2. The tumor is poorly marginated and large.
3. Most lesions are trabeculated or sclerotic.
4. Periosteal new bone and soft tissue mass are usually absent.

5. The overall appearance may suggest benignity, with only a small region showing features that suggest malignancy.

RADIOGRAPHIC DIFFERENTIAL DIAGNOSIS

1. Fibrous dysplasia.
2. Giant cell tumor.
3. Ordinary (conventional) osteosarcoma.
4. Fibrosarcoma.
5. Malignant fibrous histiocytoma.

MAJOR PATHOLOGIC FEATURES

Gross

1. These lesions are firm and fibrous, lacking the fleshy appearance of high-grade sarcomas.

209

2. A gritty quality, somewhat like that of fibrous dysplasia, may be noted.
3. The tumor is most commonly confined to the medullary cavity without an associated soft tissue mass; however, the cortex is destroyed, at least focally.

Microscopic

1. The low-magnification appearance of this tumor mimics that of fibrous dysplasia.
2. The lesional tissue is composed of disordered or irregular bony trabeculae, between which is a hypocellular spindle cell proliferation. (The pattern is essentially identical with that seen in parosteal osteosarcoma.)
3. At higher magnification, the spindle cells show little pleomorphism or anaplasia, and mitotic activity is extremely low. The spindle cells may be arranged in a "herringbone" or a storiform pattern.
4. The osteoid appears "normalized" as in parosteal osteosarcoma.

PATHOLOGIC DIFFERENTIAL DIAGNOSIS

Benign lesions:

1. Fibrous dysplasia.
2. Osteofibrous dysplasia.

Malignant lesions:

1. Osteosarcoma, ordinary intramedullary type.
2. Parosteal osteosarcoma (if location is not considered).

TREATMENT

Primary Modality: surgical resection with a wide margin and skeletal reconstruction with osteochondral allograft, custom prosthesis, or resection arthrodesis, depending upon the location of the lesion and the patient's needs.

Other Possible Approaches: amputation if an adequately wide margin cannot be achieved by surgical resection. Chemotherapy is not indicated unless there has been recurrence and "dedifferentiation" of the tumor.

References

Bertoni F, Bacchini P, Fabbri N, et al: Osteosarcoma. Low-grade intraosseous-type osteosarcoma, histologically resembling parosteal osteosarcoma, fibrous dysplasia and desmoplastic fibroma. Cancer 71:338–345, 1993.
Choong PF, Pritchard DJ, Rock MG, et al: Low grade central osteogenic sarcoma. A long-term follow up of 20 patients. Clin Orthop Rel Res (322):198–206, 1996.
Ellis JH, Siegel CL, Martel W, et al: Radiologic features of well-differentiated osteosarcoma. Am J Radiol 151:739–742, 1988.
Franceschina MJ, Hankin RC, and Irwin RB: Low-grade central osteosarcoma resembling fibrous dysplasia. A report of two cases. Am J Orthop 26(6):432–440, 1997.
Iemoto Y, Ushigome S, Fukunaga M, et al: Case report 679. Central low-grade osteosarcoma with foci of dedifferentiation. Skeletal Radiol 20:379–382, 1991.
Kurt AM, Unni KK, McLeod RA, and Pritchard DJ: Low-grade intraosseous osteosarcoma. Cancer 65(6):1418–1428, 1990.
Unni KK, Dahlin DC, McLeod RA, and Pritchard DJ: Intraosseous well-differentiated osteosarcoma. Cancer 40:1337–1347, 1977.

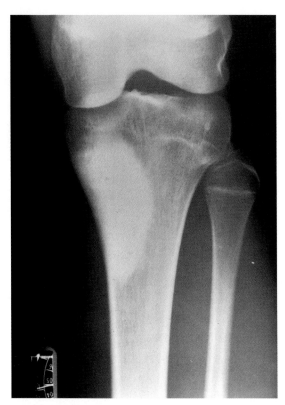

Figure 36–1. This radiograph illustrates a low-grade central osteosarcoma of the medulla of the upper tibia. The lesion is densely sclerotic.

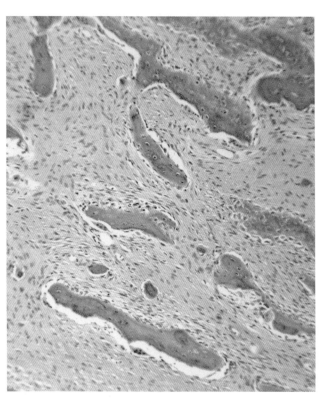

Figure 36–3. This low-power photomicrograph illustrates the parallel arrangements of bony trabeculae that can be seen in low-grade central osteosarcomas. This appearance is nearly identical with that of parosteal osteosarcoma.

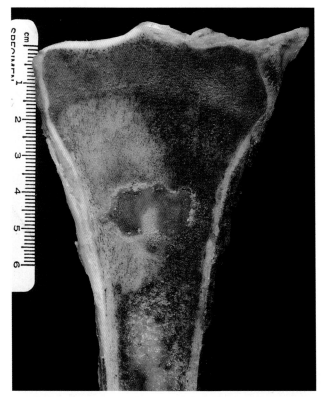

Figure 36–2. This photograph of a gross specimen of the proximal tibial lesion seen in Figure 36–1 shows the homogeneous nature of most low-grade central osteosarcomas. The central defect is the biopsy site. These tumors are frequently gritty when cut.

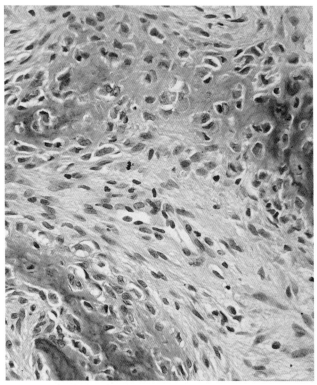

Figure 36–4. At higher magnification, low-grade central osteosarcomas show minimal cytologic atypia. The lesions are also less cellular than conventional osteosarcomas.

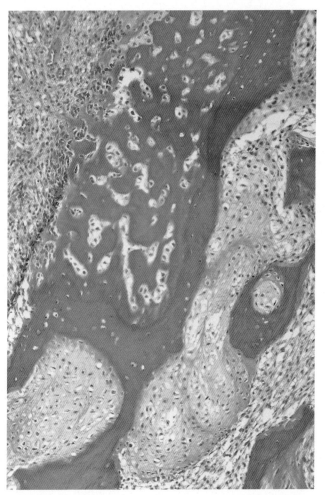

Figure 36–5. The osteoid produced by low-grade central osteosarcoma may grow in an appositional manner onto pre-existing bony trabeculae.

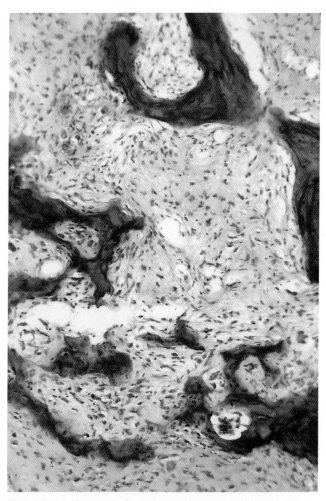

Figure 36–6. The histologic pattern of low-grade central osteosarcoma may also mimic that seen in fibrous dysplasia, as illustrated in this photomicrograph.

CHAPTER 37

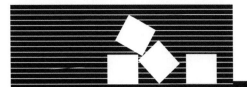

Small Cell Osteosarcoma

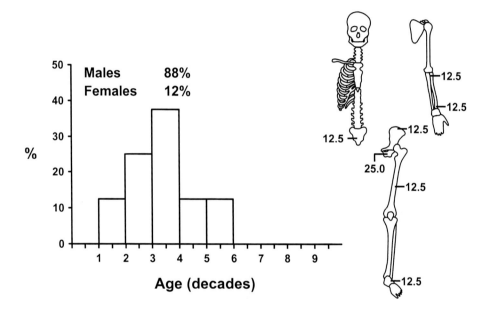

CLINICAL SIGNS

1. A painful mass may be present.
2. A neurologic deficit may be seen if the tumor involves a vertebra.

CLINICAL SYMPTOMS

1. Approximately two thirds of patients complain of pain in the region of the tumor.
2. Approximately 15 per cent of patients complain of a mass or swelling in the region of the tumor, and 25 per cent complain of both pain and swelling.

3. Neurologic symptoms may be present in patients with vertebral tumors.
4. Symptoms may be present from days to years before diagnosis of the tumor.

MAJOR RADIOGRAPHIC FEATURES

1. The tumor most commonly involves the metaphyseal region of long bones.
2. Epiphyseal extension is present in about a third of cases.
3. Approximately 15 per cent of tumors are purely diaphyseal.

213

4. All tumors have a lytic component, and associated medullary sclerosis is present in approximately half the tumors.
5. Approximately 60 per cent of tumors have an associated soft tissue mass.
6. Twenty-five per cent of tumors have an identifiable mineralized soft tissue mass.
7. All tumors have an indistinct margin, and periosteal reaction is present in approximately half the tumors.

RADIOGRAPHIC DIFFERENTIAL DIAGNOSIS

1. Conventional osteosarcoma.
2. Ewing's sarcoma.

MAJOR PATHOLOGIC FEATURES

Gross

1. Tumors are generally poorly circumscribed and infiltrative.
2. Soft tissue extension is ordinarily present.
3. The tumors are most commonly soft and gray-white.

Microscopic

1. Although the designation "small cell" is subjective, the nuclei are relatively uniform in shape (with a mean nuclear diameter of approximately 8.4 μm).
2. Nuclei are round to oval and generally hyperchromatic.
3. The shape of cells varies from round (most common) to short-spindled.
4. Osteoid is variably present but most commonly is scanty (approximately half the tumors).

5. The osteoid shows a lace-like pattern.
6. A hemangiopericytomatous pattern is present in about a third of tumors.
7. Glycogen is identified in approximately a third of tumors (periodic acid–Schiff [PAS] positivity).

PATHOLOGIC DIFFERENTIAL DIAGNOSIS

Benign lesions: none.

Malignant lesions:

1. Ewing's sarcoma.
2. Hemangiopericytoma.
3. Osteosarcoma.
4. Metastatic small cell carcinoma.
5. Malignant lymphoma.

TREATMENT

Primary Modality: limb-sparing surgery with adjuvant chemotherapy.

Other Possible Approaches: amputation.

References

Ayala AG, Ro JY, Raymond AK, et al: Small cell osteosarcoma. A clinicopathologic study of 27 cases. Cancer *64*:2162–2173, 1989.

Bertoni F, Present D, Bacchini P, et al: the Istituto Rizzoli experience with small cell osteosarcoma. Cancer *64*:2591–2599, 1989.

Nakajima H, Sim FH, Bond JR, and Unni KK: Small cell osteosarcoma of bone. Review of 72 cases. Cancer *79(11)*:2095–2106, 1977.

Sim FH, Unni KK, Beabout JW, and Dahlin DC: Osteosarcoma with small cells simulating Ewing's tumor. J Bone Joint Surg (Am) *61*:207–215, 1979.

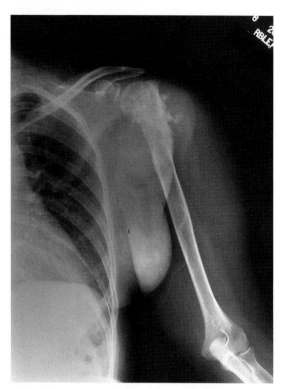

Figure 37–1. This radiograph shows small cell osteosarcoma involving the proximal humerus. The metaphysis of long bones is the most common site of small cell osteosarcoma.

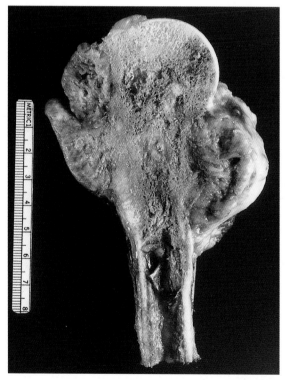

Figure 37–2. This photograph demonstrates the gross pathologic features of a small cell osteosarcoma (the specimen corresponds to the tumor illustrated in Fig. 37–1). There are no distinctive gross pathologic features of small cell osteosarcoma. Most tumors show a permeative destructive pattern of growth with soft tissue extension, as in this case.

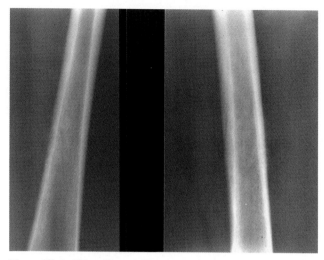

Figure 37–3. This radiograph illustrates the bony destruction associated with a small cell osteosarcoma involving the femoral diaphysis. Tumors such as this likely suggest a radiographic differential diagnosis of "small round cell tumor." Needle biopsy in such cases may be confusing, as the cytologic features of small cell osteosarcoma overlap with those of Ewing's sarcoma.

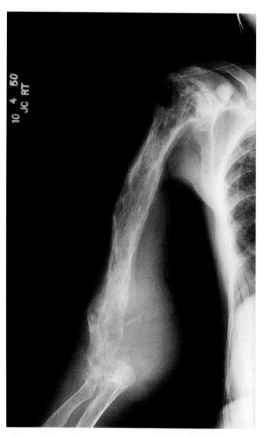

Figure 37–4. This radiograph shows the humerus of a patient with Paget's disease. Small cell osteosarcoma has developed in the humerus affected by Paget's disease.

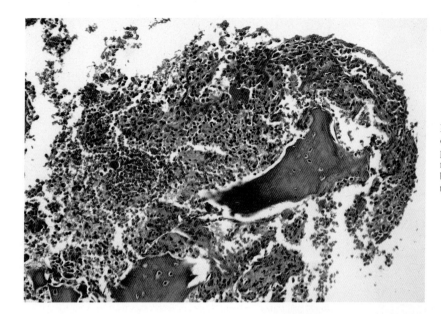

Figure 37–5. This photomicrograph of a small cell osteosarcoma involving a rib shows the permeative pattern of bony invasion commonly seen in malignant bony neoplasms. At low magnification, it may be difficult to determine whether such a small cell tumor is producing a matrix.

Figure 37–6. This photomicrograph illustrates the marked "crush artifact" that is commonly seen in needle biopsies of small cell tumors, including small cell osteosarcoma. Irregular fragments of osteoid are present, admixed with the small cell neoplasm, helping to identify this tumor as a small cell osteosarcoma.

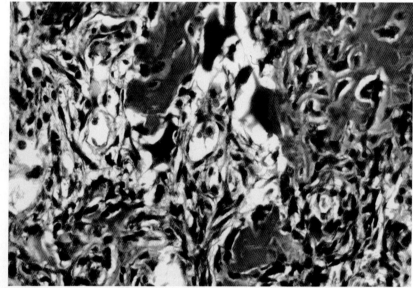

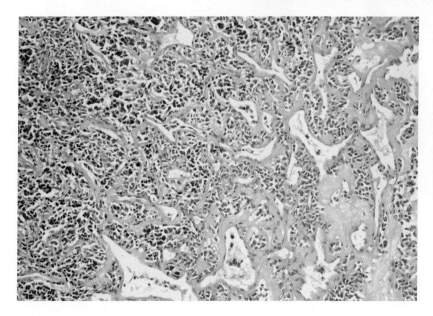

Figure 37–7. This photomicrograph illustrates the hemangiopericytomatous pattern that is commonly present in regions of small cell osteosarcoma. A similar pattern can be seen in the small cell areas of mesenchymal chondrosarcoma, and therefore these two tumors are usually in the same differential diagnosis.

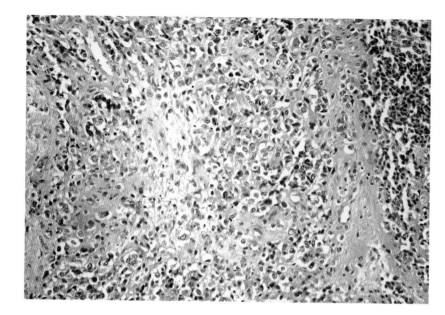

Figure 37–8. It may be necessary to search multiple sections to find tumor osteoid in cases of small cell osteosarcoma. When found, the bone produced by the tumor shows a lace-like pattern similar to that seen in conventional osteosarcoma.

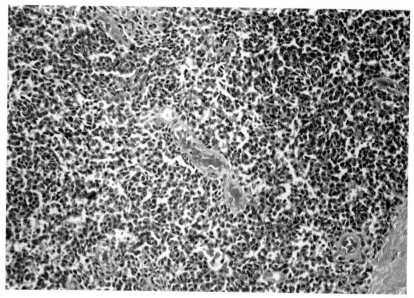

Figure 37–9. In this photomicrograph, this small cell osteosarcoma of the femur displays a low-power histologic pattern mimicking that of Ewing's sarcoma. The cytologic features of small cell osteosarcoma can also mimic those of Ewing's sarcoma (see Fig. 37–10).

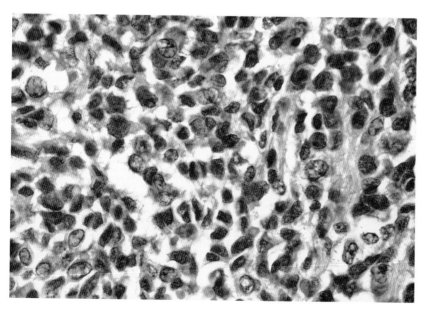

Figure 37–10. The cytologic features of small cell osteosarcoma, illustrated in this photomicrograph, mimic those of Ewing's sarcoma. Careful search for osteoid matrix is important to identify the tumor as an osteosarcoma.

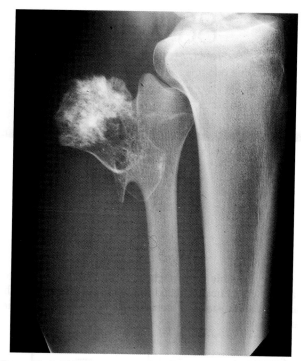

Figure 38–1. This radiograph of the proximal tibia and fibula shows a heavily mineralized osteochondroma projecting posteriorly from the upper fibular metaphysis. The continuity of the cortical and cancellous bone of the fibula with the lesion is characteristic of osteochondroma.

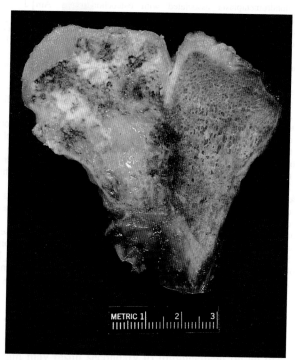

Figure 38–2. Grossly, the resected osteochondroma illustrated in Figure 38–1 shows a cartilaginous cap with regions of extensive calcification (white areas) corresponding to the heavily mineralized regions seen radiographically. The thickness of the cartilage cap is a gross pathologic feature that helps identify lesions that should be carefully assessed histologically for malignant transformation of the cartilage.

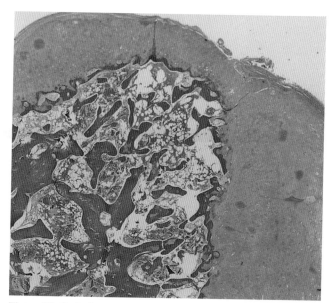

Figure 38–3. At low magnification, osteochondromas show a well-circumscribed periphery. The hyaline cartilage matures into the underlying trabecular bone.

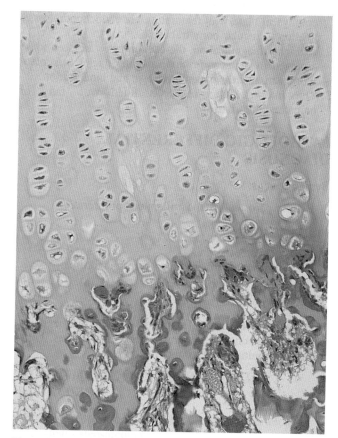

Figure 38–4. At higher magnification, the transition between the cartilage and the osseous trabeculae is identical with a normal growth plate, with columns of chondrocytes and ossification of the matrix material.

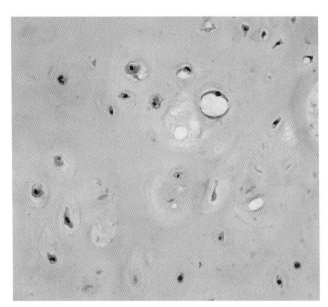

Figure 38–5. At high magnification, the chondrocytes in the cartilage cap have small, dark-staining nuclei that lack cytologic atypia.

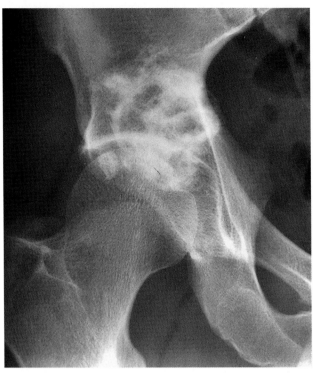

Figure 38–7. This radiograph of the pelvis demonstrates a mineralized lesion above the acetabulum. Flat bone osteochondromas such as this may be difficult to localize and characterize with plain radiographs. Computed tomographic (CT) scans are particularly helpful in this situation.

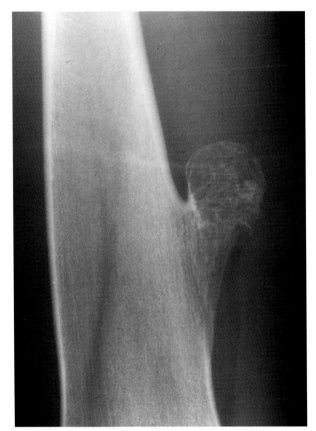

Figure 38–6. This radiograph shows an osteochondroma projecting from the lower femur. The continuity of cortical and cancellous bone is evident. In general, pedunculated osteochondromas point away from the closest joint.

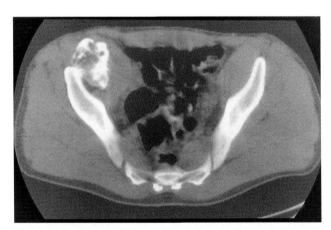

Figure 38–8. An axial CT scan of the patient in Figure 38–7 demonstrates the typical appearance of an osteochondroma projecting from the anterior iliac bone.

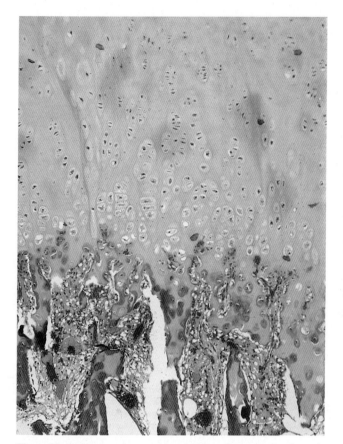

Figure 38–9. Between the osseous trabeculae of an osteochondroma is fatty or hematopoietic marrow, as shown in this photomicrograph. In contrast, parosteal osteosarcoma, which may also have a cartilaginous cap, has a spindle cell proliferation between the "normalized trabeculae" of bone.

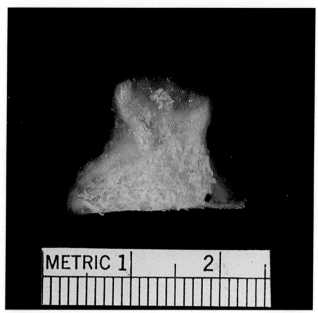

Figure 38–11. Subungual exostoses, as shown in this photograph, share some gross and microscopic features with osteochondromas.

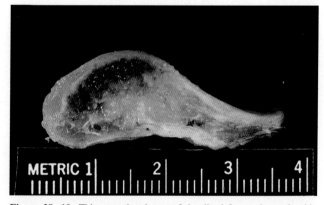

Figure 38–10. This osteochondroma of the distal femur shows the thin cartilage cap and the continuity of the cortical and cancellous bone that characterize these lesions.

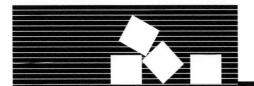

CHAPTER 39

Chondroma

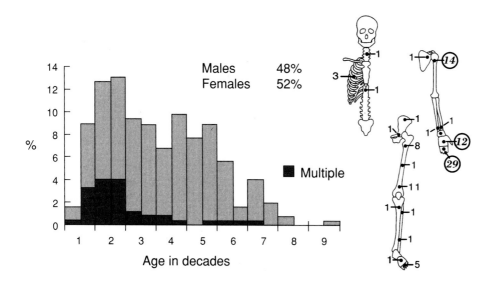

Males 48%
Females 52%

%

Age in decades

■ Multiple

CLINICAL SIGNS

1. Frequently, chondromas are diagnosed incidentally on radiographic examination.
2. Chondromas are frequently "hot" on bone scan and may be incidentally identified in this way as well.

CLINICAL SYMPTOMS

1. The majority of patients are asymptomatic.
2. Pain is rarely a presenting complaint but may occur in patients with pathologic fractures. This is commonly the case with lesions of the small bones. If pain exists in the absence of pathologic fracture, a low-grade chondrosarcoma should be suspected.

MAJOR RADIOGRAPHIC FEATURES

1. The lesion has a medullary location.
2. The features are benign, showing sharp margination and expansion of the affected bone.
3. Punctate calcification frequently is present.
4. Multiple lesions may be seen.

RADIOGRAPHIC DIFFERENTIAL DIAGNOSIS

1. Bone infarct.
2. Chondrosarcoma.

MAJOR PATHOLOGIC FEATURES

Gross

1. Lesional tissue is characteristically translucent and blue-gray.
2. Whitish-yellow calcific foci may be scattered throughout the tissue.
3. The tumors vary in consistency, but most are relatively firm. Myxoid foci should arouse suspicion that the tumor is a low-grade chondrosarcoma.

Microscopic

1. At low magnification, the tumor is hypocellular, with a blue-gray aura to the cartilaginous matrix.
2. The nuclei are inconspicuous at low magnification.
3. At higher magnification, the nuclei are uniform in their cytologic characteristics. Each is small, regular, and darkly stained.
4. Binucleated cells are rare.

PATHOLOGIC DIFFERENTIAL DIAGNOSIS

Benign lesions:

1. Fibrocartilaginous dysplasia with prominent chondroid regions.
2. The cartilage of a prominent costochondral junction.

Malignant lesions:

1. Low-grade (well-differentiated) chondrosarcoma.
2. Chondroblastic osteosarcoma.

TREATMENT

Primary Modality: A benign appearing, asymptomatic enchondroma that is not structurally weakening the bone warrants observation.

Other Possible Approaches: If the lesion is symptomatic, curettage and bone grafting usually are curative. If there is an associated pathologic fracture, curettage and grafting should be delayed until the fracture has healed and the continuity of the bone has been restored.

References

Bauer TW, Dorfman HD, and Lathan JT Jr: Periosteal chondroma: a clinicopathologic study of 23 cases. Am J Surg Pathol 6:631–637, 1982.

Boriani S, Bacchini P, Bertoni F, and Campanacci M: Periosteal chondroma: a review of twenty cases. J Bone Joint Surg (Am) 65:205–212, 1983.

DeSantos LA, and Spjut HJ: Periosteal chondroma: a radiographic spectrum. Skeletal Radiol 6:15–20, 1981.

Kocher MS, and Jupiter JB: Enchondroma versus chondrosarcoma of the phalanx. Orthopedics 23(5):493–494, 2000.

Ostrowski ML, and Spjut HJ: Lesions of the bones of the hands and feet. Am J Surg Pathol 21(6):676–690, 1997.

Schreuder HW, Pruszczynski M, Veth RP, and Lemmens JA: Treatment of benign and low-grade malignant intramedullary chondroid tumours with curettage and cryosurgery. Eur J Surg Oncol 24(2):120–126, 1998.

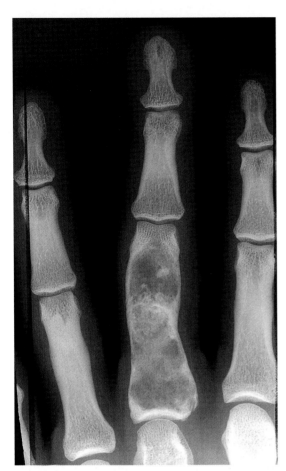

Figure 39–1. This radiograph shows an enchondroma in its most common location, a phalanx of the hand. The lesion is well marginated and expansile. The typical punctate calcification of a cartilaginous lesion is present.

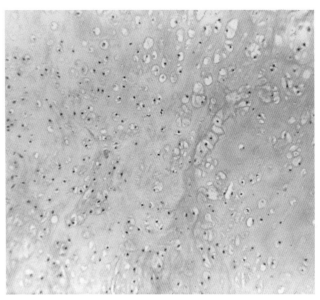

Figure 39–3. At low magnification, hyaline cartilage lesions are blue-gray. Benign lesions are hypocellular, as illustrated in this photomicrograph of a chondroma involving the femoral diaphysis.

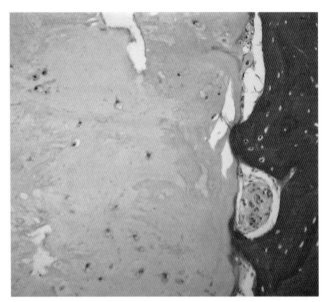

Figure 39–4. The periphery of a chondroma is well-circumscribed, both grossly and microscopically, as seen in this photomicrograph of a fibular chondroma. The lesion does not show significant endosteal erosion.

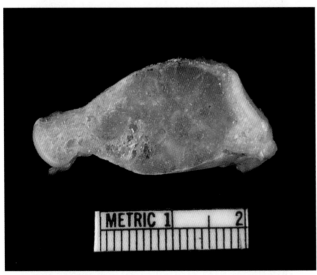

Figure 39–2. The gross appearance of hyaline cartilage lesions is shown in this photograph of a phalangeal chondroma. The lesion is well circumscribed, glistening, and gray-white. The small bones may be expanded by such a lesion, as in this case.

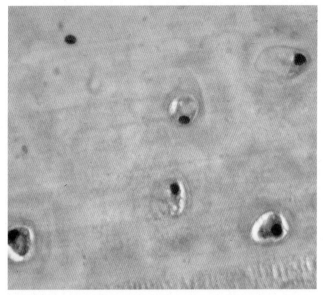

Figure 39–5. At higher magnification, the cytologic features of the chondrocytes are apparent. In a chondroma, the nuclei are uniformly small and darkly stained. Although binucleated cells may be seen occasionally, they are not common.

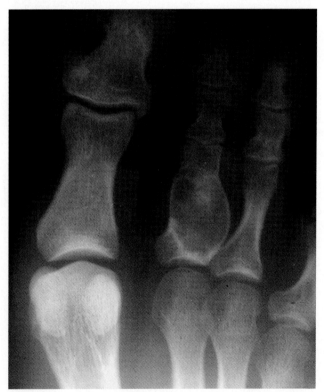

Figure 39–6. This radiograph illustrates a chondroma involving the proximal phalanx of the second toe. The lesion expands the affected bone, is calcified, and shows a sclerotic margin.

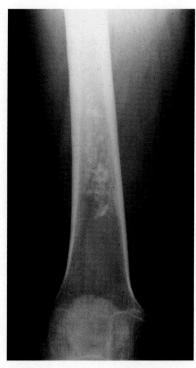

Figure 39–7. When chondromas involve the long bones, the lesions generally show an intramedullary collection of stippled calcification. Ring-like calcification may also be present. The endosteal surface of the affected bone does not show any irregularity. Endosteal erosion is a worrisome feature for a low-grade malignant cartilage tumor.

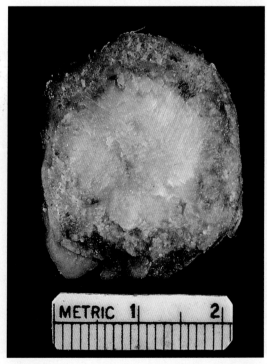

Figure 39–8. Grossly, chondromas in long bone locations are no different from those involving the small bones of the hands and feet. This chondroma of the upper fibular shows the well-marginated, glistening, gray-white aura of a hyaline cartilage tumor.

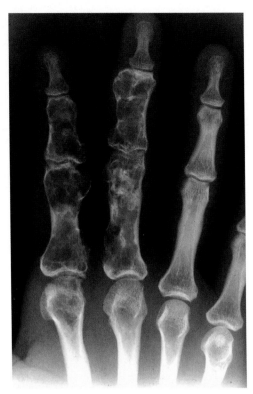

Figure 39–9. Multiple chondromas have the same radiographic features as solitary lesions, as in this case with multiple lesions involving the small bones of the hand.

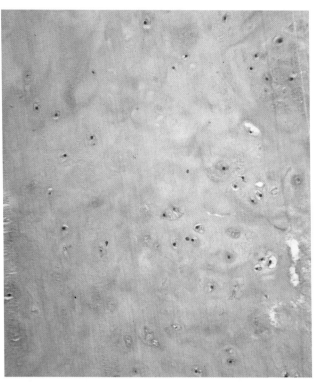

Figure 39–11. At low magnification, the nuclei of the chondrocytes are inconspicuous, appearing as small dark dots, as seen in this chondroma involving the distal femur in a male adult.

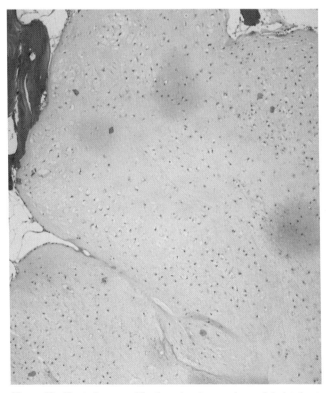

Figure 39–10. At low magnification, chondromas show a lobulated pattern, as illustrated in this photomicrograph. Many cartilage tumors share this low-power histologic feature.

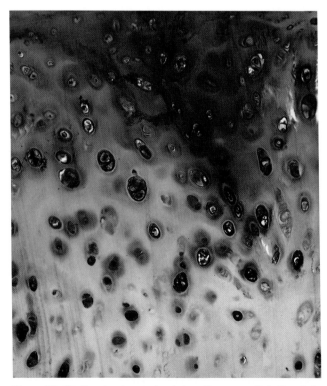

Figure 39–12. Prominent costochondral cartilage may clinically mimic the appearance of a neoplasm. If biopsy is performed, a mistaken diagnosis of a cartilage tumor may be made. However, the regular and orderly appearance of the chondrocytes is a clue that the tissue represents normal anatomy rather than neoplasm.

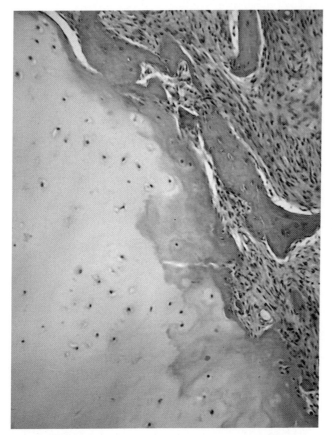

Figure 39–13. Some examples of fibrous dysplasia may demonstrate a chondroid component and thus be mistaken for a cartilage tumor. This case of fibrocartilaginous dysplasia involving the femur in a patient with Albright's syndrome shows such prominent chondroid differentiation.

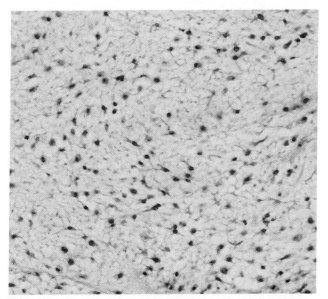

Figure 39–14. This photomicrograph shows a cartilage tumor in the thumb of a patient with Ollier's disease. Although the lesion is hypercellular and shows mild cytologic atypia, it is within the spectrum of a benign cartilage tumor of the small bones of the hands and feet.

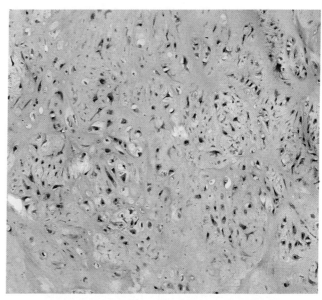

Figure 39–15. This photomicrograph illustrates the histologic features of a periosteal chondroma. The lesion is hypercellular, the degree of cellularity similar to that seen in small bone enchondromas. Periosteal chondromas are generally less than 5 cm in their greatest dimension.

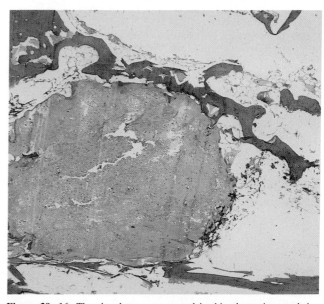

Figure 39–16. The chondroma represented in this photomicrograph involved the proximal fibula. Such lesions may show a more infiltrative pattern similar to that seen in small bone enchondromas.

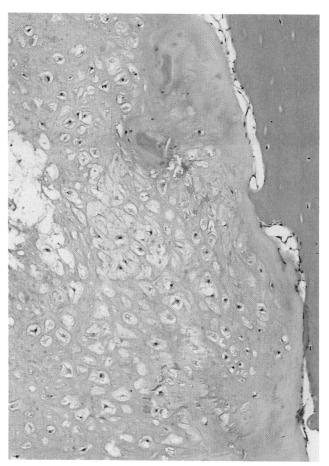

Figure 39–17. This low-power photomicrograph shows the sharp circumscription characteristic of benign hyaline cartilage tumors. A mild degree of endosteal scalloping may be allowed in enchondromas, but such lesions should be thoroughly curetted to ensure complete removal.

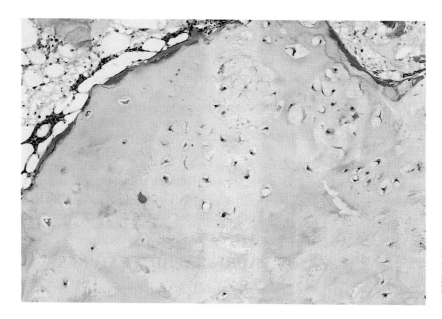

Figure 39–18. Chondromas, like this one from the femoral neck, frequently show reactive bone at the periphery of the cartilage lobules. This feature is helpful in distinguishing benign from low-grade malignant hyaline cartilage tumors.

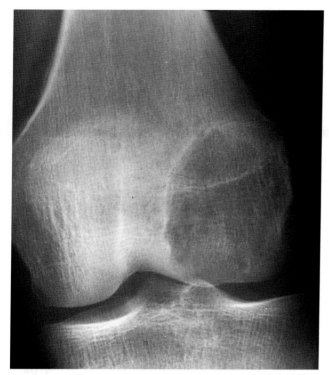

Figure 40–1. This radiograph shows a well-marginated lytic chondroblastoma located eccentrically in the distal femur. The knee region is the most common location for chondroblastoma, and this lesion involves the epiphysis, as is nearly always the case with chondroblastoma. The tumor also extends to involve the metaphysis.

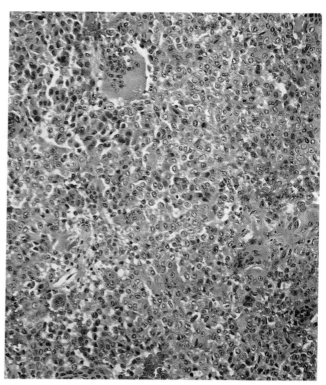

Figure 40–3. Chondroblastoma was originally thought to be a "calcifying giant cell tumor." The solid portion of the lesion may show numerous benign multinucleated giant cells, as illustrated in this photomicrograph.

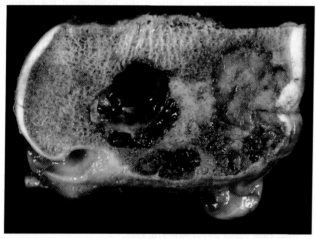

Figure 40–2. The gross characteristics of this chondroblastoma correlate well with its radiographic appearance in Figure 40–1. The lesion is fleshy and whitish in its solid regions. A hemorrhagic cystic region is also grossly evident. Secondary aneurysmal bone cyst frequently accompanies chondroblastoma.

Figure 40–4. In contrast to giant cell tumor, chondroblastoma contains zones of eosinophilic to amphophilic fibrochondroid matrix, as shown in this photomicrograph. These zones are typically hypocellular when compared with the surrounding regions.

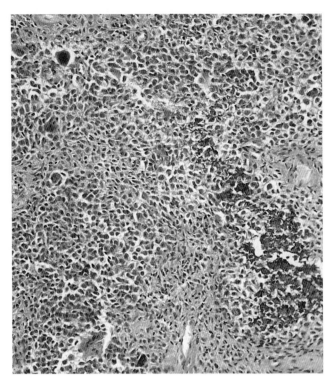

Figure 40–5. Calcification helps distinguish chondroblastoma from giant cell tumor. The calcification may be regional and identifiable radiographically, as in this tumor. At times, the calcification forms a "chicken wire" type of pattern.

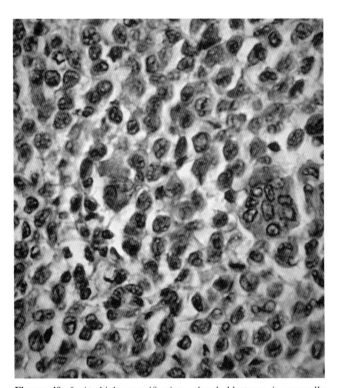

Figure 40–6. At high magnification, chondroblastoma is generally loosely organized, as seen in this photomicrograph. The nuclei are uniform and characteristically bean-shaped, with a central groove. This cytologic appearance is similar to that of the nuclei of Langerhans' cells in Langerhans' cell histiocytosis.

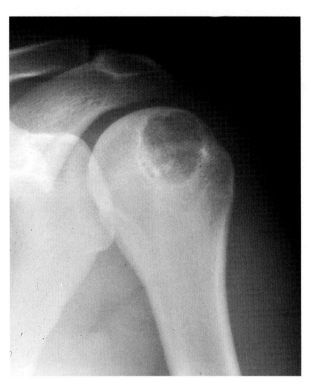

Figure 40–7. This radiograph illustrates a chondroblastoma involving the humeral head. In this region, the lesion may involve the epiphysis or apophysis. Chondroblastomas are characteristically lytic, but this tumor shows partial calcification. A thin rim of sclerosis at the periphery attests to the lesion's slow growth.

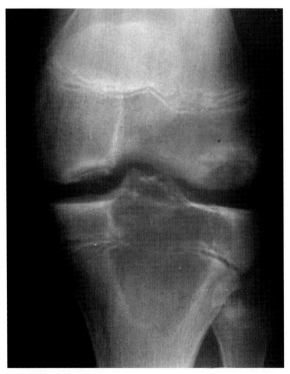

Figure 40–8. A sharply marginated chondroblastoma involving the proximal tibia is shown in this radiograph. The tumor crosses the open physis; this is a feature rarely seen in other tumors. Peripheral sclerosis is also present.

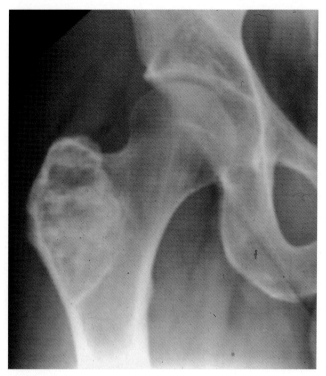

Figure 40–9. Chondroblastomas show mineralization to varying degrees. This example involving the greater trochanter (apophyseal location) is heavily mineralized.

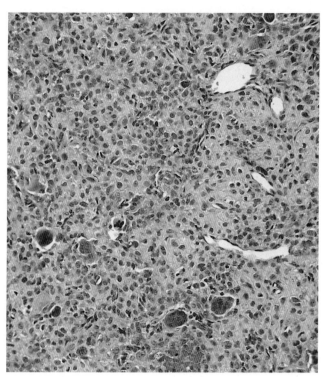

Figure 40–11. Although chondroblastoma most commonly involves the epiphyseal region of a long bone in a skeletally immature patient, some tumors occur in flat bones as well. This tumor involved the temporal bone in a three-year-old girl. The temporal bone is the most common location for lesions involving the skull.

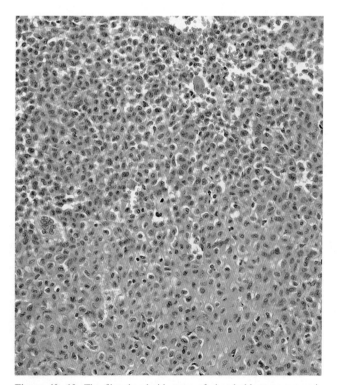

Figure 40–10. The fibrochondroid zones of chondroblastoma are variably scattered through the tumor and may not be a prominent component of the lesion, as in this photomicrograph.

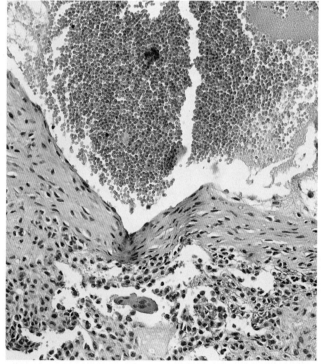

Figure 40–12. This photomicrograph illustrates the presence of a secondary aneurysmal bone cyst complicating a chondroblastoma. Such a secondary aneurysmal bone cyst may be so prominent as to mask the appearance of the chondroblastoma component and lead to a misdiagnosis.

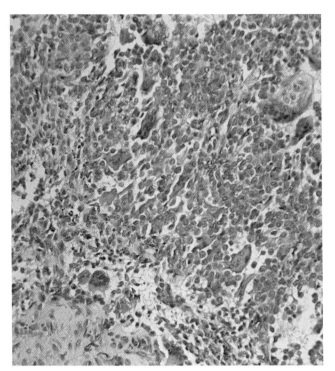

Figure 40–13. Chondroblastoma may recur within bone and soft tissue, and rarely such lesions may metastasize to the lungs. As this photomicrograph illustrates, such rare pulmonary metastases are histologically indistinguishable from their osseous primary lesions.

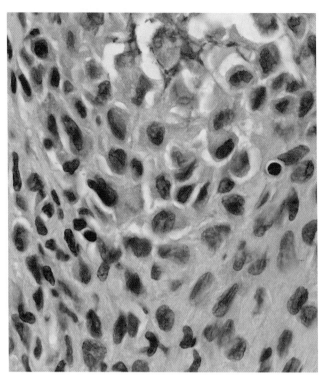

Figure 40–15. This high-power photomicrograph reveals the cytologic features of the mononuclear cells of chondroblastoma. These cells may appear epithelioid, with abundant eosinophilic cytoplasm and eccentric nuclei, as shown here.

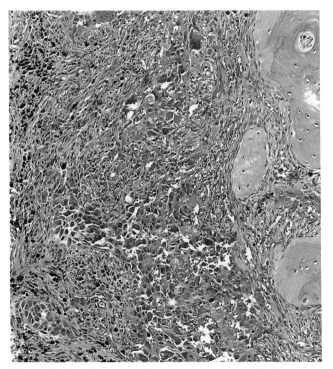

Figure 40–14. This pigmented lesion from the temporal bone contains multinucleated giant cells within a sea of mononuclear cells that have cytologic features similar to those of chondroblastoma. The differential diagnosis for such lesions includes pigmented villonodular synovitis of the temporomandibular joint and chondroblastoma.

CHAPTER 41

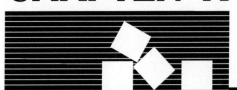

Chondromyxoid Fibroma

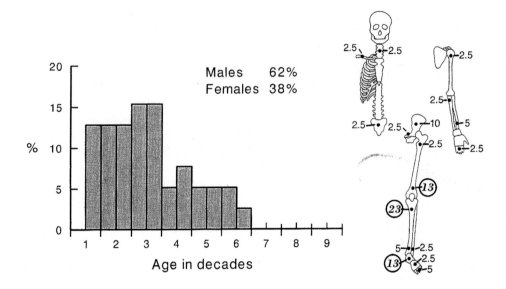

Males 62%
Females 38%

%

Age in decades

CLINICAL SIGNS

1. Regional tenderness is usually the only finding on physical examination.
2. Tumefaction is more commonly found when the tumor involves bones of the hands or feet.

CLINICAL SYMPTOMS

1. Pain is the most common presenting complaint.
2. Local swelling may be noted on rare occasions and is more frequently a presenting complaint when the tumor involves a small bone.
3. Occasionally, the lesion may be an asymptomatic, incidental radiographic abnormality.

MAJOR RADIOGRAPHIC FEATURES

1. The lesion has an eccentric metaphyseal location.
2. It shows sharp, sclerotic, and scalloped margins.
3. Matrix calcification is rare.

RADIOGRAPHIC DIFFERENTIAL DIAGNOSIS

1. Fibroma (metaphyseal fibrous defect).
2. Aneurysmal bone cyst.
3. Chondroblastoma.
4. Fibrous dysplasia.

MAJOR PATHOLOGIC FEATURES

Gross

1. Being translucent and bluish-gray, this tumor may grossly resemble hyaline cartilage; however, it is not soft and "runny" as in myxoid areas of chondrosarcoma.
2. The tumor is usually very well marginated and therefore may be lobulated grossly.
3. Bone surrounding the tumor usually shows sclerotic changes.

Microscopic

1. At low magnification, the tumor shows a distinctly lobulated pattern of growth, with peripheral hypercellularity of the lobules.
2. The tumor cells are spindled and stellate. Rarely, the nuclei may appear "bizarre." Benign giant cells are usually seen between the lobules of the tumor.
3. The stroma is myxoid, but only rarely is well-formed hyaline cartilage present.
4. More solidly cellular areas containing cells identical with those found in chondroblastoma may be seen.

PATHOLOGIC DIFFERENTIAL DIAGNOSIS

Benign lesions:

1. Chondroblastoma.
2. Chondroma.

Malignant lesions:

1. Chondrosarcoma.
2. Chondroblastic osteosarcoma.

TREATMENT

Primary Modality: curettage and bone grafting.

Other Possible Approaches: en bloc resection with a marginal margin if the tumor's location makes it amenable to removal without significant loss of function.

References

Durr HR, Lienemann A, Nerlich A, et al: Chondromyxoid fibroma of bone. Arch Orthop Trauma Surg *120(1–2)*:42–47, 2000.
Gherlinzoni F, Rock M, and Picci P: Chondromyxoid fibroma: the experience at the Istituto Ortopedico Rizzoli. J Bone Joint Surg (Am) *65*:198–204, 1983.
Nielsen GP, Keel SB, Dickersin GR, et al: Chondromyxoid fibroma: a tumor showing myofibroblastic, myochondroblastic, and chondrocytic differentiation. Mod Pathol *12(5)*:514–517, 1999.
Kyriakos M: Soft tissue implantation of chondromyxoid fibroma. Am J Surg Pathol *3*:363–372, 1979.
Rahimi A, Beabout JW, Ivins JC, and Dahlin DC: Chondromyxoid fibroma: a clinicopathologic study of 76 cases. Cancer *30*:726–736, 1972.
Schajowicz F, and Gallardo J: Chondromyxoid fibroma (fibromyxoid chondroma) of bone: a clinicopathological study of thirty-two cases. J Bone Joint Surg (Br) *53*:198–216, 1971.
Wu CT, Inwards CY, O'Laughlin S, et al: Chondromyxoid fibroma of bone: a clinicopathologic review of 278 cases. Hum Pathol *29(5)*:438–446, 1998.
Yamaguchi T, and Dorfman HD: Radiographic and histologic patterns of calcification in chondromyxoid fibroma. Skeletal Radiol *27(10)*:559–564, 1998.

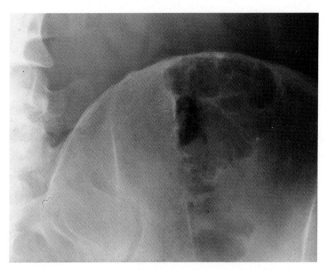

Figure 41–1. This radiograph shows a well-marginated lesion in the iliac bone. The periphery is scalloped and has a partially sclerotic rim. Although the majority of chondromyxoid fibromas are metaphyseal in long bones, approximately 10 per cent occur in the ilium (as in this case).

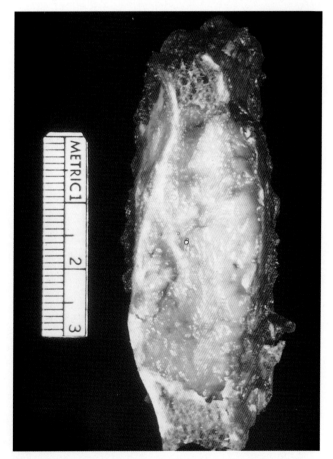

Figure 41–2. The gross features in this case correlate well with the radiograph shown in Figure 41–1. The lesion is whitish and well marginated. The lesion may show myxoid change.

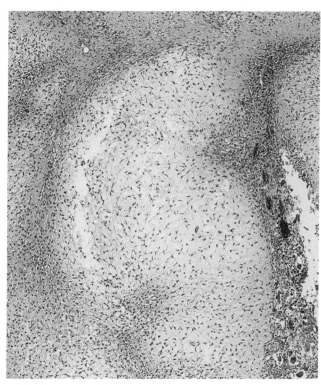

Figure 41–3. At low magnification, chondromyxoid fibromas are characteristically lobulated, as this photomicrograph illustrates. The lesion is relatively hypocellular toward the center of the lobules.

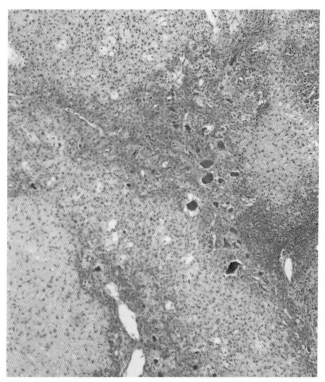

Figure 41–4. At the periphery of the lobules of tumor is a "condensation" of cellularity. In these regions, the tumor tends to show more spindling, and benign multinucleated giant cells are present. These foci may mimic the appearance of chondroblastoma.

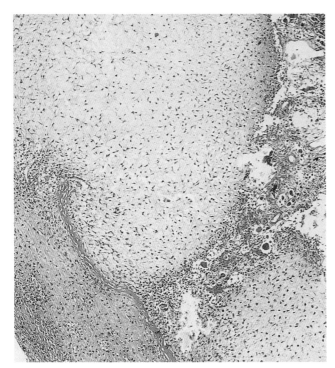

Figure 41–5. At higher magnification, chondromyxoid fibroma has a chondroid appearance in the central portion of the tumor lobules. A small sampling of this portion of the lesional tissue may mimic the appearance of a chondroma or chondrosarcoma.

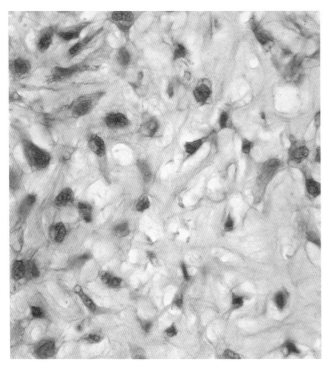

Figure 41–6. At high magnification, the central portion of the tumor is chondromyoid (well-developed hyaline cartilage is unusual in chondromyoid fibroma). Cytologically, the cells are stellate in these regions. However, the nuclei are uniform and do not show significant atypia. Longitudinal grooves and a bean shape to the nucleus may simulate the cytologic features seen in chondroblastoma or Langerhans' cell histiocytosis.

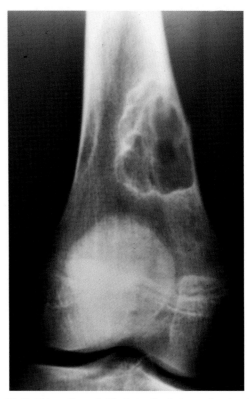

Figure 41–7. This radiograph illustrates the features of a chondromyxoid fibroma in the distal femur. The metaphyseal location is typical, and the lesion is eccentric. The sclerotic and scalloped rim is clearly visible in this case.

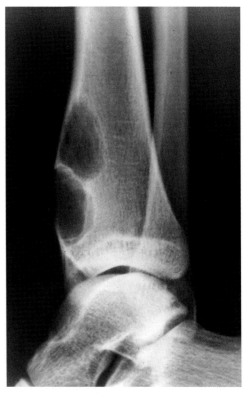

Figure 41–8. The lobulated radiographic appearance of a chondromyxoid fibroma is demonstrated here. The differential diagnosis in such a case includes a metaphyseal fibrous defect (fibroma).

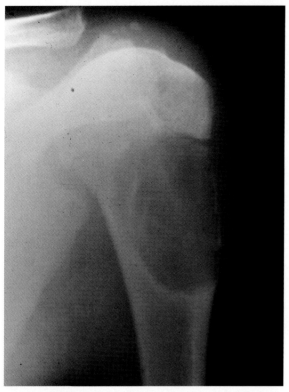

Figure 41–9. This chondromyxoid fibroma of the upper humerus has a lytic and well-marginated radiographic appearance. The lesion abuts but does not cross the physis.

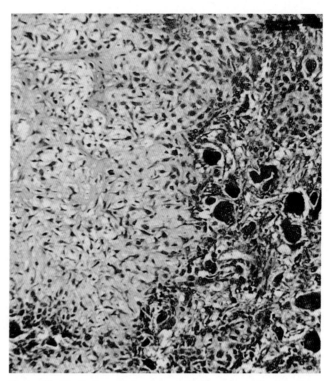

Figure 41–11. Regions of chondromyxoid fibroma may simulate chondroblastoma, as in this photomicrograph. The cytologic features also overlap, suggesting that the two lesions are closely related.

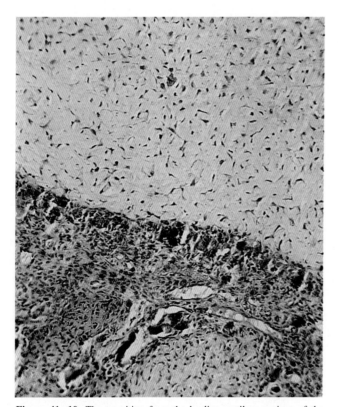

Figure 41–10. The transition from the hyaline cartilage regions of the tumor to the more cellular areas may be quite abrupt, as shown in this photomicrograph. The tumor may thus exhibit a "bimorphic" histologic pattern.

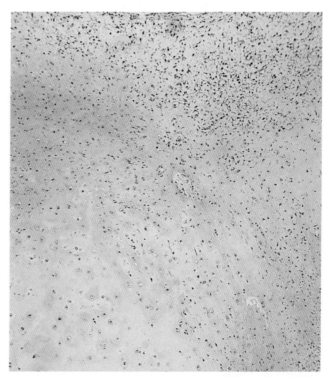

Figure 41–12. Foci within a chondromyxoid fibroma may be markedly chondroid and thus simulate a chondroma or chondrosarcoma. Chondromyxoid fibromas were commonly mistaken for chondrosarcomas in the past, but the publication of this fact has resulted in more mistaken identification of chondrosarcomas as chondromyxoid fibromas in recent years.

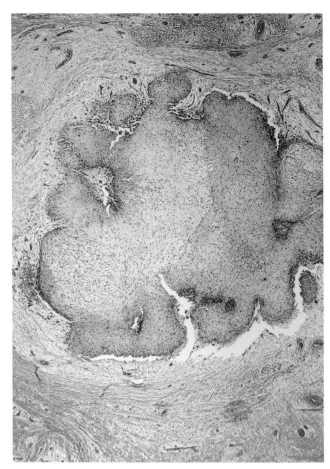

Figure 41–13. As with chondroblastoma, chondromyxoid fibroma may recur if inadequately treated. The recurrence may be within the bone or soft tissues, as shown in this photomicrograph. Such soft tissue recurrences frequently exhibit a rim of calcification radiographically.

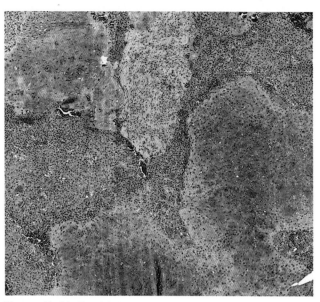

Figure 41–14. The lobulated nature of chondromyxoid fibroma is nicely illustrated in this low-power photomicrograph of a proximal tibial tumor.

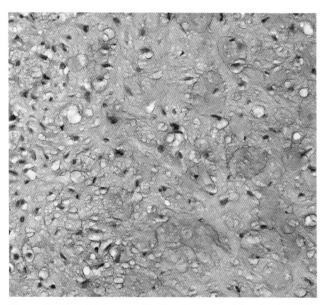

Figure 41–15. At higher magnification, the center of the chondroid lobules in chondromyxoid fibroma may be relatively cellular. This tumor is the same as that illustrated in Figure 41–14. Taken out of context, such regions may lead the pathologist to consider a diagnosis of low-grade chondrosarcoma.

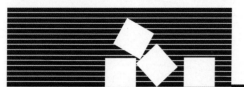

CHAPTER 42

Multiple Chondromas

Males 54%
Females 46%

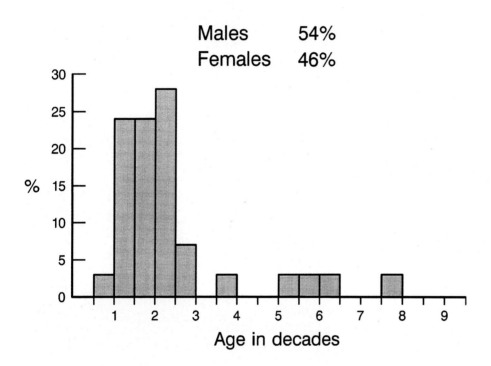

% (y-axis), Age in decades (x-axis)

CLINICAL SIGNS

1. Multiple mass lesions are palpable.
2. Deformity and shortness of stature are often present because of epiphyseal involvement.
3. There is a tendency to unilaterality in Ollier's disease.
4. Hemangiomas are associated with Maffucci's syndrome.

CLINICAL SYMPTOMS

1. Symptoms are similar to those of the solitary lesion, with pain and associated pathologic fracture.

MAJOR RADIOGRAPHIC FEATURES

1. Most cases are bilateral, but involvement usually predominates on one side.
2. Affected bones are shortened and deformed.
3. Cartilage masses extend linearly from the physis into the metaphysis.
4. Cartilage masses often have no overlying cortex and may contain stippled calcification.
5. There is a tendency to spare the epiphysis and diaphysis except in severe cases.
6. Affected bones cannot tubulate, and the ends may have a clubbed appearance.
7. The disease tends to regress after puberty.

RADIOGRAPHIC DIFFERENTIAL DIAGNOSIS

1. Fibrous dysplasia.
2. Multiple hereditary exostoses.

MAJOR PATHOLOGIC FEATURES

Gross

1. The lesional tissue is blue-gray and translucent.
2. No myxoid or cystic change is evident grossly.

Microscopic

1. At low magnification, these lesions are composed predominantly of blue-gray hyaline cartilage matrix.
2. The lesions are generally more cellular than is seen in solitary chondromas. No myxoid stromal change is evident.
3. At higher magnification, the nuclei may be hyperchromic, and binucleated cells may be identified.

PATHOLOGIC DIFFERENTIAL DIAGNOSIS

Benign lesions:

1. Solitary chondroma.
2. Synovial chondromatosis.

Malignant lesions:

1. Chondrosarcoma, ordinary type

TREATMENT

Primary Modality: Treatment is similar to that for solitary enchondromas, with observation of the lesions if they are asymptomatic.

Other Possible Approaches: If the lesion is symptomatic, curettage and bone grafting are performed.

References

Ben-Itzhak I, Denolf FA, Versfeld G, and Noll BJ: The Maffucci syndrome. J Pediatr Orthop 8(3):345–348, 1988.
Gruning T, and Franke WG: Bone scan appearances in a case of Ollier's disease. Clin Nucl Med 24(11):886–887, 1999.
Liu J, Hudkins PG, Swee RG, and Unni KK: Bone sarcomas associated with Ollier's disease. Cancer 59(7):1376–1385, 1987.
Loewinger RJ, Lichtenstein JR, Dodson WE, et al: Maffucci's syndrome: a mesenchymal dysplasia and multiple tumour syndrome. Br J Dermatol 96:317–322, 1977.
Nardell SG: Ollier's disease: dyschondroplasia. Br Med J 2:555–557, 1950.
Phelan EM, Carty HM, and Kalos S: Generalised enchondromatosis associated with haemangiomas, soft-tissue calcifications and hemihypertrophy. Br J Radiol 59(697):69–74, 1986.
Sun TC, Swee RG, Shives TC, and Unni KK: Chondrosarcoma in Maffucci's syndrome. J Bone Joint Surg (Am) 67(8):1214–1219, 1985.

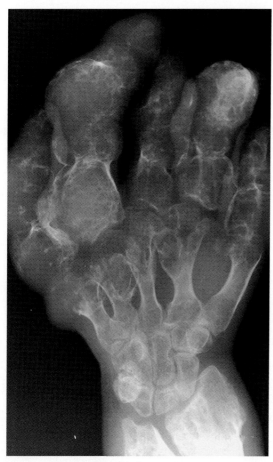

Figure 42–1. This radiograph illustrates extreme deformity of the bones of the hand and wrist by numerous masses of cartilage.

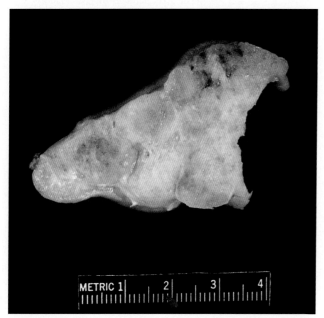

Figure 42–2. This photograph shows the gross features of multiple chondromas in Ollier's disease involving the fifth finger. The disease had resulted in such bony deformity that amputation was done.

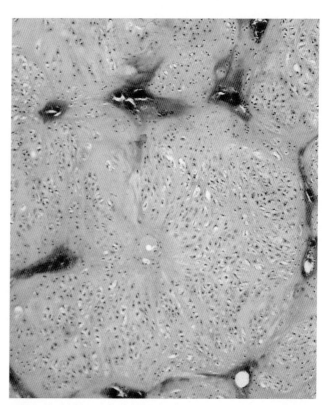

Figure 42–3. This low-power photomicrograph illustrates the lobulated appearance of a chondroma in Ollier's disease. This lesion of the humerus shows somewhat greater cellularity than is seen in many solitary chondromas of the long bones.

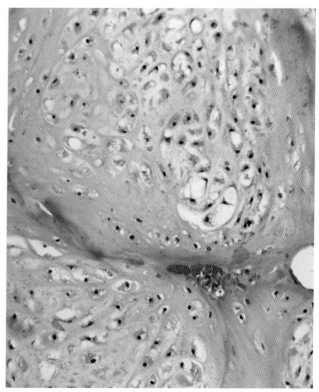

Figure 42–4. The lobulated nature of the chondromas in Ollier's disease is shown at higher magnification in this photomicrograph. Some mild cytologic atypia is also evident in this humeral lesion.

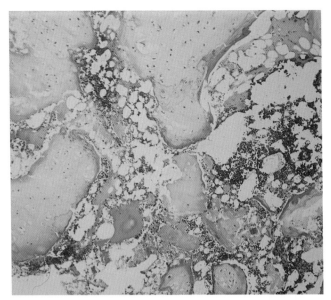

Figure 42–5. The multifocal nature of the chondroma in Ollier's disease is sometimes appreciable histologically, as in this photomicrograph.

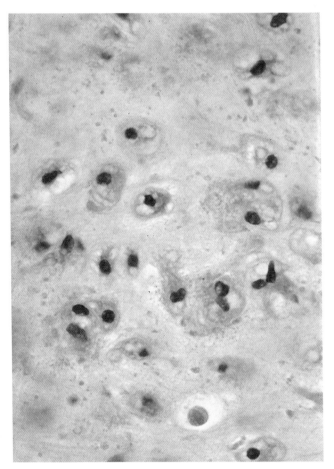

Figure 42–6. The cytologic atypia commonly seen in chondromas of the small bones of the hands and feet can also be seen in Ollier's disease, as demonstrated in this lesion of the thumb.

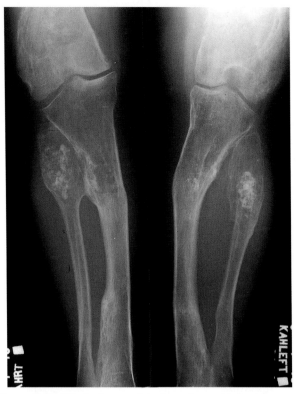

Figure 42–7. Ollier's disease of the lower legs, with bowing, expansion, and deformity of the tibia and fibula, is illustrated in this radiograph. Multiple cartilage masses containing stippled calcification are evident.

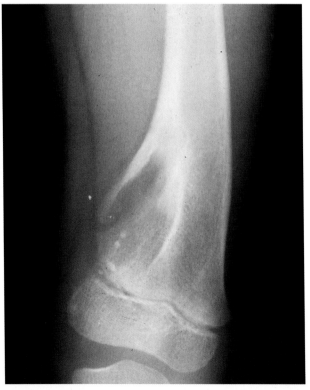

Figure 42–8. Cartilage mass extending linearly from the physis into the metaphysis is noted in this example of Ollier's disease in a four-year-old male patient. There is absence of overlying cortex, and stippled calcification is present.

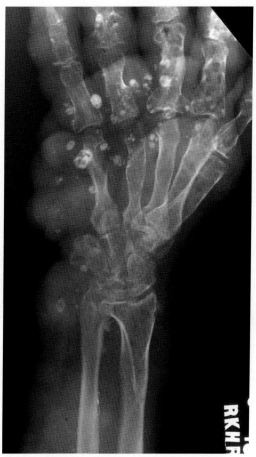

Figure 42–9. Typical changes of Ollier's disease in the bones, associated with soft tissue hemangiomas containing phleboliths, are shown in this example of Maffucci's syndrome.

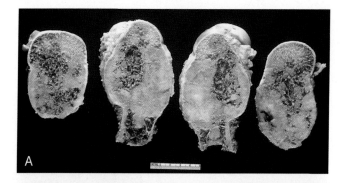

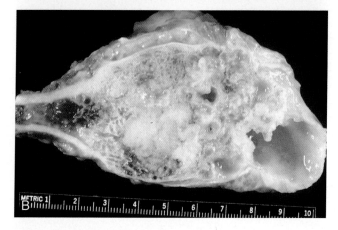

Figure 42–10. Chondrosarcomas can be seen in association with the multiple chondroma syndromes of Ollier's disease (distal femoral tumor shown in *A*) and Maffucci's syndrome (proximal fibular chondrosarcoma shown in *B*).

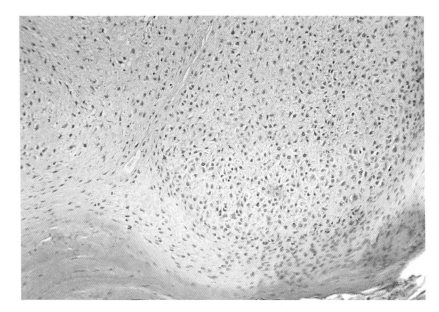

Figure 42–11. Chondrosarcomas in Ollier's disease and Maffucci's syndrome show the cellularity typical of low-grade chondrosarcomas not associated with multiple chondroma syndromes. This Grade 1 chondrosarcoma is from the proximal ulna in a patient with Ollier's disease.

Figure 42–12. The cytologic atypia seen in ordinary chondrosarcomas is also evident in chondrosarcomas complicating Ollier's disease, as illustrated in this case involving the tibia.

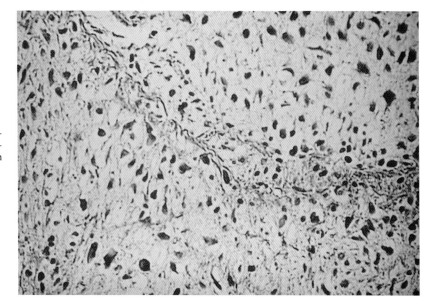

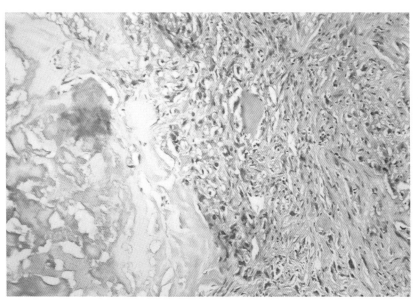

Figure 42–13. Rarely, chondrosarcomas with a dedifferentiated histologic appearance have been identified arising in the background of Ollier's disease, as shown in this case involving the femur.

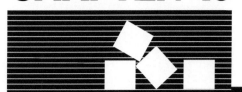

CHAPTER 43

Periosteal Chondroma

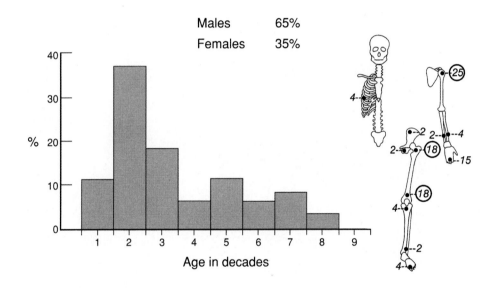

Males   65%
Females   35%

CLINICAL SIGNS

1. The lesion may be palpable on physical examination.
2. The lesion is usually not painful to palpation.

CLINICAL SYMPTOMS

1. Patients usually are asymptomatic.
2. The lesion is most commonly an incidental finding on radiographic examination.

MAJOR RADIOGRAPHIC FEATURES

1. The lesion consists of a small surface mass (less than 3 cm) with saucerization of the underlying bone.
2. The location of the lesion is metaphyseal or diaphyseal.
3. Marginal spicules or "buttresses" are present.
4. Approximately 33 per cent are calcified.

RADIOGRAPHIC DIFFERENTIAL DIAGNOSIS

1. Periosteal chondrosarcoma.
2. Periosteal osteosarcoma.
3. Soft tissue neoplasm secondarily involving the cortical bone.

MAJOR PATHOLOGIC FEATURES

Gross

1. The tumor is gray-blue and translucent, like all tumors with a prominent hyaline cartilage component.
2. If the margin is present in the specimen, it shows sharp circumscription.
3. The medullary portion of the bone is not involved.
4. The tumor is firm and lacks liquefaction or cystic change.

Microscopic

1. The low-power histologic appearance is that of a lobulated hyaline cartilage tumor that is well circumscribed.
2. The lesion is usually hypercellular.
3. The lesion usually contains binucleated chondrocytes.
4. Nuclear atypia may be prominent.

PATHOLOGIC DIFFERENTIAL DIAGNOSIS

Benign lesions:

1. Synovial chondromatosis.
2. Chondroma.

Malignant lesions:

1. Periosteal chondrosarcoma.
2. Periosteal osteosarcoma.

TREATMENT

Primary Modality: These lesions should be excised en bloc with a marginal or wide margin. Depending upon the size of the defect, bone grafting may be necessary.

Other Possible Approaches: Observation may be sufficient if a diagnosis is secure and the patient is asymptomatic.

References

Bauer TW, Dorfman HD, and Latham JT Jr: Periosteal chondroma: a clinicopathologic study of 23 cases. Am J Surg Pathol 6:631–637, 1982.

Boriani S, Bacchini P, Bertoni F, and Campanacci M: Periosteal chondroma: a review of twenty cases. J Bone Joint Surg (Am) 65:205–212, 1983.

Desantos LA, and Spjut JH. Periosteal chondroma: a radiographic spectrum. Skeletal Radiol 6:15–20, 1981.

Lewis MM, Kenan S, Yabut SM, et al: Periosteal chondroma: A report of ten cases and review of the literature. Clin Orthop 256:185–192, 1990.

Nojima T, Unni KK, McLeod RA, and Pritchard DJ: Periosteal chondroma and periosteal chondrosarcoma. Am J Surg Pathol 9:666–677, 1985.

Varma DG, Kumar R, Carrasco CH, et al: MR imaging of periosteal chondroma. J Comput Assist Tomogr 15:1008–1010, 1991.

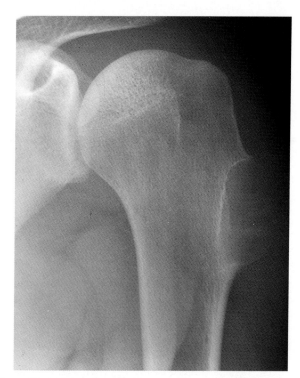

Figure 43–1. This radiograph shows a small periosteal chondroma arising on the lateral surface of the upper humeral metaphysis. The sharp margination and thin sclerotic rim, as well as the marginal spicules of calcification, are typical of periosteal chondroma. An incomplete rim of calcification surrounds the soft tissue component of this lesion.

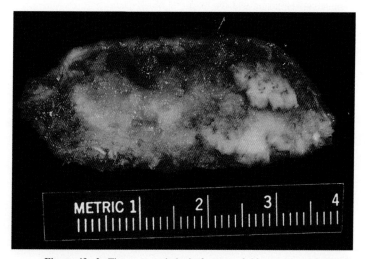

Figure 43–2. The gross pathologic features of this tumor correlate well with its radiographic appearance in Figure 43–1. The small size of the lesion supports a benign diagnosis. As with other hyaline cartilage lesions, the tumor is blue-gray and glistening.

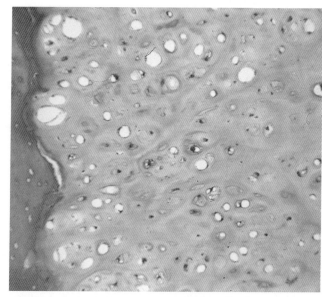

Figure 43–3. At low magnification, a periosteal chondroma is hypocellular and well circumscribed. This photomicrograph shows that the tumor has not penetrated the underlying cortical bone.

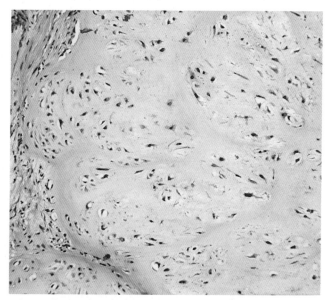

Figure 43–4. The lobulated pattern of a hyaline cartilage tumor is revealed in this photomicrograph. Although periosteal chondromas are benign, they may show greater cellularity at low magnification than their intramedullary counterparts.

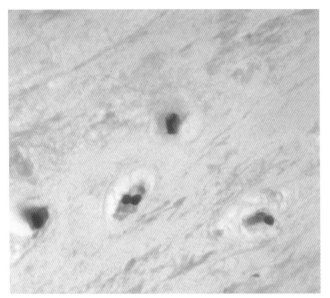

Figure 43–5. At high magnification, the cytologic features of the chondrocytes are uniform. Binucleation, as seen in this photomicrograph, should not dissuade the pathologist from making a diagnosis of periosteal chondroma if the gross and radiographic features are typical.

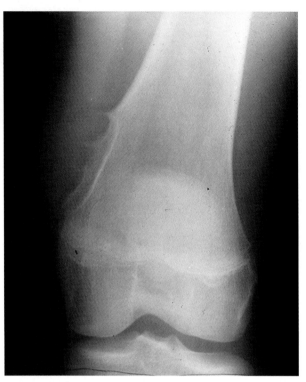

Figure 43–7. Mineralization need not be present in periosteal chondromas, as shown by this example of a distal femoral lesion, which otherwise exhibits radiographic features typical of periosteal chondroma.

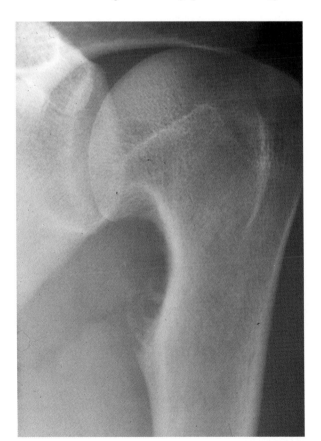

Figure 43–6. This radiograph illustrates a periosteal chondroma of the proximal humerus. The lesion shows a sharp sclerotic margin indicative of slow growth. The marginal spicules and buttresses are typical of periosteal chondroma.

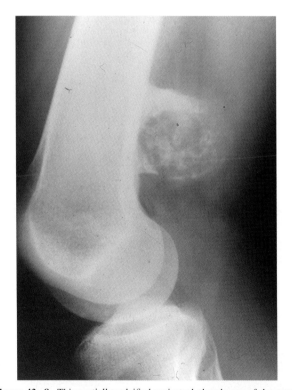

Figure 43–8. This partially calcified periosteal chondroma of the posterior distal femur occupies the most common location of a parosteal osteosarcoma. However, the mineralization present is typical of a hyaline cartilage lesion.

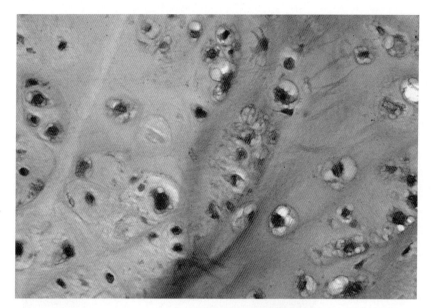

Figure 43–9. At high magnification, periosteal chondromas frequently show greater nuclear pleomorphism and more numerous occurrences of binucleation than intramedullary chondromas. Thus, the histologic features of periosteal chondroma are closer to those of chondromas of the small bones and synovial chondromatosis.

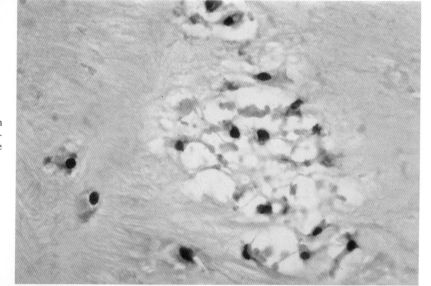

Figure 43–10. Focal myxoid change may be seen in a periosteal chondroma, as in this photomicrograph. Such a feature, however, should alert the pathologist to evaluate the lesion carefully.

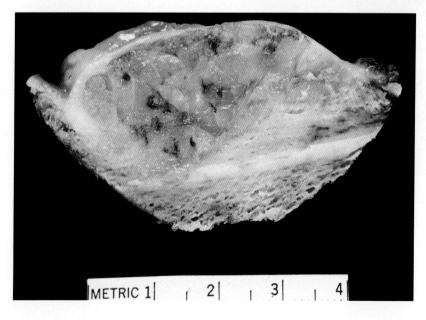

Figure 43–11. This gross specimen shows a periosteal chondrosarcoma. In contrast to periosteal chondromas, which are 3 cm or less, periosteal chondrosarcomas are 5 cm or larger, as is this femoral lesion.

CHAPTER 44

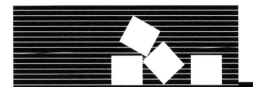

Chondrosarcoma

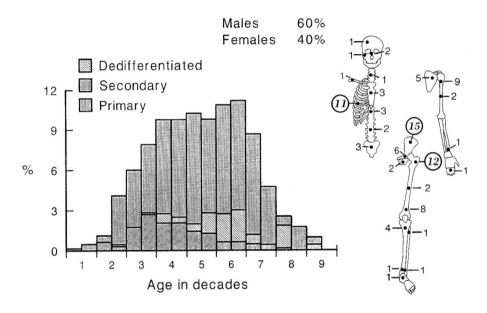

Males 60%
Females 40%

- Dedifferentiated
- Secondary
- Primary

CLINICAL SIGNS

1. Local tenderness is present.
2. A mass may be found on physical examination. The mass is generally hard.

CLINICAL SYMPTOMS

1. Pain is the usual presenting complaint. The pain is usually local; however, when tumors involve the pelvic girdle or vertebra, referred pain may be the initial manifestation.
2. A mass lesion may be noted but is more commonly present in patients who have tumors involving the appendicular skeleton.

3. A long duration of clinical symptoms—even of one or two decades—is frequently seen, since these tumors almost invariably are slow-growing.

MAJOR RADIOGRAPHIC FEATURES

1. There is a predilection for the central skeleton and for the metaphysis or diaphysis of the affected bone.
2. Sixty-six per cent of lesions are partially calcified.
3. Cortical erosion or destruction is usually present.
4. The cortex is often thickened, but periosteal reaction is scant or absent.
5. Soft tissue extension is commonly seen in large lesions.

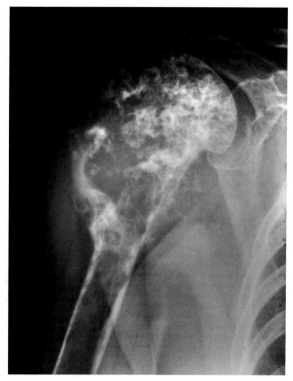

Figure 44–1. This radiograph shows a destructive lesion in the proximal humerus in an adult patient. The lesion is partially calcified, with multiple areas of ring-like calcification. These features are indicative of a hyaline cartilage tumor. The extensive cortical destruction and associated soft tissue extension of the tumor support a malignant diagnosis.

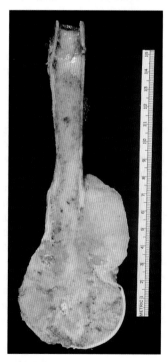

Figure 44–2. The bisected gross specimen of the tumor correlates well with its radiographic appearance shown in Figure 44–1. The tumor has the characteristic blue-gray aura of a hyaline cartilage tumor on cross-section. The cortex has been destroyed, and an associated soft tissue mass is present.

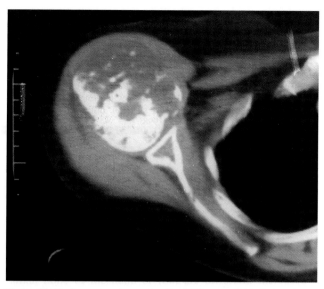

Figure 44–3. A computed tomographic (CT) scan of this lesion shows extensive calcification. CT and magnetic resonance imaging (MRI) are particularly helpful in defining the extent of soft tissue involvement and the relationship of any soft tissue extension to regional neurovascular structures.

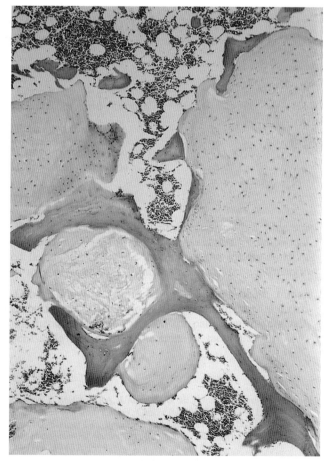

Figure 44–4. At low magnification, chondrosarcomas are blue-gray with hematoxylin-eosin–stained sections. The tumors are generally not highly cellular but are often arranged in a lobulated manner. Adjacent lobules at the periphery of the lesion show an invasive quality of growth, as in this photomicrograph.

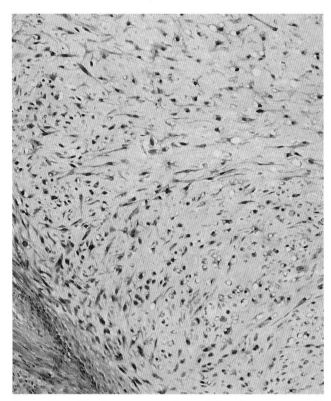

Figure 44–5. Chondrosarcomas are hypercellular when compared with chondromas, as in this example of a chondrosarcoma of the distal femur. The nuclei show greater pleomorphism and hyperchromasia as well.

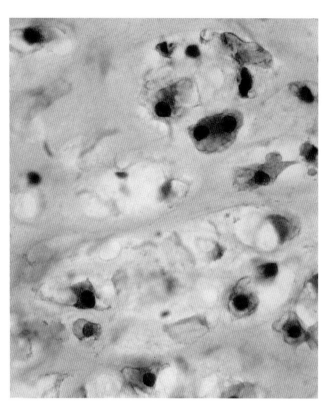

Figure 44–7. Binucleation is commonly stated to be an important feature in the differentiation of chondrosarcoma from chondroma. Binucleated chondrocytes are identifiable in this example of a chondrosarcoma involving the sacroiliac region.

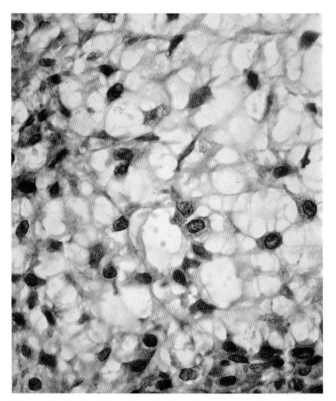

Figure 44–6. At higher magnification, the nuclear pleomorphism is more evident. This tumor also shows a myxoid stromal quality, a feature frequently seen in chondrosarcomas.

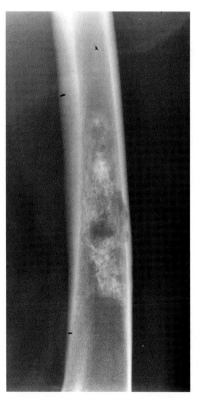

Figure 44–8. This radiograph shows a calcified intramedullary chondrosarcoma of the femoral diaphysis. Central lysis and cortical erosion are present and constitute the major radiographic evidence that the lesion is malignant.

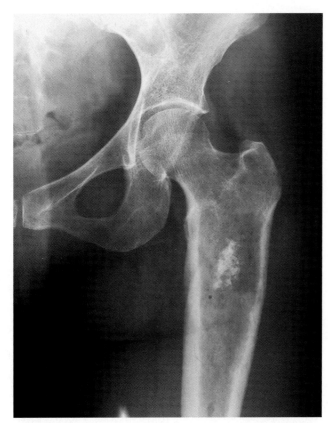

Figure 44–9. This chondrosarcoma is large, partially calcified, and poorly marginated. Expansion of the bone in combination with cortical thickening, as in this example, is unusual in any tumor other than chondrosarcoma.

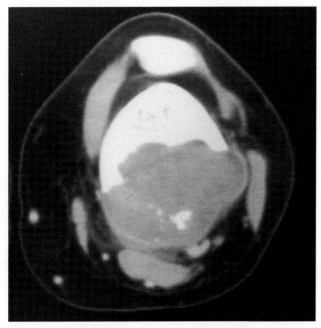

Figure 44–10. Destruction of the cortex is associated with a bulky soft tissue mass in this case. An area of central calcification is also present. CT and MRI are essential for preoperative staging. This CT scan demonstrates the extent of this chondrosarcoma and the presence of subtle calcification, which help identify the tumor as most likely a chondrosarcoma.

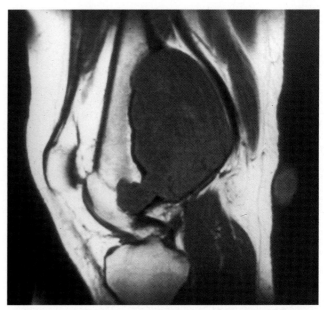

Figure 44–11. MRI provides superior contrast between the tumor and normal marrow as well as between the tumor and adjacent soft tissues, as demonstrated in this image of the same tumor seen in the CT scan in Figure 44–10. Sagittal images are useful in showing the longitudinal extent of the tumor in a single slice. Calcification is not demonstrated.

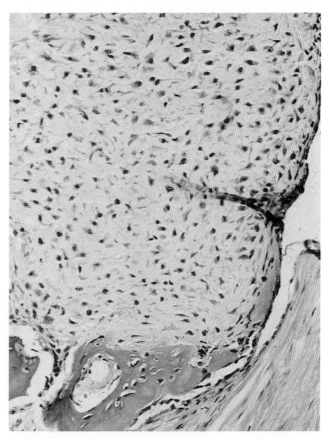

Figure 44–12. This low-power photomicrograph illustrates the lobulated pattern of growth in a chondrosarcoma.

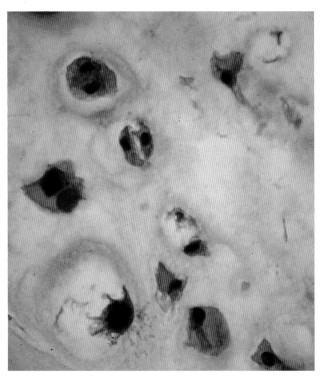

Figure 44–13. Multiple binucleated chondrocytes are identifiable in this high-power photomicrograph of a chondrosarcoma. Nuclear pleomorphism is also evident. Although chondromas of the small bones, periosteal chondromas, and synovial chondromatosis may also share these features, they are not present to the extent illustrated here.

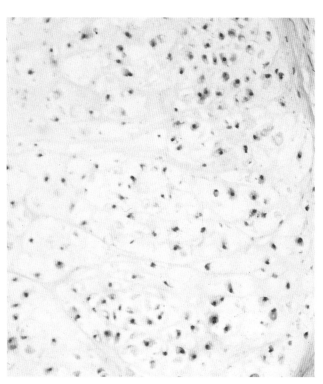

Figure 44–15. As the majority of chondrosarcomas are low-grade, the histologic features alone may not be sufficient to support a malignant diagnosis. Although the tumor is slightly hypercellular, its location (non–small bone and not periosteal) and the radiographic features showing endosteal erosion would be particularly helpful in classifying this tumor as malignant.

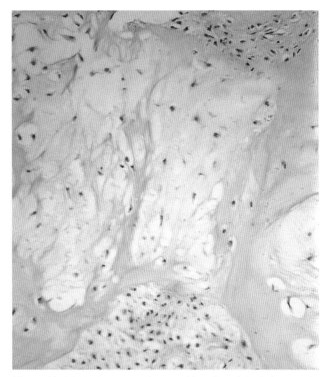

Figure 44–14. At low power, the myxoid quality of the lesion may be the first clue that the hyaline cartilage tumor is not a chondroma. This photomicrograph shows such a stromal myxoid change.

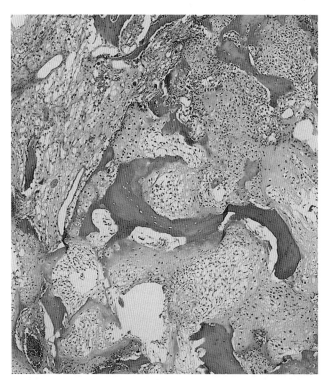

Figure 44–16. This low-power photomicrograph of a low-grade chondrosarcoma from the acetabular region shows the characteristic permeative pattern of medullary bone involvement.

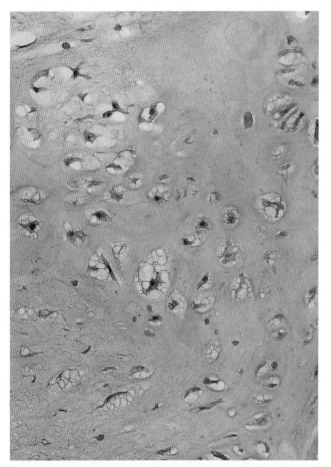

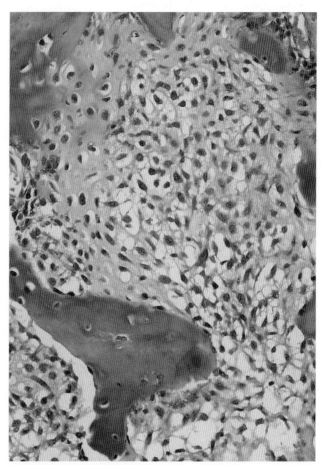

Figure 44–17. Low-grade chondrosarcomas, like this tumor that involved the acetabular region, can be difficult to distinguish from enchondroma. Careful correlation with the radiographic appearance of the tumor is generally helpful in such cases.

Figure 44–18. Higher-grade chondrosarcomas, like this example from the region of the acetabulum, may be difficult to distinguish from chondroblastic osteosarcomas.

CHAPTER 45

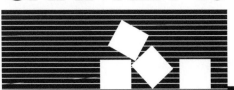

Chondrosarcoma Arising in Osteochondroma

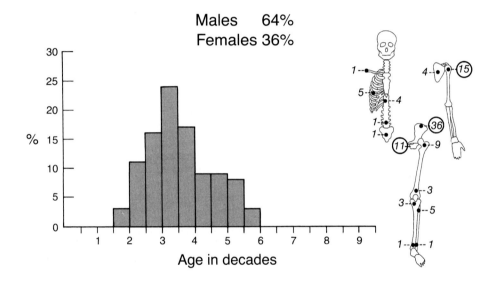

Males   64%
Females 36%

%

Age in decades

CLINICAL SIGNS

1. A tender mass lesion is present.

CLINICAL SYMPTOMS

1. A mass lesion that may have recently increased in size is found.
2. Pain is present in the region of the lesion.

MAJOR RADIOGRAPHIC FEATURES

1. A thick and indistinct cartilage cap may be seen on a lesion that otherwise has the features of an osteochondroma.

2. When present, radiolucent regions in the lesion are a useful indicator of secondary chondrosarcoma.
3. Destruction of the underlying osteochondroma or adjacent bone is evident in advanced cases.
4. Magnetic resonance imaging (MRI) and computed tomography (CT) are the most sensitive diagnostic techniques for assessing these radiographic features.

RADIOGRAPHIC DIFFERENTIAL DIAGNOSIS

1. Osteochondroma with secondary bursa formation.
2. Atypical benign osteochondroma.

MAJOR PATHOLOGIC FEATURES

Gross

1. Masses of cartilaginous tissue greater than 1 cm in thickness are present.
2. The cartilaginous tissue may show liquefaction or frank cystification.
3. There is extension into the surrounding soft tissues.

Microscopic

1. On low-power examination, the tumor is composed predominantly of hyaline cartilage.
2. Most tumors are hypocellular but show greater cytologic atypia than is seen in an osteochondroma.
3. The cartilage cap is not arranged in the orderly columnar manner of an osteochondroma but rather is disorganized, with clusters of cells scattered in the cartilage matrix.
4. Myxoid change characterized by a loose, watery appearance of the cartilage matrix or by a stringing of the matrix is evident.

PATHOLOGIC DIFFERENTIAL DIAGNOSIS

Benign lesions:

1. Osteochondroma.
2. Periosteal chondroma.

Malignant lesions:

1. Perisoteal chondrosarcoma.
2. Periosteal osteosarcoma.

TREATMENT

Primary Modality: surgical resection with a wide margin. Bone grafting of the cortical defect is usually necessary. Other bone and joint reconstructive procedures may be indicated, depending upon the size of the defect.

Other Possible Approaches: amputation, if a wide margin cannot be achieved by resection owing to soft tissue or neurovascular involvement.

References

Garrison RC, Unni KK, McLeod RA, et al: Chondrosarcoma arising in osteochondroma. Cancer 49:1890–1897, 1982.

Kilpatrick SE, Pike EJ, Ward WG, and Pope TL: Dedifferentiated chondrosarcoma in patients with multiple osteochondromatosis: report of a case and review of the literature. Skeletal Radiol 26(6):370–374, 1997.

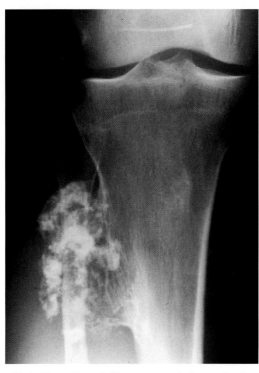

Figure 45–1. The radiograph illustrates a typical osteochondroma arising from the diametaphyseal region of the proximal tibia. The surface is indistinct and irregular, with some areas lacking calcification. These features suggest the possibility of a chondrosarcoma arising in the osteochondroma.

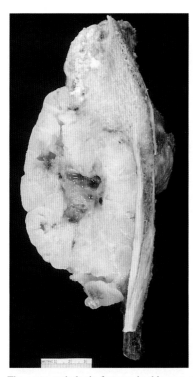

Figure 45–2. The gross pathologic features in this case mirror the radiographic appearance of the lesion (Fig. 45–1). The thickness of the cartilage (more than 2 cm) indicates that the tumor may be malignant. In addition, the central portion of the hyaline cartilage tumor has undergone myxoid degeneration, a gross pathologic feature commonly associated with malignancy.

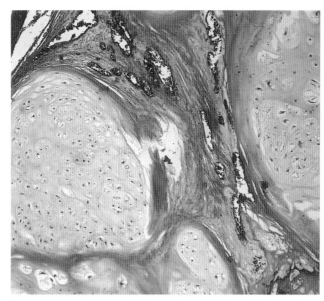

Figure 45–3. At low magnification, the periphery of a chondrosarcoma arising in an osteochondroma may show invasion, as in this photomicrograph. The lobulated nature of the lesion is also evident at low power, and the tumor is more cellular than the cartilage cap of an osteochondroma.

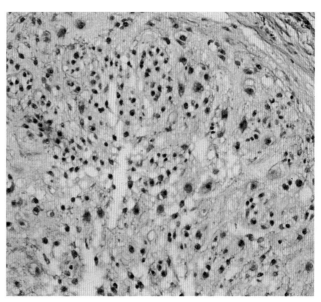

Figure 45–4. At higher magnification, the cellularity of the lesion and the cytologic atypia are evident. The nuclear pleomorphism and cellularity are equivalent to that seen in intramedullary chondrosarcoma.

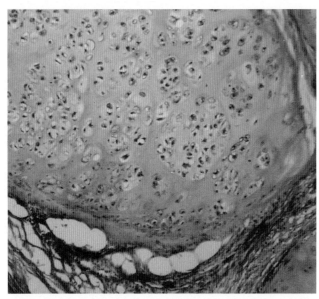

Figure 45–5. Invasion of the soft tissues adjacent to the lesion is helpful in identifying the tumor as malignant. However, bursa formation can occur in the region of an osteochondroma and radiographically mimic the appearance of soft tissue invasion.

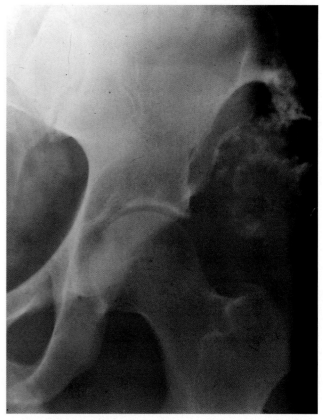

Figure 45–7. Eight years after the initial radiographic evaluation (see Fig. 45–6), the lesion is markedly enlarged, and the periphery is indistinct. A secondary chondrosarcoma has developed in the lesion.

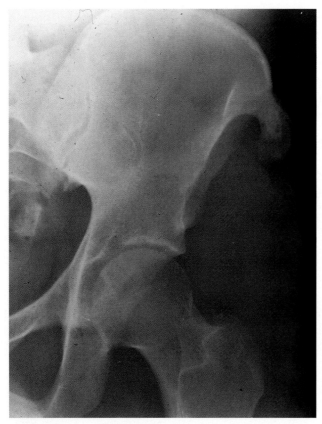

Figure 45–6. This radiograph demonstrates the typical features of an osteochondroma involving the iliac bone.

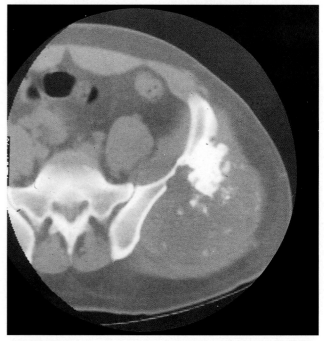

Figure 45–8. This computed tomographic (CT) scan shows a chondrosarcoma arising in an osteochondroma of the iliac bone. Soft tissue masses may be more easily evaluated with this imaging modality. Note that the soft tissue component of this lesion shows scanty calcification.

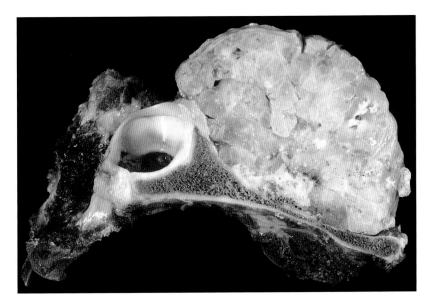

Figure 45–9. This gross specimen shows a secondary chondrosarcoma arising in an osteochondroma of the pelvis. The chondrosarcoma has become so large as to obscure the original osteochondroma.

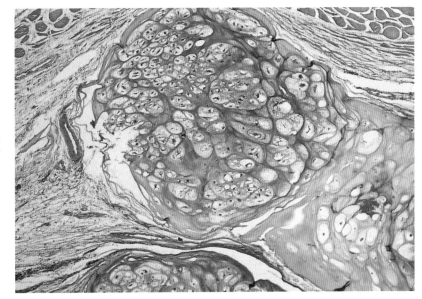

Figure 45–10. This low-power photomicrograph shows the invasion of skeletal muscle adjacent to the secondary chondrosarcoma.

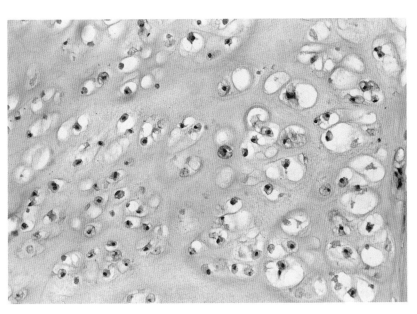

Figure 45–11. Higher magnification of this secondary chondrosarcoma shows the characteristic features of a low-grade hyaline cartilage malignancy: (1) hypercellularity, (2) pleomorphism, and (3) binucleation of the chondrocytes.

MAJOR PATHOLOGIC FEATURES

Gross

1. This tumor shows a bimorphic gross appearance; areas of lobulated gray-white hyaline cartilage coexist with regions of more fleshy yellow-brown soft tumor.
2. There is an abrupt transition from the hyaline cartilage component of the tumor, which is usually centrally located, to the spindle cell component.
3. The anaplastic component of the tumor nearly always dominates the gross lesion and usually has caused cortical destruction of the affected bone with associated production of a soft tissue mass.

Microscopic

1. The grossly evident bimorphic pattern is also appreciable histologically.
2. The low-grade hyaline cartilage component shows the typical features of ordinary chondrosarcoma.
3. Immediately adjacent to the lobules of well-differentiated chondrosarcoma are sheet-like regions of high-grade spindle cell malignancy.
4. Osteoid matrix may be identified in the spindle cell component of the lesion.
5. The spindle cell component of the lesion may show the histologic features of fibrosarcoma or malignant fibrous histiocytoma.

PATHOLOGIC DIFFERENTIAL DIAGNOSIS

Benign lesions:

1. Chondroma, if incompletely sampled.

Malignant lesions:

1. Chondrosarcoma, ordinary type.
2. Osteosarcoma.
3. Fibrosarcoma.
4. Malignant fibrous histiocytoma.

TREATMENT

Primary Modality: Surgical ablation by amputation is usually necessary because of aggressive soft tissue invasion by the tumor.

Other Possible Approaches: Limb-saving resection and oncologic reconstruction can be done if an adequately wide margin can be achieved. Adjuvant chemotherapy may be used.

References

Dahlin DC, and Beabout JW: Dedifferentiation of low-grade chondrosarcomas. Cancer 28:461–466, 1971.

Kalil RK, Inwards CY, Unni KK, et al: Dedifferentiated clear cell chondrosarcoma. Am J Surg Pathol 24(8):1079–1086, 2000.

McCarthy EF, and Dorfman HD: Chondrosarcoma of bone with dedifferentiation: a study of eighteen cases. Hum Pathol 13:36–40, 1982.

Mirra JM, and Marcove RC: Fibrosarcomatous dedifferentiation of primary and secondary chondrosarcoma: review of five cases. J Bone Joint Surg (Am) 56:285–296, 1974.

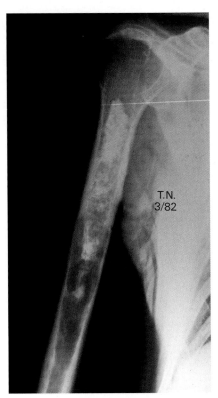

Figure 46–1. This radiograph illustrates a large diaphyseal dedifferentiated chondrosarcoma of the humerus. The aggressive destruction of the area, inferiorly superimposed on an otherwise typical appearance of chondrosarcoma, suggests the correct diagnosis.

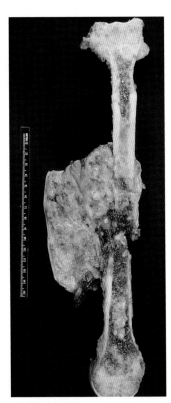

Figure 46–2. The gross appearance of the lesion correlates well with the radiographic evidence of cortical destruction and associated soft tissue extension.

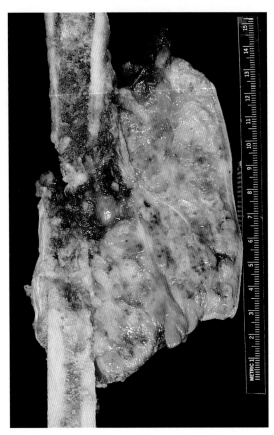

Figure 46–3. Although the majority of the lesion is fleshy and distinctly different grossly from the usual hyaline cartilage tumor, the medullary portion of the tumor shows the characteristic glistening blue-gray aura of the underlying low-grade chondrosarcoma.

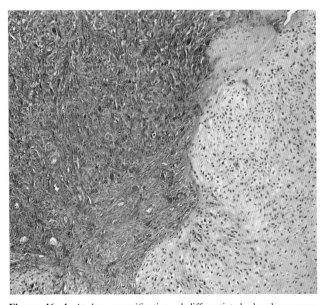

Figure 46–4. At low magnification, dedifferentiated chondrosarcoma shows a bimorphic pattern consisting of a hypocellular cartilage tumor juxtaposed with a high-grade spindle cell sarcoma.

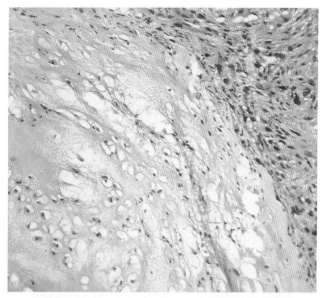

Figure 46–5. At higher magnification, the hyaline cartilage portion of the tumor is indistinguishable from a low-grade chondrosarcoma. In contrast, the hypercellular spindle cell portion of the tumor may be identical with a fibrosarcoma, malignant fibrous histiocytoma, or fibroblastic osteosarcoma.

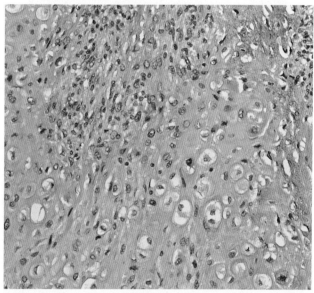

Figure 46–6. At higher magnification, the cytologic atypia associated with the high-grade portion of the tumor is evident. Osteoid may be identified, as in this photomicrograph.

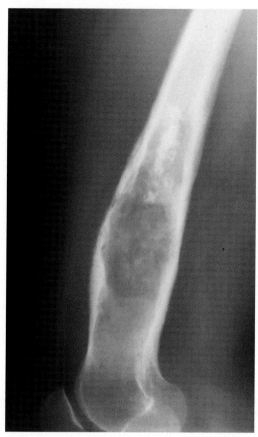

Figure 46–7. This radiograph illustrates the typical features of chondrosarcoma superiorly but shows a very aggressive appearance inferiorly, which is worrisome for a dedifferentiated chondrosarcoma.

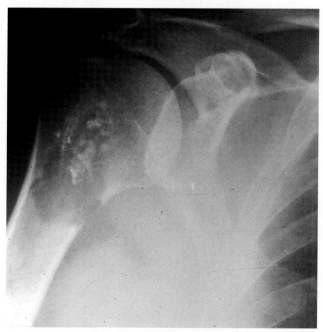

Figure 46–8. This dedifferentiated chondrosarcoma of the proximal humerus shows an aggressive lytic region inferiorly superimposed on an otherwise typical radiographic appearance for chondrosarcoma. The medial cortical destruction is particularly worrisome for dedifferentiation.

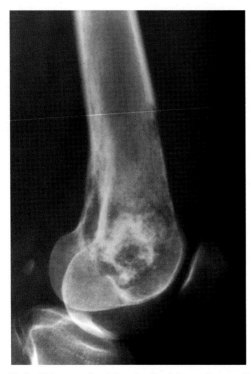

Figure 46–9. This tumor involving the distal femur shows radiographic features typical of chondrosarcoma distally. Again, however, a permeative destructive pattern of growth, seen proximally in the lesion, suggests that the tumor is a dedifferentiated chondrosarcoma.

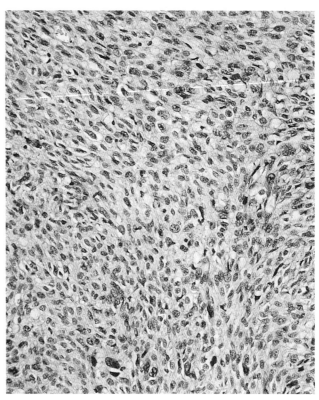

Figure 46–11. At higher magnification, the spindle cell portion of the tumor shows a "herringbone" pattern of growth, as seen in fibrosarcoma.

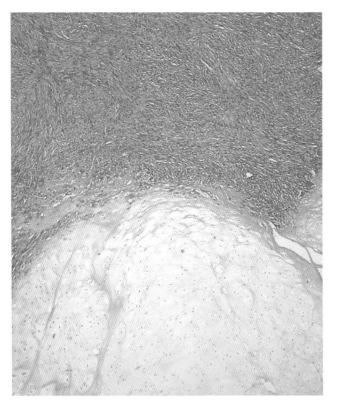

Figure 46–10. The low-power pattern of juxtaposition of hypocellular hyaline cartilage tumor and hypercellular spindle cell sarcoma is characteristic of dedifferentiated chondrosarcoma.

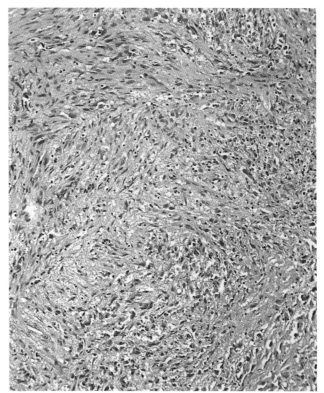

Figure 46–12. A storiform pattern of growth, characteristically associated with malignant fibrous histiocytoma, may also be seen in the dedifferentiated portion of the tumor.

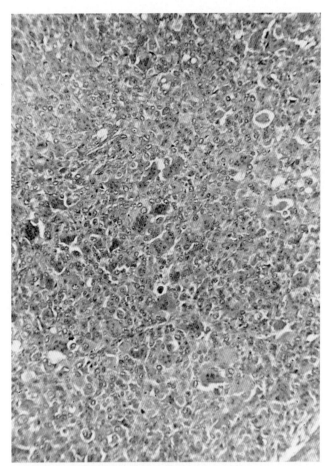

Figure 46–13. Numerous benign multinucleated giant cells may also be seen in the hypercellular portion of the tumor. Such a pattern may histologically mimic the appearance of malignant fibrous histiocytoma or malignant giant cell tumor.

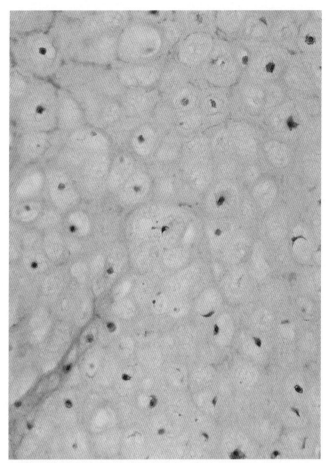

Figure 46–14. Although dedifferentiated chondrosarcoma is a high-grade malignancy, the chondroid portion of the tumor histologically may mimic a benign enchondroma, as in this photomicrograph.

CHAPTER 47

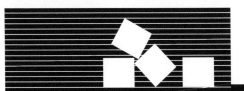

Mesenchymal Chondrosarcoma

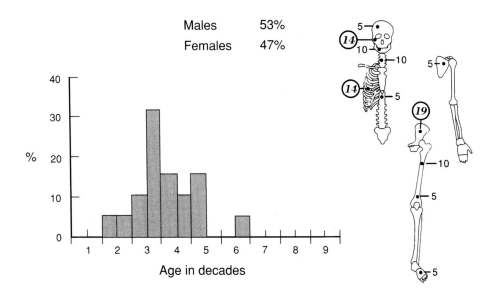

Males	53%
Females	47%

CLINICAL SIGNS

1. A mass lesion is usually the only clinical sign.

CLINICAL SYMPTOMS

1. Pain and swelling are usually the only symptoms.
2. Approximately one third of patients have had symptoms for longer than one year at the time of diagnosis.

MAJOR RADIOGRAPHIC FEATURES

1. Most mesenchymal chondrosarcomas have a malignant radiographic appearance but no specific diagnostic features, or the radiographic features are suggestive of ordinary chondrosarcoma.
2. The tumor usually shows calcification.

3. Poor margination and cortical destruction are present.
4. Frequently there is an associated soft tissue mass.

RADIOGRAPHIC DIFFERENTIAL DIAGNOSIS

1. Chondrosarcoma.
2. Osteosarcoma.
3. Fibrosarcoma.

MAJOR PATHOLOGIC FEATURES

Gross

1. These tumors are typically gray to pink and vary in consistency from firm to soft.
2. The border of the tumor is usually well defined.

3. Hard calcific foci are usually scattered throughout the tumor.
4. Necrosis and hemorrhage may be evident.

Microscopic

1. The low-power pattern shows a bimorphic appearance with islands of benign-appearing hyaline cartilage embedded within highly cellular zones of small, round-to-slightly spindled cells.
2. Chondroid zones vary in size and may be more calcified or even ossified.
3. The pattern at low-power magnification in the cellular regions is usually hemangiopericytomatous, with numerous thin-walled branching vessels coursing through the tumor.
4. At higher magnification, the cells within the cellular regions have uniform cytologic characteristics, being round to oval with uniform round to oval nuclei.

PATHOLOGIC DIFFERENTIAL DIAGNOSIS

Benign lesions:

1. Benign hemangiopericytoma.

Malignant lesions:

1. Ewing's sarcoma.
2. Dedifferentiated chondrosarcoma.
3. Osteosarcoma.
4. Malignant hemangiopericytoma.

TREATMENT

Primary Modality: Surgical resection with a wide margin is performed, and reconstruction is individualized according to the location and the patient. This tumor's aggressive behavior with extensive involvement often mandates amputation to achieve an adequate margin.

Other Possible Approaches: Adjuvant chemotherapy may be useful. Therapeutic radiation is indicated for surgically inaccessible lesions.

References

Bertoni F, Picci P, Bacchini P, et al: Mesenchymal chondrosarcoma of bone and soft tissues. Cancer 52:533–541, 1983.

Dabska M, and Huvos A: Mesenchymal chondrosarcoma in the young: a clinicopathologic study of 19 patients with explanation of histogenesis. Virchows Arch (Pathol Anat) Histopathol 399:89–104, 1983.

Huvos AG, Rosen G, Dabska M, and Marcove RC: Mesenchymal chondrosarcoma: a clinicopathologic analysis of 35 patients with emphasis on treatment. Cancer 51:1230–1237, 1983.

Nakashima Y, Unni KK, Shives TC, et al: Mesenchymal chondrosarcoma of bone and soft tissue. A review of 111 cases. Cancer 57(12):2444–2453, 1986.

Salvador AH, Beabout JW, and Dahlin DC: Mesenchymal chondrosarcoma—observations on 30 new cases. Cancer 28:605–615, 1971.

Steiner GC, Mirra JM, and Bullough PG: Mesenchymal chondrosarcoma: a study of the ultrastructure. Cancer 32:926–939, 1973.

Swanson PE, Lillemoe TJ, Manivel JC, and Wick MR: Mesenchymal chondrosarcoma. An immunohistochemical study. Arch Pathol Lab Med 114:943–948, 1990.

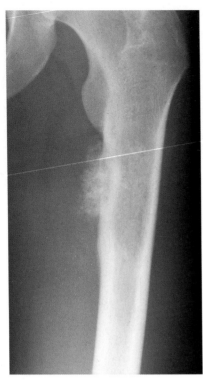

Figure 47–1. This radiograph illustrates the poorly marginated appearance of a mesenchymal chondrosarcoma. The lesion exhibits calcification, a feature suggesting that this is a cartilage tumor. The cortical destruction and associated soft tissue mass are radiographic indications of the malignancy of the process.

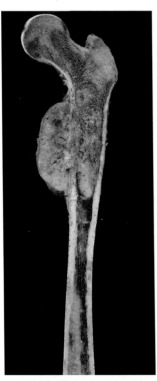

Figure 47–2. The gross pathologic features of the tumor correlate well with the radiographic appearance shown in Figure 47–1. The tumor is fleshy, in contrast with a hyaline cartilage tumor. However, the lesional tissue may be gritty owing to foci of calcification within the tumor.

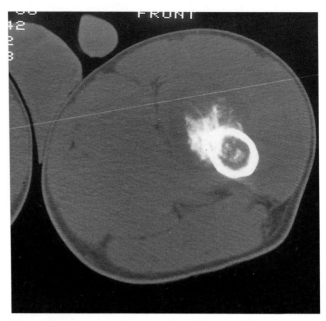

Figure 47–3. A computed tomographic (CT) scan of the tumor shows the soft tissue extent of the lesion as well as the medullary involvement.

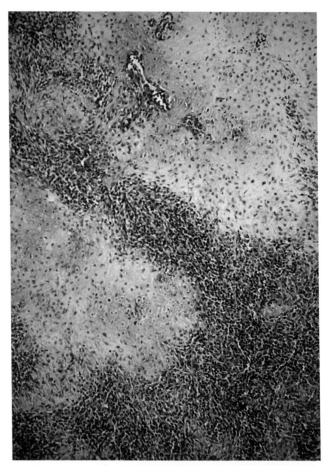

Figure 47–4. At low magnification, mesenchymal chondrosarcomas are bimorphic tumors, composed of relatively hypocellular chondroid zones and hypercellular regions. The hypercellular regions consist of small cells.

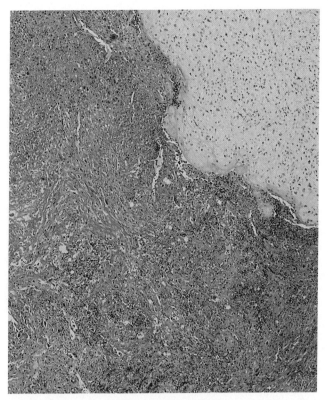

Figure 47–5. Chondroid zones within the tumor are variable in size, some being quite small, as in this photomicrograph.

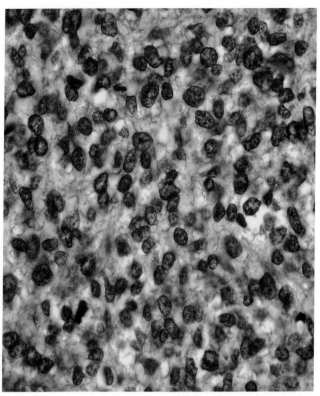

Figure 47–7. At high magnification, the hypercellular portion of the tumor is composed of small cells, which are round to oval. The cytologic features are similar to those of small cell osteosarcoma and hemangiopericytoma.

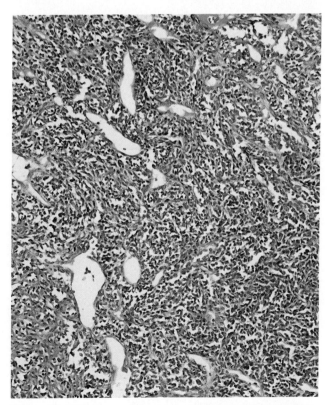

Figure 47–6. The hypercellular zones of the tumor characteristically have a hemangiopericytomatous pattern of growth, as illustrated in this photomicrograph. "Stag horn"–like vascular spaces are evident at low magnification.

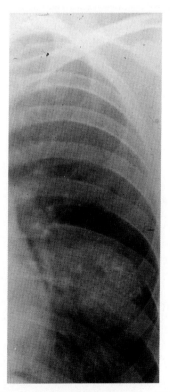

Figure 47–8. Mesenchymal chondrosarcomas are common in flat bone locations, as in this case involving the rib. There is an associated large, partially calcified soft tissue mass with apparent underlying cortical destruction of the affected rib.

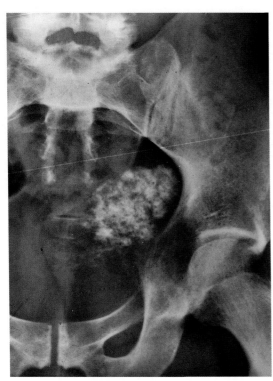

Figure 47–9. This mesenchymal chondrosarcoma involves the acetabular region, a location often involved in ordinary chondrosarcoma. The bone shows lytic destruction, and there is associated calcification in the soft tissue portion of the tumor.

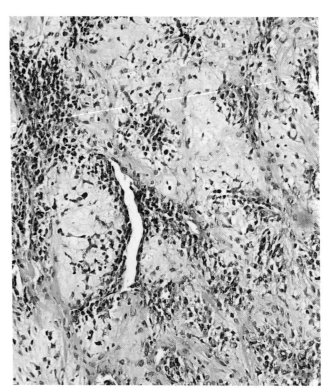

Figure 47–11. This photomicrograph, at low magnification, shows a mesenchymal chondrosarcoma in which the hyaline cartilage portion of the lesion predominates. The small cell portion of the tumor persists in a perivascular pattern.

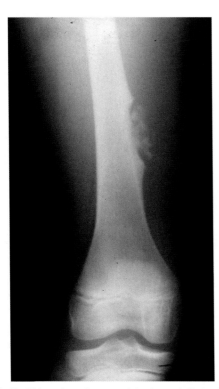

Figure 47–10. This periosteal tumor of the femoral diaphysis proved to be a mesenchymal chondrosarcoma. The buttresses and periosteal location are atypical of mesenchymal chondrosarcoma, as the majority of these lesions are centrally located.

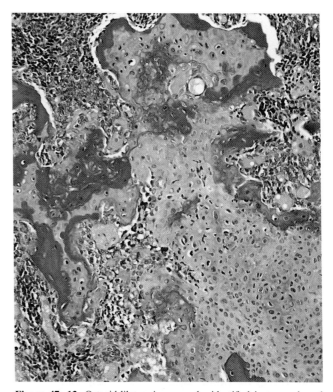

Figure 47–12. Osteoid-like regions may be identified in mesenchymal chondrosarcoma. The differential diagnosis in such cases includes small cell osteosarcoma, a lesion that probably is closely related to mesenchymal chondrosarcoma.

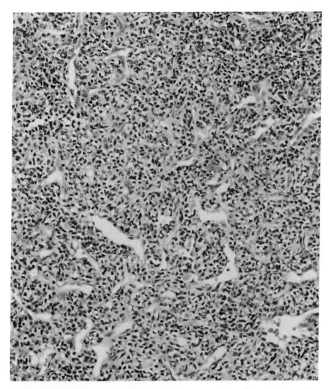

Figure 47–13. The hemangiopericytomatous pattern of growth is particularly prominent in this mesenchymal chondrosarcoma that involves the mandible, a common primary location for the tumor.

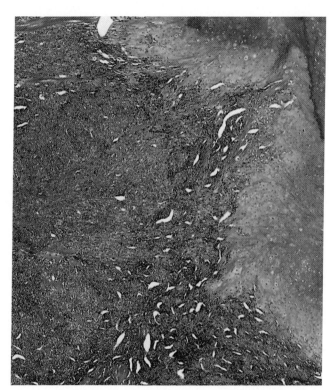

Figure 47–15. This photomicrograph illustrates a mesenchymal chondrosarcoma of the soft tissue of the thigh. Approximately one third of mesenchymal chondrosarcomas are of soft tissue origin.

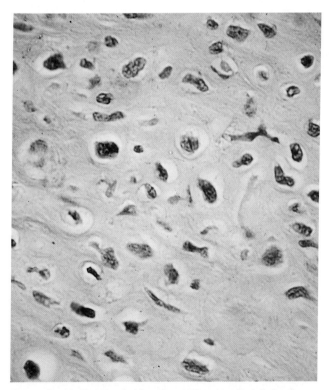

Figure 47–14. The chondroid portions of a mesenchymal chondrosarcoma are indistinguishable from ordinary chondrosarcoma. A small sample from such a region would be identified as an ordinary chondrosarcoma.

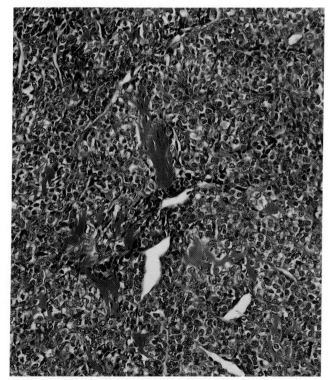

Figure 47–16. This photomicrograph demonstrates the morphology of the tumor shown in Figure 47–15. This tumor has the small cell hemangiopericytomatous pattern commonly present in mesenchymal chondrosarcoma. Foci of pink osteoid formation may rarely also be seen in this tumor.

CHAPTER 48

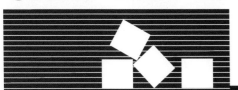

Clear Cell Chondrosarcoma

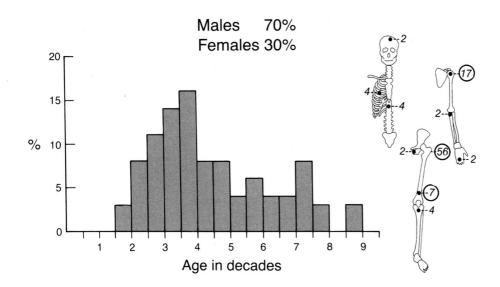

Males   70%
Females 30%

CLINICAL SIGNS

1. Regional tenderness is present.
2. A mass lesion may be found on physical examination.

CLINICAL SYMPTOMS

1. Pain is the most common symptom at the time of presentation.
2. These tumors are slow-growing; as such, the symptoms may be of long duration. Eighteen per cent of patients in the Mayo Clinic series had symptoms for longer than five years.

MAJOR RADIOGRAPHIC FEATURES

1. The lesion has an epiphyseal location in the proximal femur or humerus.

2. Early lesions look benign, with sharp margination, sclerosis at the periphery, and expansion of the affected bone.
3. Twenty-five per cent are calcified on plain radiograph.
4. Larger lesions look malignant, with poor margination and cortical destruction.

RADIOGRAPHIC DIFFERENTIAL DIAGNOSIS

1. Chondroblastoma.
2. Chondrosarcoma, ordinary type.
3. Giant cell tumor.

MAJOR PATHOLOGIC FEATURES

Gross

1. The curetted fragments are frequently found to contain a cartilaginous bluish-gray translucent matrix.

2. Cystic spaces may be identified; these may represent secondary aneurysmal bone cyst formation.

Microscopic

1. At low magnification, these tumors are faintly lobulated and variable from region to region. Foci of obvious cartilage matrix production may lie adjacent to zones containing numerous mononuclear and multinucleated giant cells.
2. Bony trabeculae are usually identified in this tumor at low power. These are either at the center of lobules of tumor or scattered within the zones of mononuclear cells.
3. At higher magnification, the tumor cells have vesicular nuclei and characteristically show abundant clear cytoplasm. The cell boundaries between such cells are usually distinct.
4. About 50 per cent of the tumors show regions of ordinary chondrosarcoma; in these regions, the multinucleated giant cells are not identified.

PATHOLOGIC DIFFERENTIAL DIAGNOSIS

Benign lesions:

1. Chondroblastoma.
2. Osteoblastoma.
3. Aneurysmal bone cyst.

Malignant lesions:

1. Chondrosarcoma, ordinary type.
2. Chondroblastic osteosarcoma.

TREATMENT

Primary Modality: En bloc resection with a wide surgical margin is performed, with reconstruction of the joint by custom prosthesis, osteochondral allograft, or resection arthrodesis, depending upon the location and the needs of the patient.

Other Possible Approaches: Amputation may be necessary with large lesions, recurrent lesions, or lesions associated with local contamination due to a pathologic fracture or where a wide margin cannot be achieved with resection.

References

Bjornsson J, Unni KK, Dahlin DC, et al: Clear cell chondrosarcoma of bone: observations in 47 cases. Am J Surg Pathol 8:223–230, 1984.

Cohen EK, Kresell HY, Frank TS, et al: Hyaline-cartilage origin bone and soft tissue neoplasms: MR appearance and histologic correlation. Radiology 167:477–481, 1988.

Faraggiana T, Sender B, and Glicksman P: Light- and electron-microscopic study of clear cell chondrosarcoma. Am J Clin Pathol 75:117–121, 1981.

Leggon RE, Unni KK, Beabout JW, and Sim FH: Clear cell chondrosarcoma. Orthopedics 13:593–596, 1990.

Weiss AP, and Dorfman HD: Clear-cell chondrosarcoma: a report of ten cases and review of the literature. Surg Pathol 1:123–129, 1988.

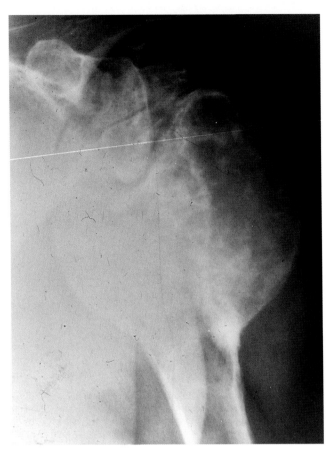

Figure 48–1. This radiograph shows a clear cell chondrosarcoma of the proximal humerus causing marked expansion of the bone and cortical thinning. Mottled calcification is present. At this point in the evolution of the tumor, a radiographic diagnosis of chondrosarcoma, ordinary type, would be most likely. The radiographic features of the lesion ten years earlier (see Fig. 48–3) are more characteristic of clear cell chondrosarcoma.

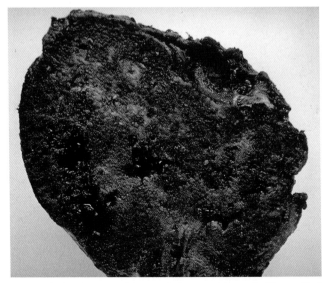

Figure 48–2. The gross features of the tumor shown in Figure 48–1 correlate well with its radiographic appearance. Hemorrhagic cystic spaces are evident in this tumor. Such regions of secondary aneurysmal bone cyst are frequently seen in cases of clear cell chondrosarcoma.

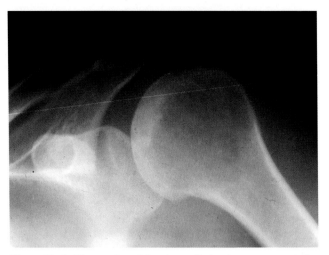

Figure 48–3. The margins of the clear cell chondrosarcoma are better defined in this radiograph of the proximal humerus ten years prior to definitive surgery. There is only mild expansion of the bone, and no calcification is present. These radiographic features are nonspecific but suggestive of a benign lesion. Early in their evolution, clear cell chondrosarcomas frequently mimic benign conditions.

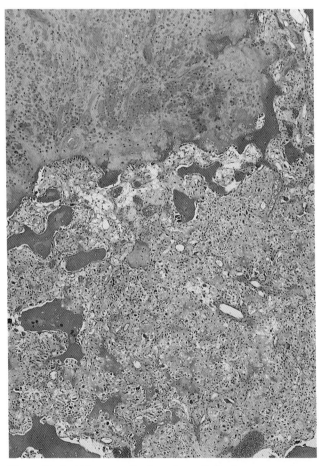

Figure 48–4. At low magnification, clear cell chondrosarcomas show a variable histologic pattern of growth. Hyaline cartilage regions interdigitate with more cellular regions, as shown in this case involving the proximal femur.

Figure 48–5. Calcification similar to that seen in chondroblastoma may be found in clear cell chondrosarcoma. This feature, in combination with the histologic variability and the presence of benign multinucleated giant cells, may result in a mistaken diagnosis of chondroblastoma.

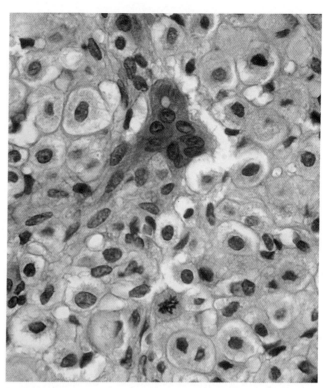

Figure 48–7. At high magnification, the cytologic features of clear cell chondrosarcoma may be deceptively bland. Tumor cells show abundant cytoplasm, as in this photomicrograph. The occurrence of such polygonal cytoplasm, the bland nuclear features, and the presence of multinucleated giant cells mimic the features of chondroblastoma.

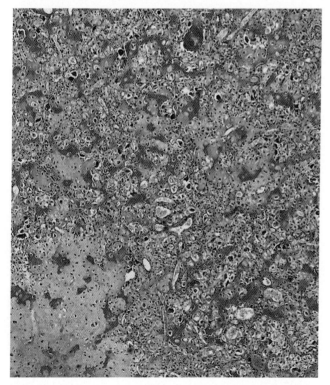

Figure 48–6. Clear cell chondrosarcoma shows an invasive pattern of growth at the periphery of the lesion. In this photomicrograph, permeation through the adjacent medullary bone is evident.

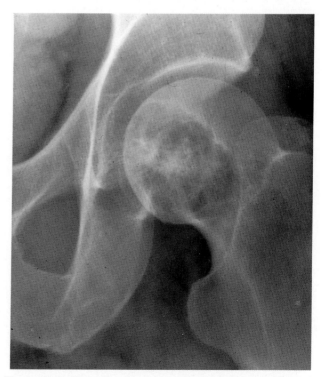

Figure 48–8. This radiograph illustrates the benign features commonly seen in clear cell chondrosarcoma. The sharp sclerotic margin of this tumor is compatible with the appearance of chondroblastoma.

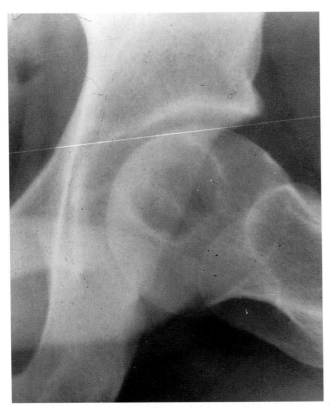

Figure 48–9. Like chondroblastoma, clear cell chondrosarcoma frequently involves the epiphysis of the affected bone. Such is the case with this tumor, which is partially calcified, has sclerotic margins, and involves the epiphysis of the proximal femur.

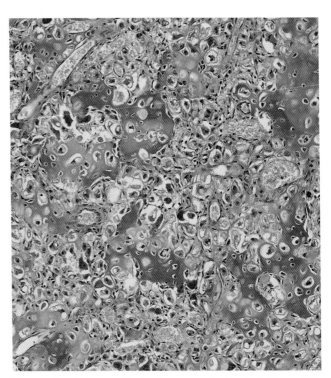

Figure 48–11. Clear cell chondrosarcoma is histologically variable from region to region, as seen in this low-power photomicrograph. Foci may show pure hyaline cartilage differentiation, whereas other regions may show bone production. Thus, the differential diagnosis may include ordinary chondrosarcoma as well as chondroblastic osteosarcoma.

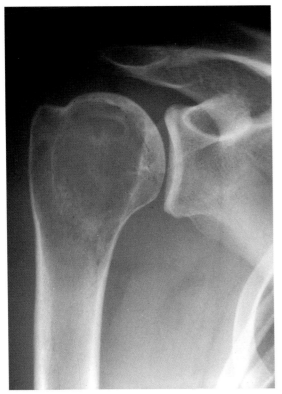

Figure 48–10. This radiograph shows a more advanced lesion in the proximal humerus, presenting as a purely lytic and poorly marginated tumor.

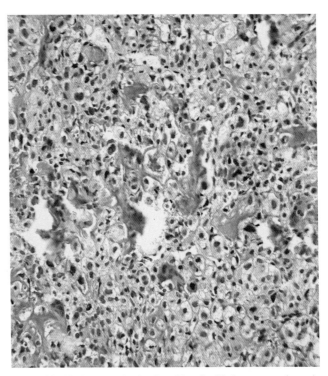

Figure 48–12. Bone production is evident in this low-power photomicrograph. Such foci may mimic the appearance of a chondroblastic osteosarcoma. However, the cytologic atypia is much less pronounced in clear cell chondrosarcoma than in chondroblastic osteosarcoma.

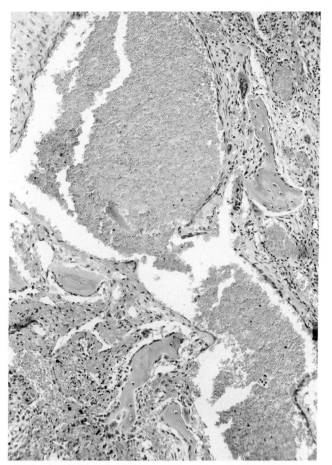

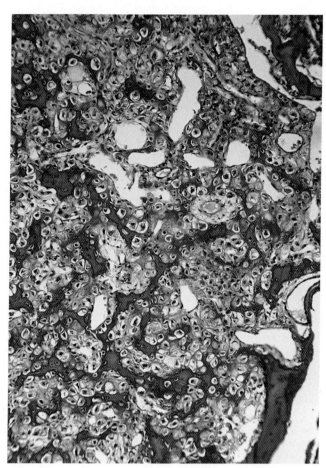

Figure 48–13. This photomicrograph shows a region of secondary aneurysmal bone cyst complicating clear cell chondrosarcoma. Although such secondary aneurysmal bone cysts are more commonly encountered in benign tumors, they quite frequently occur as a component in clear cell chondrosarcoma.

Figure 48–14. Although clear cell chondrosarcoma is a well-differentiated or low-grade tumor, it can recur locally or in other osseous locations or metastasize to the lung. The histologic features of the pulmonary metastases are identical with those of the primary tumor, as illustrated in this photomicrograph.

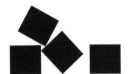

C

FIBROUS AND
FIBROHISTIOCYTIC
TUMORS

CHAPTER 49

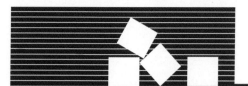

Benign Fibrous Histiocytoma

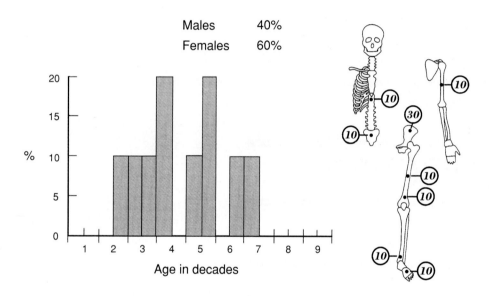

Males   40%
Females   60%

Age in decades

CLINICAL SIGNS

1. These lesions are generally asymptomatic, and there are no common findings on physical examination.

CLINICAL SYMPTOMS

1. Local pain is the most common symptom associated with these lesions.
2. A mass may be found if the lesion involves a superficial bone.

MAJOR RADIOGRAPHIC FEATURES

1. The lesion is lytic, without matrix mineralization.
2. The lesion has a sharp margin, often with a sclerotic rim and expansion of the affected bone.

3. Larger lesions may destroy the cortex and extend into soft tissues, suggesting a malignant process.

RADIOGRAPHIC DIFFERENTIAL DIAGNOSIS

1. Fibroma.
2. Fibrous dysplasia.
3. Chondromyxoid fibroma.

MAJOR PATHOLOGIC FEATURES

Gross

1. Curetted fragments have most frequently been described as firm.
2. Lesional tissue varies from red-brown to yellow, as does the tissue of a fibroma.

Microscopic

1. The light microscopic appearance of this lesion is identical with that of a fibroma.
2. At low magnification, a storiform arrangement of the spindling cells is evident.
3. Hemosiderin and lipid-laden histiocytes are commonly identifiable.
4. At higher magnification, the tumor shows a uniform cytologic appearance of the nuclei, and mitotic figures are rare.

PATHOLOGIC DIFFERENTIAL DIAGNOSIS

Benign lesions:

1. Fibroma (metaphyseal fibrous defect).
2. Giant cell tumor of the tendon-sheath type.
3. Pigmented villonodular synovitis.

Malignant lesions:

1. Malignant fibrous histiocytoma.

TREATMENT

Primary Modality: Curettage and bone grafting are performed.

Other Possible Approaches: Lesions with a favorable location, such as the ilium, may be removed by en bloc resection with a marginal or wide margin when this can be performed without significant loss of function.

References

Bjornsson J, Unni KK, Dahlin DC, et al: Clear cell chondrosarcoma of bone: observations in 47 cases. Am J Surg Pathol 8:223–230, 1984.

Cohen EK, Kresell HY, Frank TS, et al: Hyaline-cartilage origin bone and soft tissue neoplasms: MR appearance and histologic correlation. Radiology 167:477–481, 1988.

Faraggiana T, Sender B, and Glicksman P: Light- and electron-microscopic study of clear cell chondrosarcoma. Am J Clin Pathol 75:117–121, 1981.

Leggon RE, Unni KK, Beabout JW, and Sim FH: Clear cell chondrosarcoma. Orthopedics 13:593–596, 1990.

Weiss AP, and Dorfman HD: Clear-cell chondrosarcoma: a report of ten cases and review of the literature. Surg Pathol 1:123–129, 1988.

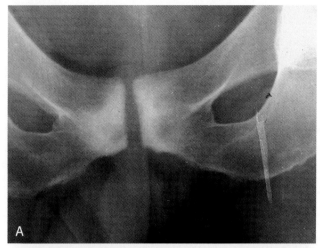

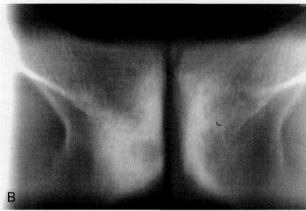

Figure 49–1. This radiograph *(A)* and tomogram *(B)* illustrate a benign fibrous histiocytoma of the pubis. A small, oval lytic tumor with sharp margination and surrounding sclerosis indicates the benign nature of the process.

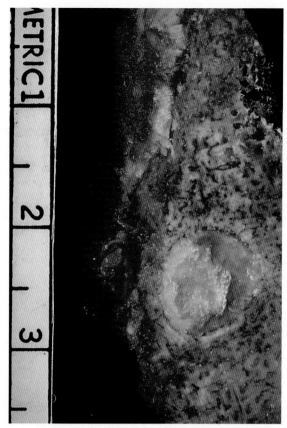

Figure 49–2. This photograph of a gross specimen reveals the well-circumscribed, fibrous appearance of a benign fibrous histiocytoma involving the pubis.

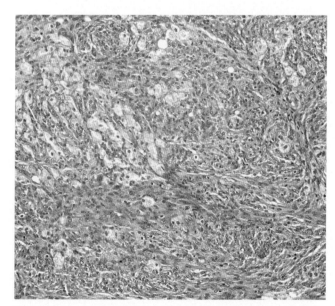

Figure 49–3. Histologically, benign fibrous histiocytomas are indistinguishable from metaphyseal fibrous defects (fibromas). This lesion from the tibia of a 28-year-old woman shows the admixture of lipid-laden histiocytes and spindle cells, which may be arranged in a storiform pattern.

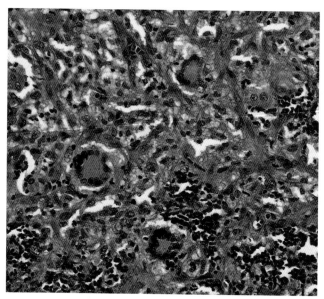

Figure 49–4. Multinucleated giant cells, illustrated in this photomicrograph, are commonly seen in cases classified as benign fibrous histiocytoma. This tumor was in the sacrum.

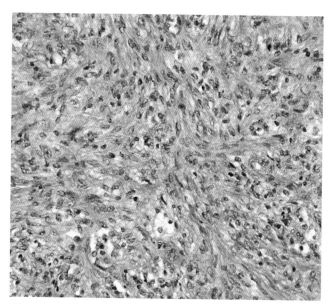

Figure 49–5. Like fibromas, benign fibrous histiocytomas demonstrate variability from region to region. This region in a lesion from the sacrum contains few lipid-laden cells and no giant cells.

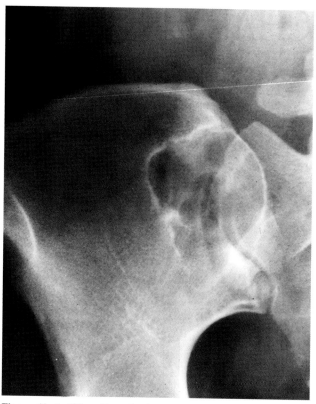

Figure 49–6. This radiograph shows a radiographically benign lytic lesion of the iliac bone. The sharp margination, expansion, and sclerotic rim support a benign diagnosis. On biopsy, the lesion was found to be a benign fibrous histiocytoma.

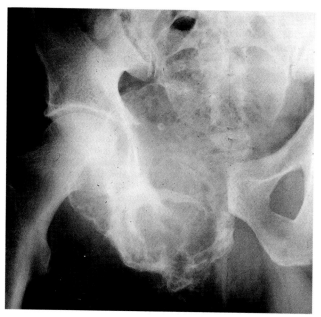

Figure 49–7. This large, benign fibrous histiocytoma of the ischium and pubis shows cortical destruction and soft tissue extension.

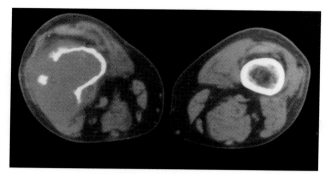

Figure 50–1. This computed tomographic (CT) scan shows a large lytic and eccentric defect in the distal femur. Cortical destruction and soft tissue extension of the lesion attest to its malignant nature; however, the tumor is otherwise nondescript.

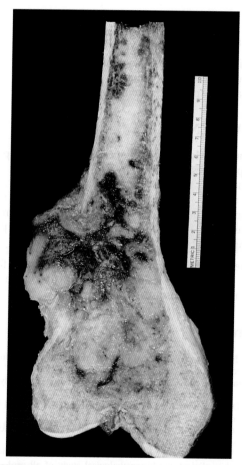

Figure 50–2. The gross pathologic features of the fibrosarcoma in Figure 50–1 are shown in this photograph. The lesional tissue is soft and gray-white to tan. The cortical destruction and soft tissue extension evident radiographically are illustrated grossly in this cross-section of the tumor.

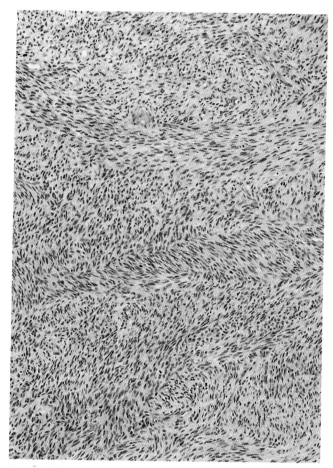

Figure 50–3. At low magnification, fibrosarcomas are composed of spindle cells in a "herringbone" pattern of growth. The high-grade tumors show greater cellularity, mitotic activity, and cytologic pleomorphism.

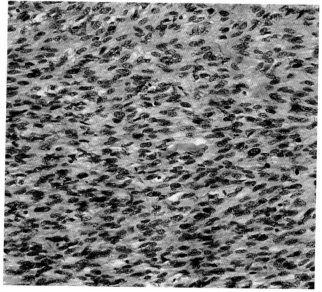

Figure 50–4. At higher magnification, fibrosarcomas vary in their degree of cytologic atypia and mitotic activity. This tumor that involved the maxilla resulted in pulmonary metastasis 34 months after diagnosis, attesting to its high-grade nature.

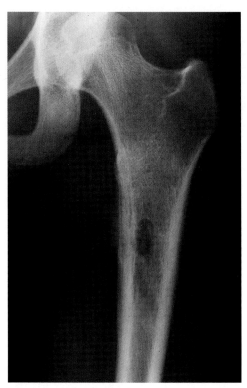

Figure 50–5. This radiograph shows a poorly marginated lytic fibrosarcoma in the subtrochanteric diaphyseal region of the femur. Scanty periosteal reaction is present in this case.

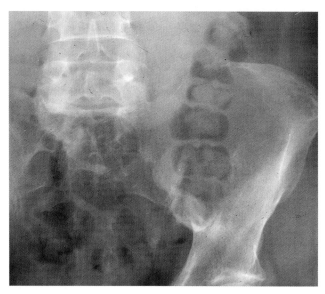

Figure 50–7. This radiograph of the pelvis illustrates a large, purely lytic fibrosarcoma of the left iliac bone and sacrum. There is extensive destruction of the bone.

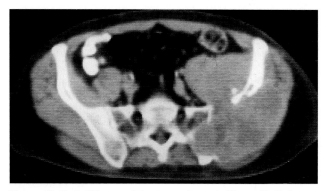

Figure 50–8. A CT scan of the tumor shown in Figure 50–7 demonstrates a large soft tissue component containing low-density areas of necrotic tumor or hemorrhage.

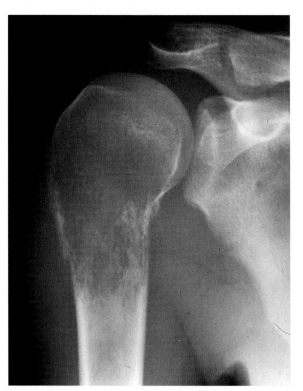

Figure 50–6. This large fibrosarcoma of the proximal humerus presented as a purely lytic metaphyseal lesion. The cortical destruction attests to the aggressiveness of the lesion, and the bone has been sufficiently weakened to have sustained a pathologic fracture.

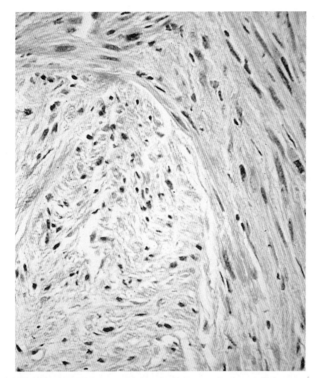

Figure 50–9. This photomicrograph illustrates the hypocellular nature of well-differentiated or low-grade fibrosarcomas. Although nuclear pleomorphism may be present, such tumors lack significant mitotic activity and generally show abundant collagenous stroma.

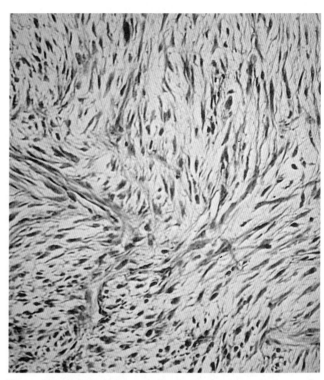

Figure 50–11. Myxoid stromal change may be present and generally accompanies low-grade fibrosarcomas.

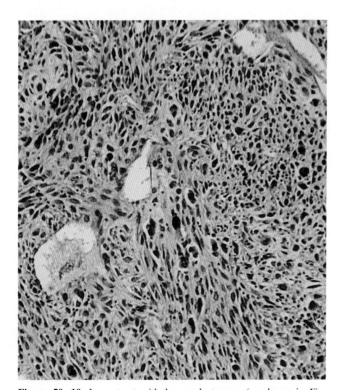

Figure 50–10. In contrast with low-grade tumors (as shown in Fig. 50–9), high-grade tumors are hypercellular and show less collagenous matrix production. Greater nuclear pleomorphism is also evident even at low magnification, as in this example of a high-grade fibrosarcoma.

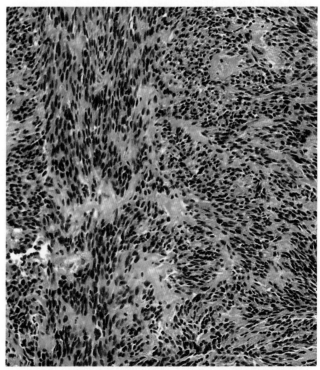

Figure 50–12. The histologic differentiation of high-grade fibrosarcoma from fibroblastic osteosarcoma is made on the basis of identifying osteoid; however, dense collagen can mimic the appearance of osteoid, as in this photomicrograph; thus, the distinction is, at times, subjective.

Figure 50–13. This photomicrograph shows a desmoplastic fibroma. These tumors are histologically identical with soft tissue aggressive fibromatosis of desmoid type.

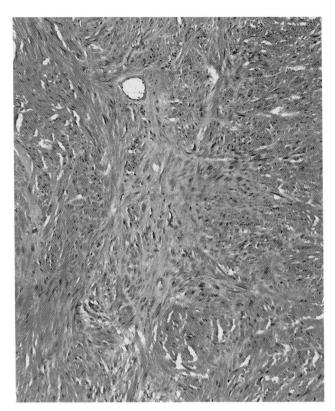

Figure 50–15. Leiomyosarcomas may arise as primary bone tumors. These tumors are commonly in the pathologic differential diagnosis with fibrosarcoma of bone.

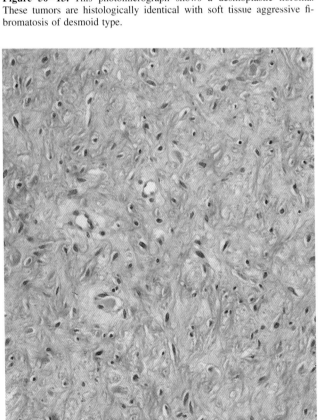

Figure 50–14. This photomicrograph illustrates the densely collagenized stroma seen in desmoplastic fibroma of bone. Such lesions are in the differential diagnosis of low-grade fibrosarcoma.

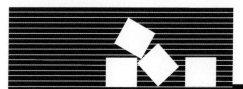

CHAPTER 51

Malignant Fibrous Histiocytoma

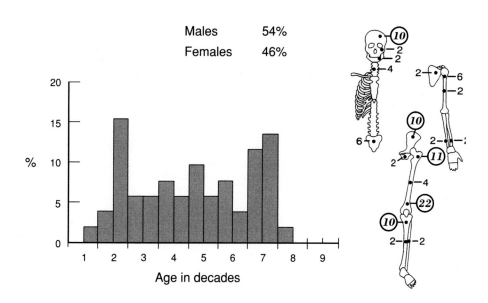

Males   54%
Females   46%

%

Age in decades

CLINICAL SIGNS

1. A painful or tender mass lesion is the most common finding on physical examination.

CLINICAL SYMPTOMS

1. Pain and swelling are the most common symptoms.
2. Symptoms may be of short duration but are generally present for six months or longer.
3. This tumor may arise after radiation therapy for an unrelated malignancy or as a malignancy complicating Paget's disease.

MAJOR RADIOGRAPHIC FEATURES

1. The lesion most often arises in a metaphyseal or diaphyseal location in the affected bone.

2. The lesion most often is purely lytic, although a few have mixed sclerosis and lysis.
3. Cortical destruction and associated soft tissue mass are common.
4. Periosteal reaction is absent or scant.
5. The tumor may be identified arising from a pre-existing lesion, e.g., a bone infarct.

RADIOGRAPHIC DIFFERENTIAL DIAGNOSIS

1. Osteosarcoma.
2. Fibrosarcoma.
3. Malignant lymphoma.
4. Metastatic carcinoma.
5. Myeloma.

MAJOR PATHOLOGIC FEATURES

Gross

1. The gross tumor varies in consistency from firm to soft, depending upon the cellularity and the amount of collagen being produced.
2. The color varies from tumor to tumor and within a given tumor; it may be yellow, brown, or tan.
3. Necrotic regions are frequently present in high-grade tumors.

Microscopic

1. At low magnification, the appearance is generally that of a spindle cell tumor arranged in a matted or storiform pattern.
2. The cytologic features tend to be quite variable, with some cells being more rounded and "histiocytic" and others spindled and "fibroblastic."
3. Multinucleated giant cells, lipid-laden histiocytes, and malignant giant cells are scattered throughout the lesion.
4. At higher magnification, the cytologic atypia can be quite variable from low-grade to high-grade tumors, as can the variability in the mitotic activity present.

PATHOLOGIC DIFFERENTIAL DIAGNOSIS

Benign lesions:

1. Fibroma (metaphyseal fibrous defect).
2. Benign fibrous histiocytoma.
3. Giant cell tumor.
4. Giant cell reparative granuloma (giant cell reaction).

Malignant lesions:

1. Metastatic sarcomatoid carcinoma (particularly hypernephroma).
2. Fibrosaromca.
3. Fibroblastic osteosarcoma.

TREATMENT

Primary Modality: Preoperative chemotherapy and wide surgical resection are used when possible. Oncologic reconstruction varies with the location. Amputation may be necessary to achieve a margin in large lesions with neurovascular involvement.

Other Possible Approaches: Adjuvant chemotherapy may be used. Thoracotomy is useful for patients with pulmonary metastases. Radiation therapy has been effective in some surgically inaccessible lesions.

References

Capanna R, Bertoni F, Bacchini P, et al: Malignant fibrous histiocytoma of bone: the experience at the Rizzoli Institute: report of 90 cases. Cancer 54:177–187, 1984

Ghandur-Mnaymneh L, Zych G, and Mnaymneh W: Primary malignant fibrous histiocytoma of bone: report of six cases with ultrastructural study and analysis of the literature. Cancer 49:698–707, 1982.

Huvos AG, Heilweil M, and Bretsky SS: The pathology of malignant fibrous histiocytoma of bone. A study of 130 patients. Am J Surg Pathol 9:853–871, 1985.

McCarthy EF, Matsuno T, and Dorfman HD: Malignant fibrous histiocytoma of bone: a study of 35 cases. Hum Pathol 10:57–70, 1979.

Mirra JM, Gold RH, and Marafiote R: Malignant (fibrous) histiocytoma arising in association with a bone infarct in sickle-cell disease: coincidence or cause and effect? Cancer 39:186–194, 1977.

Nishida J, Sim FH, Wenger DE, and Unni KK: Malignant fibrous histiocytoma of bone. A clinicopathologic study of 81 patients [see comments]. Cancer 79(3):482–493, 1997.

Ruggieri P, Sim FH, Bond JR, and Unni KK: Malignancies in fibrous dysplasia. Cancer 73(5):1411–1424, 1994.

Taconis WK, and Minder JD: Fibrosarcoma and malignant fibrous histiocytoma of long bones: radiographic features and grading. Skeletal Radiol 11:237–245, 1984.

Taconis WK, and Van Rijssel TG: Fibrosarcoma of long bones. A study of the significance of areas of malignant fibrous histiocytoma. J Bone Joint Surg (Br) 67:111–116, 1985.

Yokoyama R, Tsuneyoshi M, Enjoji M, et al: Prognostic factors of malignant fibrous histiocytoma of bone. A clinical and histopathologic analysis of 34 cases. Cancer 72:1902–1908, 1993.

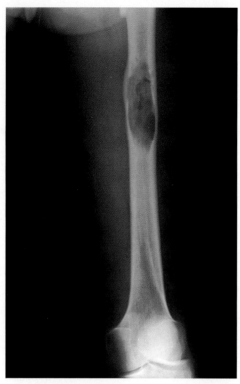

Figure 51–1. This radiograph illustrates an intramedullary malignant fibrous histiocytoma that shows a purely lytic pattern of growth. Mild expansion of the femoral diaphysis and cortical destruction are evident.

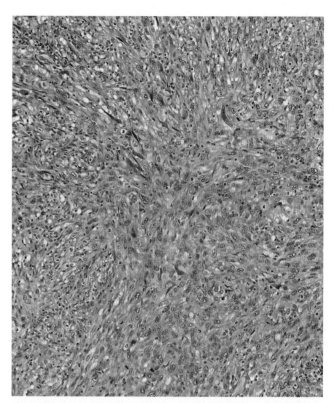

Figure 51–3. At low magnification, the histologic pattern of malignant fibrous histiocytoma may vary from region to region. Classically, the tumor grows in a storiform pattern, as shown in this photomicrograph.

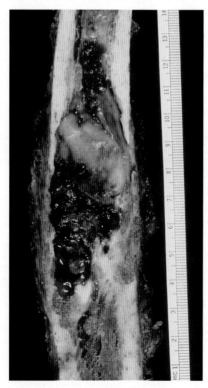

Figure 51–2. The gross pathologic features of this lesion correlate well with its radiographic appearance in Figure 51–1. Grossly, the tumor is soft, fleshy, and variable in color from gray-white to yellow. Foci of hemorrhage, as are visible in this case, may be present.

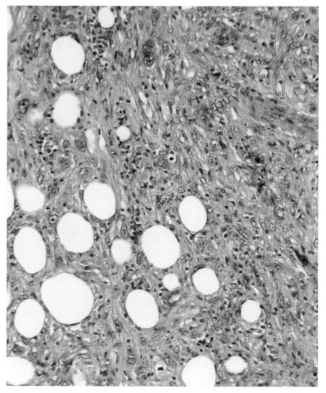

Figure 51–4. At higher magnification, the tumor is seen to be composed of a variety of cell types. Some tumors have a pronounced inflammatory component; others show lesser degrees of inflammatory reaction.

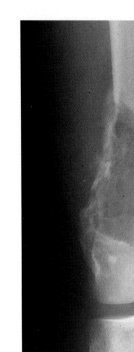

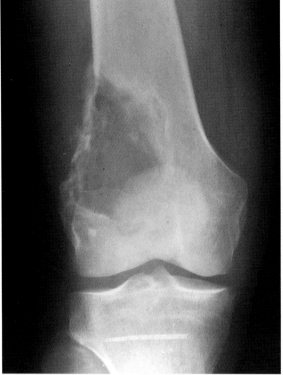

Figure 51–5. At higher magnification, the degree of cytologic atypia present in malignant fibrous histiocytomas is variable. Most commonly, significant cytologic atypia and brisk mitotic activity are present, as shown in this photomicrograph.

Figure 51–7. This radiograph illustrates a malignant fibrous histiocytoma of the distal femoral metaphysis. The tumor is eccentric and shows a permeative pattern of growth with cortical destruction.

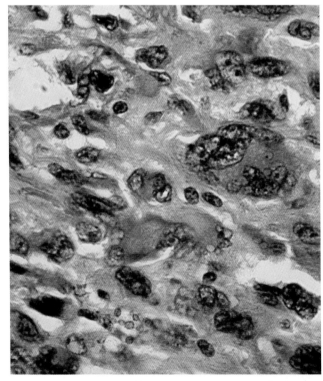

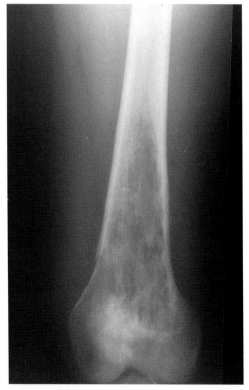

Figure 51–6. At high magnification, marked cytologic atypia characterized by nuclear pleomorphism, hyperchromasia, and an irregular chromatin pattern are common in malignant fibrous histiocytoma. Multinucleation is also common. Such tumors may simulate a giant cell tumor.

Figure 51–8. A large, poorly marginated, malignant fibrous histiocytoma of the lower femoral diametaphysis is shown in this radiograph. The lesion is irregular in contour and demonstrates a mixed lytic and sclerotic pattern of growth.

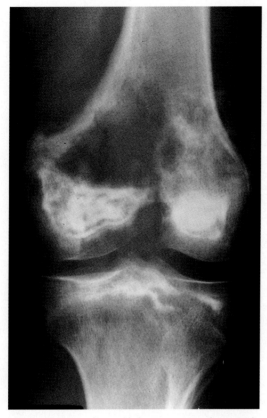

Figure 51–9. Malignant fibrous histiocytoma may arise secondary to a bone infarct, as shown in this radiograph of the distal femur. Infarct is also present in the upper tibia.

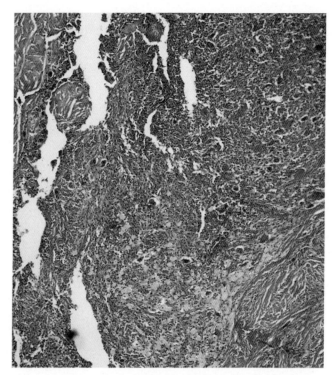

Figure 51–11. Numerous multinucleated giant cells may be present in malignant fibrous histiocytomas, resulting in a histologic appearance simulating that of giant cell tumor. This photomicrograph illustrates such a histologic pattern in a tumor that involved the distal femur.

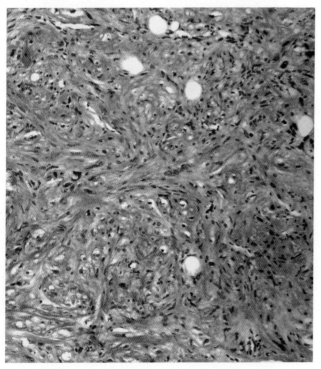

Figure 51–10. At low magnification, an ill-defined storiform pattern of growth is evident in this malignant fibrous histiocytoma of the proximal tibia. The tumor is growing in a permeative manner.

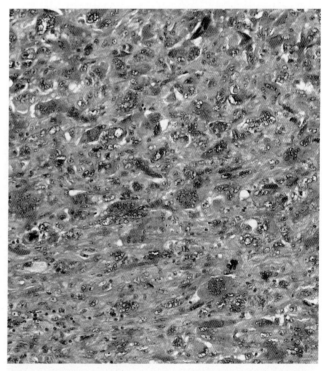

Figure 51–12. When numerous multinucleated giant cells are found in a tumor, careful assessment of the cytologic features of the mononuclear cells is necessary. At high magnification, the nuclei of the mononuclear cells of malignant fibrous histiocytoma are cytologically different from those of the multinucleated giant cells, as this photomicrograph shows.

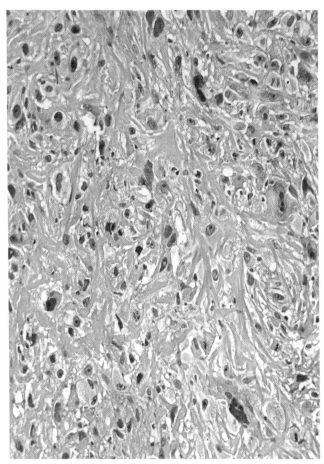

Figure 51–13. Differentiation of fibroblastic osteosarcoma (shown in this photomicrograph) from malignant fibrous histiocytoma can be extremely difficult. Demonstration of "malignant" osteoid in the lesion identifies it as an osteosarcoma; however, fracture callus and reactive new bone formation associated with malignant fibrous histiocytoma may simulate such osteoid. Such a distinction is probably only of academic importance.

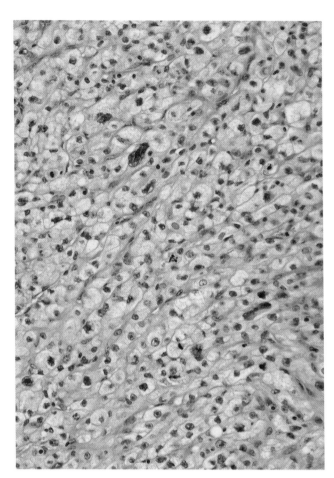

Figure 51–14. Metastatic sarcomatoid renal cell carcinoma can histologically mimic the appearance of malignant fibrous histiocytoma. This photomicrograph illustrates that malignant fibrous histiocytoma may contain clear cells that are somewhat packeted and thus mimic the appearance of renal cell carcinoma.

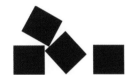

HEMATOPOIETIC
TUMORS

D

CHAPTER 52

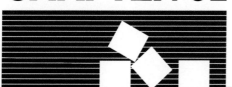

Malignant Lymphoma

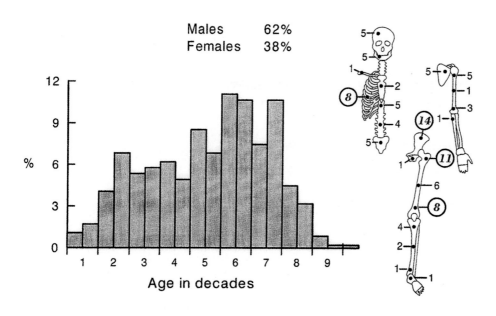

Males 62%
Females 38%

Age in decades

CLINICAL SIGNS

1. A tender mass lesion is commonly found on physical examination if the affected bone is superficial.
2. Lymphadenopathy and splenomegaly may be present in disseminated disease.
3. Extension into the soft tissues may result in an associated soft tissue mass.

CLINICAL SYMPTOMS

1. Malignant lymphoma most commonly is associated with pain and swelling.

2. Pain is variable in intensity but may have been present for years.
3. Neurologic symptoms may be present in those patients who have vertebral involvement related to cord or nerve root compression.
4. The patient may have few complaints, however, and generally feels quite well despite extensive disease.

MAJOR RADIOGRAPHIC FEATURES

1. The lesion is generally characterized by extensive diaphyseal permeative destruction of the affected bone.

2. The pattern may be one of pure lysis or sclerosis, or it may be a mixture of lysis and sclerosis.
3. Periosteal reaction is unusual.
4. The cortex may be thickened, and the lesion shows poor margination at the periphery.
5. An associated soft tissue mass is commonly present.
6. Isotope bone scan, computed tomography (CT), and magnetic resonance imaging (MRI) are frequently helpful in defining the extent of the lesion and its location.

RADIOGRAPHIC DIFFERENTIAL DIAGNOSIS

1. Ewing's sarcoma.
2. Osteosarcoma.
3. Osteomyelitis.
4. Metastatic carcinoma.

MAJOR PATHOLOGIC FEATURES

Gross

1. Viable tumor extending into the soft tissues generally shows a whitish, fish flesh–like appearance.
2. Lymphomas generally permeate the bone extensively, leaving residual bony trabeculae that may impart a gritty consistency to the medullary portion of the specimen.

Microscopic

1. At low magnification, lymphomas show a diffuse sheet-like proliferation of cells without matrix production.
2. At higher magnification, osseous lymphomas generally show a mixture of cells, with both small and large cells scattered throughout the lesional tissue.
3. The nuclear characteristics are generally quite variable, with both cleaved and noncleaved nuclei identifiable.
4. Reticulin stains generally show a fine meshwork of reticulin fibers surrounding individual cells.

5. Immunohistochemical stains for lymphoid markers are positive if optimally fixed tissue is available for analysis. (*Note:* Touch preparations may be used for immunohistochemical analysis, thereby avoiding the use of tissue that has been subjected to decalcification procedures.)

PATHOLOGIC DIFFERENTIAL DIAGNOSIS

Benign lesions:

1. Chronic osteomyelitis.

Malignant lesions:

1. Metastatic undifferentiated carcinoma.
2. Malignant fibrous histiocytoma (histiocytic variant).

TREATMENT

Primary Modality: Radiation therapy is the mainstay of treatment of the local bony lesion. Chemotherapy is used when systemic disease is identifiable.

Other Possible Approaches: Surgical intervention with internal fixation or joint replacement for pathologic fractures may be used. Resection or amputation may be required for distal extremity lesions that have failed to respond to radiation therapy.

References

Clayton F, Butlier JJ, Ayala AG, et al: Non-Hodgkin's lymphoma in bone. Pathologic and radiologic features with clinical correlates. Cancer *60*:2494–2501, 1987.

Dosoretz DE, Murphy GF, Raymond AK, et al: Radiation therapy for primary lymphoma of bone. Cancer *51*:44–46, 1983.

Dosoretz DE, Raymond AK, Murphy GF, et al. Primary lymphoma of bone: the relationship of morphologic diversity to clinical behavior. Cancer *50*:1009–1014, 1982.

Neiman RS, Barcos M, Berard C, et al: Granulocytic sarcoma: a clinicopathologic study of 61 biopsied cases. Cancer *48*:1426–1437, 1981.

Ostrowski ML, Unni KK, Banks PM, et al: Malignant lymphoma of bone. Cancer *58*:2646–2655, 1986.

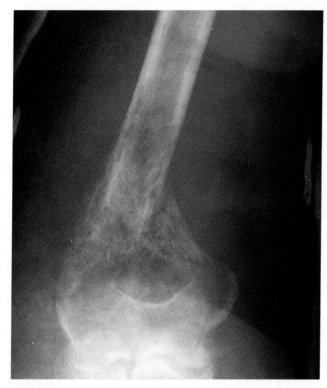

Figure 52–1. This radiograph demonstrates the permeative destructive appearance of a malignant lymphoma involving the distal humerus. An associated soft tissue mass is present, and a pathologic fracture has occurred.

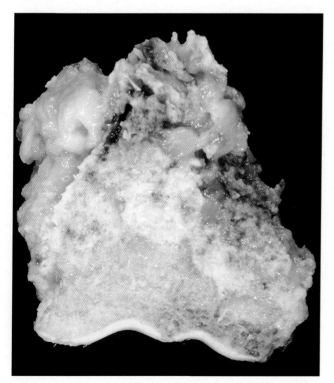

Figure 52–2. The gross pathologic features of malignant lymphoma of bone are demonstrated in this tumor, which was resected owing to the pathologic fracture and loss of bone. Classically, lymphomas are soft, "fish flesh" tumors that are gray-white.

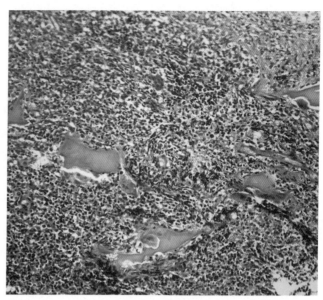

Figure 52–3. At low magnification, malignant lymphoma grows in a permeative pattern, whether it involves bone (as in this photomicrograph) or soft tissue. Residual bony trabeculae are present within the medullary portion of this non-Hodgkin's lymphoma.

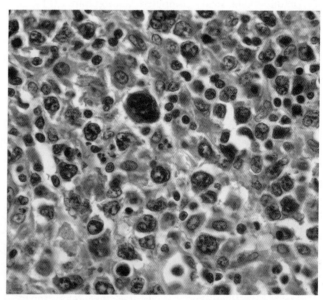

Figure 52–4. At high magnification, the cytologic variability generally present in osseous lymphomas is seen in this photomicrograph. Large and small cells are mixed and generally grow in a sheet-like, diffuse manner. "Multilobulated" cells may be seen, as in this example, and some cases represent neoplasms of T-cell origin; however, most osseous lymphomas are of B-cell lineage.

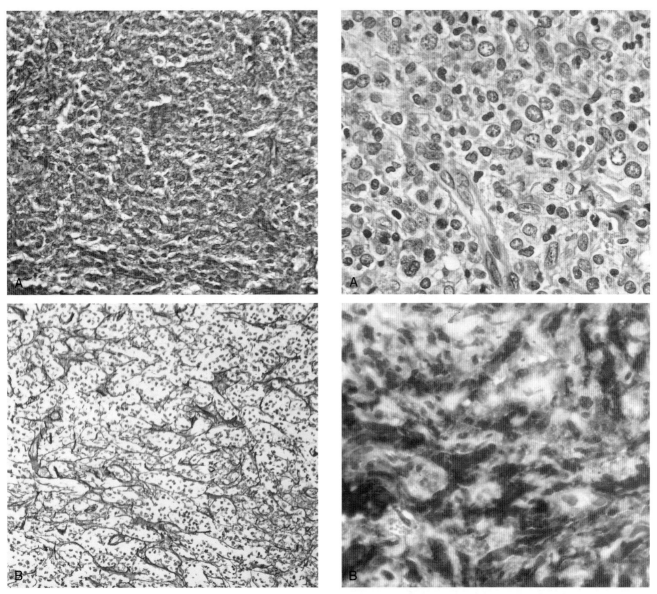

Figure 52–5. Special stains may be helpful in distinguishing malignant lymphoma from other "small round cell" tumors. The periodic acid–Schiff stain (*A*) helps to distinguish lymphoma from Ewing's sarcoma, as lymphomas are negative and most Ewing's sarcomas are positive. Lymphomas may show more reticulin fibers (*B*, reticulin stain) than do Ewing's sarcomas.

Figure 52–6. Other hematopoietic neoplasms may mimic the appearance of lymphoma. Granulocytic sarcoma is particularly notorious for resembling a diffuse mixed cell lymphoma, as shown in *A*. Special stain may be helpful in differentiating such cases from lymphoma. The chloroacetate esterase stain (*B*) is positive in granulocytic sarcomas and negative in lymphomas.

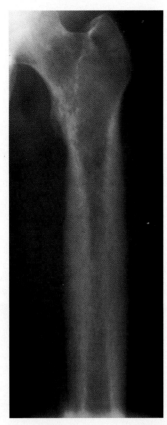

Figure 52–7. This radiograph shows an extensive diaphyseal lymphoma of the femur with poor margination and cortical thickening.

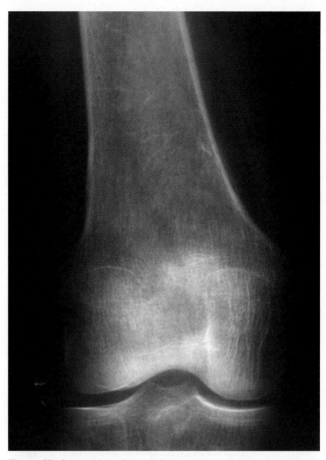

Figure 52–9. As this radiograph demonstrates, not all lymphomas are identifiable with plain radiography. This patient had a tumor involving the distal femur.

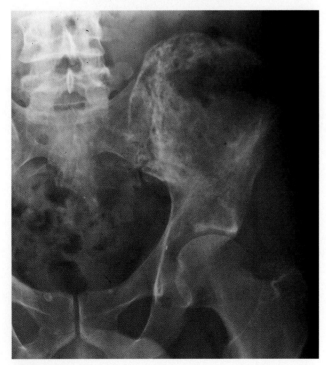

Figure 52–8. Although many lymphomas of bone show a lytic pattern radiographically, mixed lytic and sclerotic lesions, as in this tumor of the ilium, are common. The irregular, permeative pattern of growth of the tumor also favors the radiographic appearance of a malignant process.

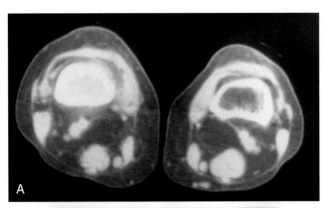

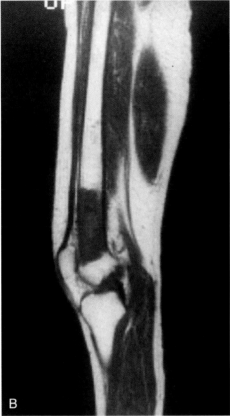

Figure 52–10. *A,* A computed tomographic (CT) scan of the distal femur seen in Figure 52–9 shows an intramedullary lymphoma. The radiographic density of the marrow in the right femur is greater than in the uninvolved left femur. Magnetic resonance imaging (MRI) may also be helpful in such cases; in *B,* the longitudinal extent of the lymphoma appears as a low-signal (black) area as compared with the normal marrow (white) in this sagittal reconstruction.

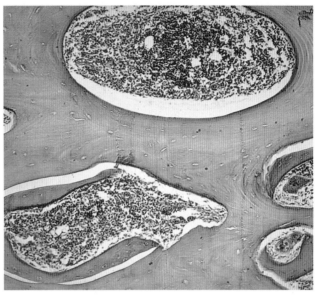

Figure 52–11. The sclerotic radiographic appearance of some lymphomas is due to the sclerotic reaction induced by the tumor. Such bony sclerosis is illustrated in this low-power photomicrograph of a calvarial lymphoma showing a permeative pattern of growth.

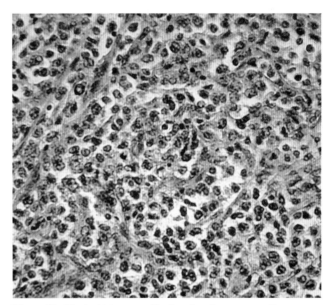

Figure 52–12. At higher magnification, lymphomas generally are seen to be composed of a pleomorphic discohesive infiltrate, as is the case with this femoral tumor.

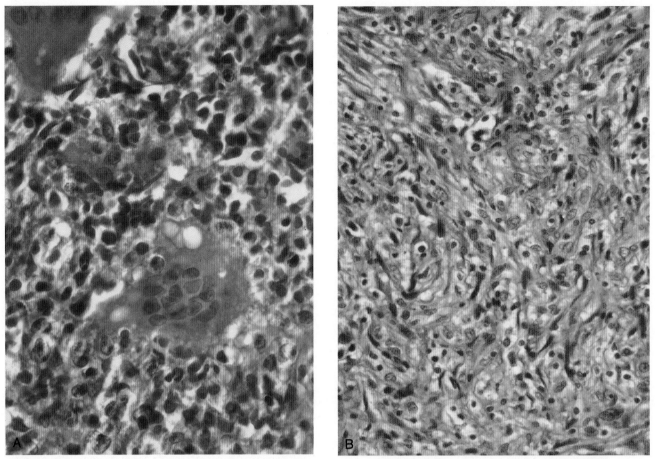

Figure 52–13. Malignant lymphoma can mimic other primary sarcomas of bone. *A* shows the presence of multinucleated giant cells in a lymphoma. The "histiocytic" appearance of the large cells in lymphoma and the presence of multinucleated giant cells may suggest the diagnosis of malignant fibrous histiocytoma. Although spindling of the cells is rare in lymphoma, such change may rarely be seen in osseous lymphomas (*B*) and may mimic histologically the appearance of a primary sarcoma.

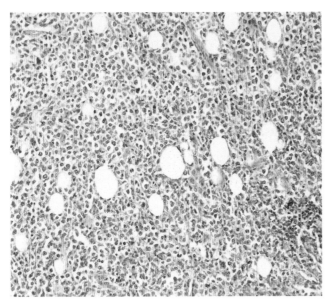

Figure 52–14. At low magnification, malignant lymphoma tends to grow in a permeative pattern that leaves behind parts of the normal architecture. The normal elements left may be bony trabeculae or fatty marrow elements, as this photomicrograph shows.

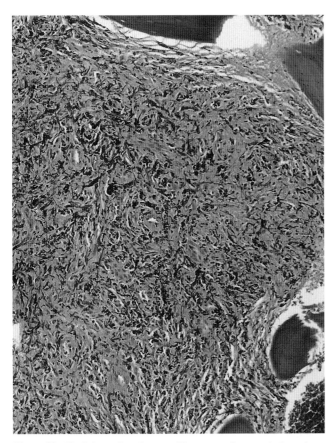

Figure 52–15. Primary lymphomas of bone may show marked crush artifact, as illustrated in this photomicrograph. Such crush artifact may be the first histologic clue that the tumor is a primary osseous lymphoma.

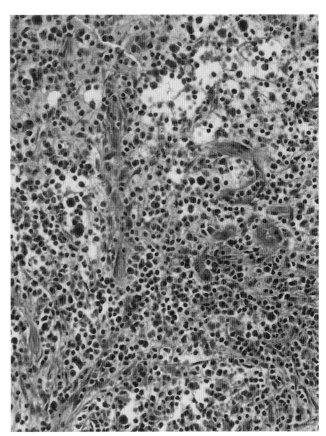

Figure 52–16. A mixed population of lymphocytes, plasma cells, and eosinophils may be appreciated at low magnification in cases of primary Hodgkin's lymphoma of bone. Careful search for Reed-Sternberg cells is essential in such cases. This photomicrograph illustrates an example of Hodgkin's lymphoma of the ilium.

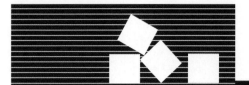

CHAPTER 53

Myeloma

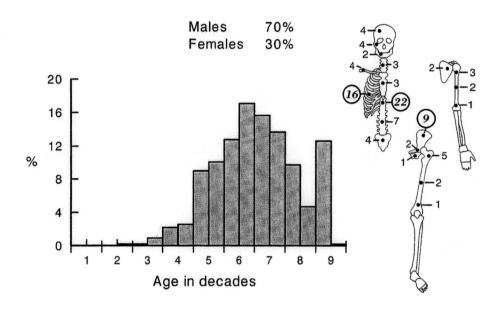

Males 70%
Females 30%

CLINICAL SIGNS

1. Local pain and tenderness are common on physical examination.
2. A palpable mass may be found that is due to extraosseous extension of the tumor or hemorrhage related to it.
3. Peripheral neuropathy may be detected in some patients.
4. Hypercalcemia occurs in fewer than 50 per cent of patients.
5. Hypergammaglobulinemia may manifest itself as rouleaux formation appreciable on peripheral blood smear.
6. Serum electrophoresis and immunoelectrophoresis generally reveal a monoclonal gammopathy, but nonsecretory myelomas rarely occur.

CLINICAL SYMPTOMS

1. Pain is the most frequent complaint at the time of diagnosis.
2. The duration of the pain is usually less than six months.
3. Constitutional symptoms of weakness and weight loss are almost uniformly present.
4. Pathologic fracture results in a sudden onset of pain in many patients.
5. Peripheral neuropathy may be present, particularly in osteosclerotic myeloma.
6. A tendency toward bleeding and fever may also be experienced.

314

MAJOR RADIOGRAPHIC FEATURES

1. Multiple small, discrete lesions involving one or several bones are identifiable.
2. The tumor occasionally may present as a solitary osseous lesion.
3. The lesion is purely lytic.
4. The surrounding bone does not show a sclerotic reaction, nor is there periosteal reaction.
5. Endosteal scalloping may be identified.
6. Expansion of the affected bone and an associated soft tissue mass are common.

RADIOGRAPHIC DIFFERENTIAL DIAGNOSIS

1. Metastatic carcinoma.
2. Malignant lymphoma.
3. Fibrosarcoma.

MAJOR PATHOLOGIC FEATURES

Gross

1. The tumor tissue is generally soft and friable.
2. The color of the tissue varies from reddish to gray-white and grossly may appear similar to that of malignant lymphoma.
3. Extension into soft tissue may be discovered at the time of biopsy.

Microscopic

1. At low magnification, the pattern is that of a cellular tumor lacking production of matrix.
2. The amount of cytoplasm on the cells varies but generally is abundant.
3. At higher magnification, the nuclei generally are eccentrically placed in the cytoplasm and show a clumped chromatin pattern.
4. A cytoplasmic clearing adjacent to the nucleus (perinuclear hof) is frequently discernible.
5. Amyloid may be present as large masses of amorphous eosinophilic material. In such cases, a foreign body giant cell reaction may be elicited by the amyloid.
6. Mitotic activity is generally not brisk.

PATHOLOGIC DIFFERENTIAL DIAGNOSIS

Benign lesions:

1. Chronic osteomyelitis.

Malignant lesions:

1. Malignant lymphoma.

TREATMENT

Primary Modality: The mainstay of treatment is chemotherapy. Radiation therapy is effective in controlling localized lesions that are causing disabling pain or limitation of activity. The patient with solitary myeloma requires high-dose radiation for control of the disease.

Other Possible Approaches: Surgical intervention with internal fixation of impending or actual pathologic fractures may be needed. Decompressive laminectomy may be indicated in patients with compressive myelopathy, and spinal stabilization is occasionally warranted.

References

Bataille R, and Sany J: Solitary myeloma: clinical and prognostic features of a review of 114 cases. Cancer 48:845–851, 1981.

Dimopoulos MA, Moulopoulos LA, Maniatis A, and Alexanian R: Solitary plasmacytoma of bone and asymptomatic multiple myeloma. Blood 96(6):2037–2044, 2000.

Frassica FJ, Beabout JW, Unni KK, and Sim FH: Myeloma of bone. Orthopedics 8(9):1184–1186, 1985.

Haferlach T, and Loffler H: Prognostic factors in multiple myeloma: practicability for clinical practice and future perspectives. Leukemia 11 (Suppl 5):S5–S9, 1997.

Kelly JJ Jr, Kyle RA, Miles JM, and Dyck PJ: Osteosclerotic myeloma and peripheral neuropathy. Neurology 33:202–210, 1983.

Kyle RA: Multiple myeloma: review of 869 cases. Mayo Clin Proc 50:29–40, 1975.

Kyle RA: Long-term survival in multiple myeloma. N Engl J Med 308:314–316, 1983.

Kyle RA, and Elveback LR: Management and prognosis of multiple myeloma. Mayo Clin Proc 51:751–760, 1976.

Ludwig H, Meran J, and Zojer N: Multiple myeloma: an update on biology and treatment. Ann Oncol 10 (Suppl 6):31–43, 1999.

Rajkumar SV, and Greipp PR: Prognostic factors in multiple myeloma. Hematol Oncol Clin North Am 13(6):1295–1314, xi, 1999.

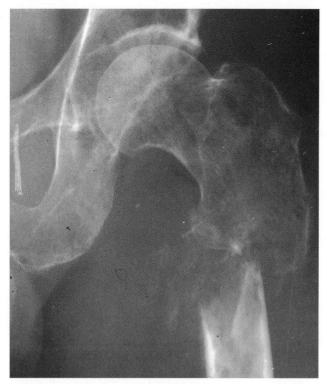

Figure 53–1. This radiograph illustrates a large, purely lytic lesion involving the proximal femur. The tumor has expanded the femur, resulting in pathologic fracture. The underlying process is myeloma.

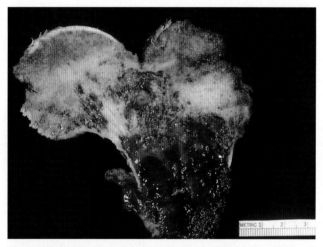

Figure 53–2. The gross pathologic features in this case correlate well with its radiographic features in Figure 53–1. Grossly, myeloma is a soft, fish flesh–like lesion, as shown here. Hemorrhage is commonly seen, in this case the result of the pathologic fracture that necessitated resection of the proximal femur.

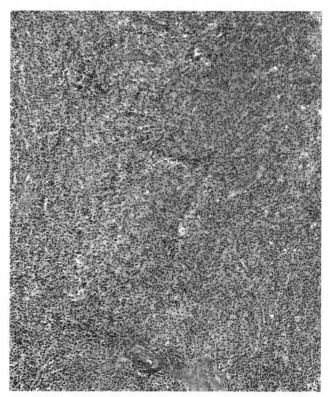

Figure 53–3. At low magnification, myeloma is a tumor that is uniform in appearance. The tumor is composed of round cells without any evidence of stromal proliferation.

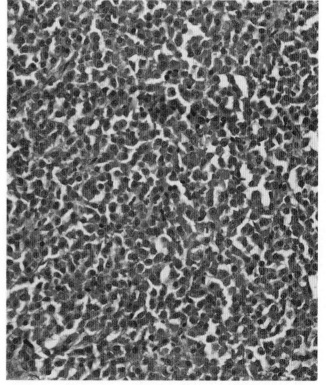

Figure 53–4. In contrast with most cases of malignant lymphoma, myeloma is generally composed of a homogeneous population of cells. This case illustrates such a proliferation of uniform cells.

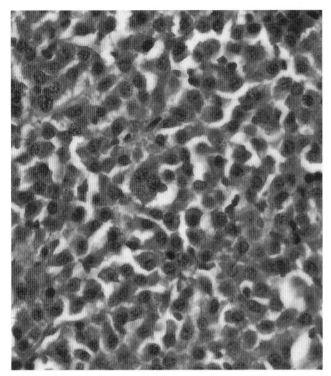

Figure 53–5. At high magnification, the proliferating plasma cells show abundant cytoplasm and an eccentrically located nucleus. Well-differentiated myelomas have cytologic features that deviate minimally from benign plasma cells; in such cases, chronic osteomyelitis may be included in the histologic differential diagnosis.

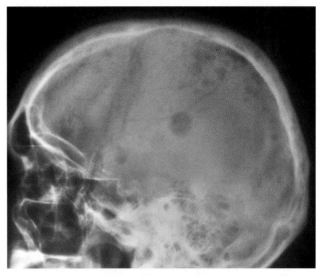

Figure 53–7. Multiple discrete lytic calvarial lesions, seen in this radiograph, are the hallmark of multiple myeloma.

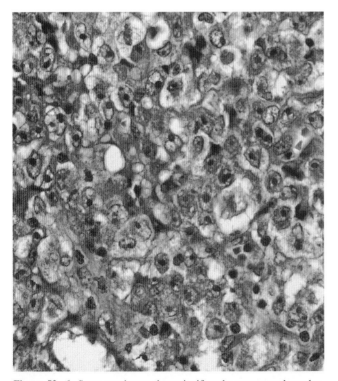

Figure 53–6. Some myelomas show significantly greater nuclear pleomorphism. In such cases, the differential diagnosis includes immunoblastic lymphoma. However, some evidence of plasmacytic differentiation, as illustrated in this case, usually is seen.

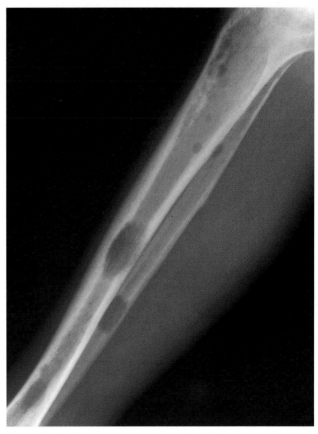

Figure 53–8. The long bone lesions of multiple myeloma show the same general radiographic features as lesions of flat bones, as in this radiograph illustrating tibial and fibular involvement.

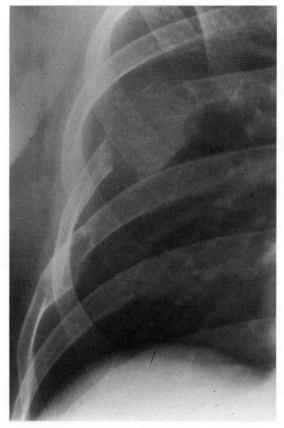

Figure 53–9. When myeloma involves the flat bone, a soft tissue mass may be evident, as in this example of myeloma involving two ribs.

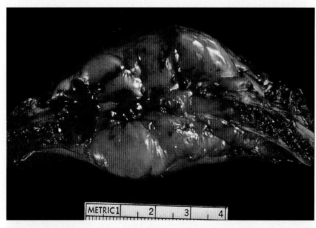

Figure 53–10. The gross appearance of myeloma is similar to that of malignant lymphoma, as in this case involving the rib. Extension of the tumor into the soft tissues, as seen in Figure 53–9, is present.

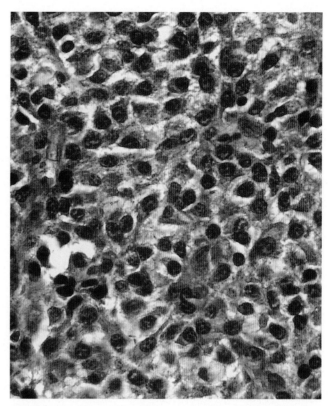

Figure 53–11. At high magnification, the nuclei of myeloma cells are eccentrically placed and lie within abundant cytoplasm. A perinuclear clearing is frequently evident in the cytoplasm, as this photomicrograph illustrates.

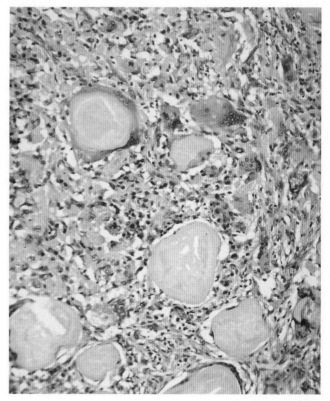

Figure 53–12. Amyloid may be formed in cases of myeloma. Such deposits of amyloid may result in a foreign body type of giant cell reaction, as shown in this photomicrograph.

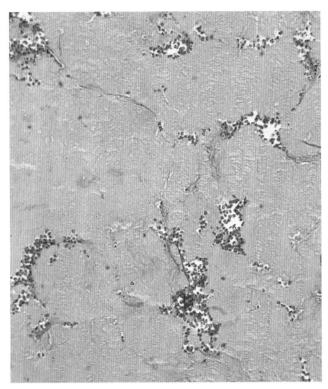

Figure 53–13. In some cases of myeloma, amyloid formation may be so prominent as to overwhelm the plasmacytic proliferation. Such is the case in this tumor involving the fourth thoracic vertebra.

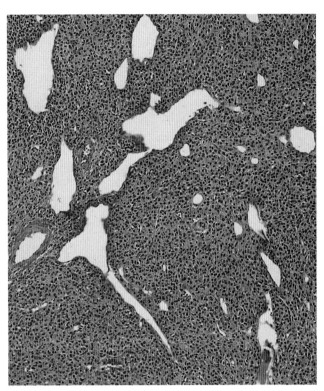

Figure 53–15. Some myelomas may show a prominent vascular pattern, as in this example from a rib lesion. Such tumors may be confused with hemangiopericytomas on initial low-power histologic evaluation.

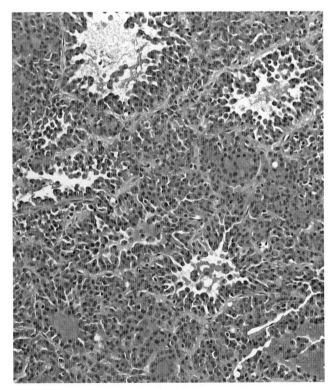

Figure 53–14. Myeloma grows in a noncohesive manner, and, in some cases, the resulting pattern may even resemble gland formation, as in metastatic adenocarcinoma. This case of myeloma shows such a pseudogland histologic pattern of growth.

CHAPTER 54

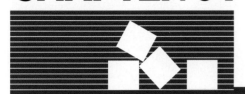

Mastocytosis (Mast Cell Disease)

CLINICAL SIGNS

1. The pigmented rash urticates when rubbed (urticaria pigmentosa).
2. Hepatosplenomegaly may be found on physical examination.

CLINICAL SYMPTOMS

1. Pigmented skin rash may be the patient's presenting complaint (urticaria pigmentosa).
2. Abdominal fullness may be experienced (hepatosplenomegaly).
3. Abdominal cramping and diarrhea may occur.
4. The lesion may be an incidental finding on radiography and is usually mistaken for metastatic carcinoma.

MAJOR RADIOGRAPHIC FEATURES

1. Skeletal involvement is most commonly diffuse; focal lesions are occasionally superimposed on diffuse disease, whereas focal lesions alone are unusual.
2. Diffuse osteopenia is the most common presentation, but diffuse sclerosis or mixed lysis and sclerosis are also seen.
3. Focal lesions are usually sclerotic or mixed.

RADIOGRAPHIC DIFFERENTIAL DIAGNOSIS

1. Osteoporosis.
2. Diffuse myeloma.
3. Lymphoma.

MAJOR PATHOLOGIC FEATURES

Gross

1. Lesional tissue may be too ossified to cut with frozen section.

Microscopic

1. At low magnification, the bone shows diffuse permeation of the medullary space by a uniform population of small, regular cells. The cells are usually concentrated around bony trabeculae and are associated with fibrosis.
2. The trabeculae may show sclerosis, with increased thickness and greater irregularity than normal.
3. At higher magnification, the cells are uniform, with a faintly granular cytoplasm.
4. The nuclei are regular, are round to oval, and have a finely stippled chromatin pattern.
5. The cells may show a tendency to spindle, and in some areas the proliferation exhibits a granuloma-like quality.
6. Eosinophils may form a prominent part of the infiltrate.
7. Special stains may be used to demonstrate the metachromatic granules within the cytoplasm of the mast cells.

PATHOLOGIC DIFFERENTIAL DIAGNOSIS

Benign lesions:

1. Histiocytosis X.
2. Granulomatous osteomyelitis.
3. Nonspecific reactive changes.

320

Malignant lesions:

1. Hairy cell leukemia.
2. Malignant lymphoma.
3. Metastatic breast carcinoma.

TREATMENT

Primary Modality: Depends upon the extent of disease. In children with limited disease, the prognosis is good. In patients with skeletal involvement, the prognosis is guarded but good. Rarely is there associated mast cell leukemia. Resection with a marginal or wide surgical margin is applicable in cases with limited disease.

Other Possible Approaches: Chemotherapy.

References

Bain BJ: Systemic mastocytosis and other mast cell neoplasms. Br J Haematol *106(1)*:9–17, 1999.

Barer M, Peterson LFA, Dahlin DC, et al: Mastocytosis with osseous lesions resembling metastatic malignant lesions in bone. J Bone Joint Surg (Am) *50*:142–152, 1968.

Havard CWH, and Scott RB: Urticaria pigmentosa with visceral and skeletal lesions. Q J Med *28*:459–470, 1959.

Horny HP, Ruck P, Krober S, Kaiserling E: Systemic mast cell disease (mastocytosis). General aspects and histopathological diagnosis. Histol Histopathol *12(4)*:1081–1089, 1997.

Webb TA, Li CY, and Yam LT: Systemic mast cell disease: a clinical and hematopathologic study of 26 cases. Cancer *49*:927–938, 1982.

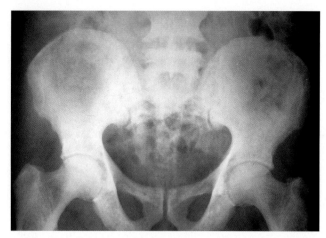

Figure 54–1. Mastocytosis may produce multifocal sclerosing lesions, as in this case involving the pelvic bones. Such lesions are commonly mistaken for metastatic osteoblastic carcinoma.

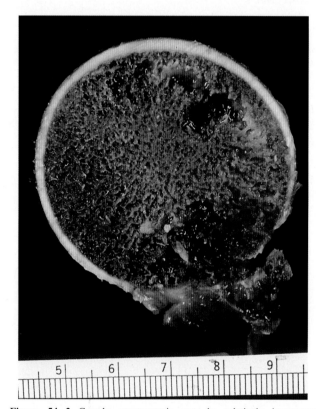

Figure 54–2. Grossly, mastocytosis may be relatively inapparent. Although this femoral head showed diffuse involvement microscopically, only some thickening of the bony trabeculae was grossly evident.

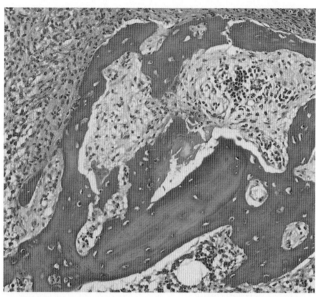

Figure 54–3. At low magnification, the marrow space may show diffuse replacement in cases of mastocytosis. Even at this level of magnification, the uniform cytologic features of the infiltrate are evident.

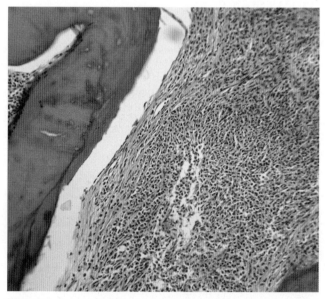

Figure 54–4. Fibrosis of the marrow space and bony sclerosis, evident in this case of mastocytosis involving the ilium, may also be seen.

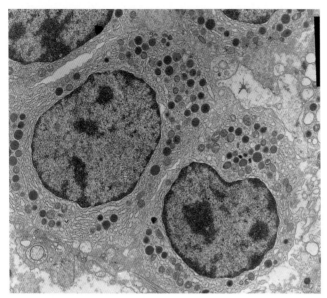

Figure 54–5. Ultrastructurally, mastocytosis is characterized by large cytoplasmic granules, as illustrated in this sample of a lesion involving the femoral head.

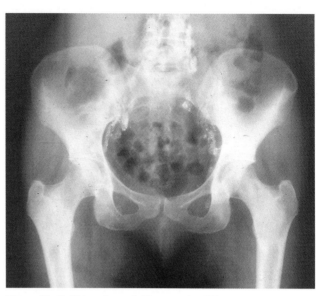

Figure 54–7. This radiograph illustrates the diffuse bony sclerosis that may be seen in mastocytosis.

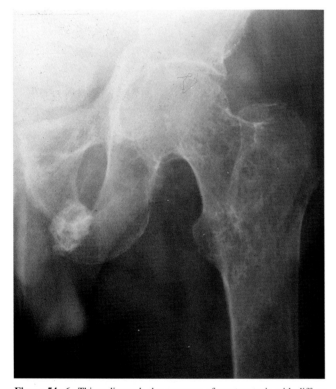

Figure 54–6. This radiograph shows a case of mastocytosis with diffuse skeletal demineralization and fracture of the pubic ramus.

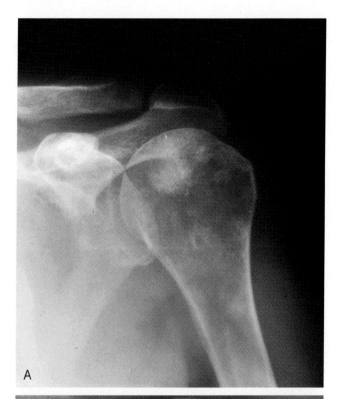

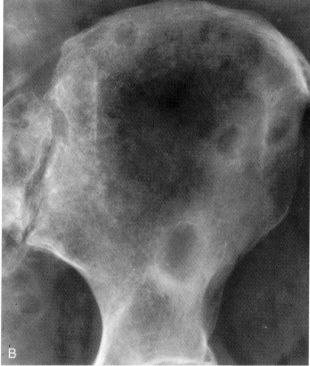

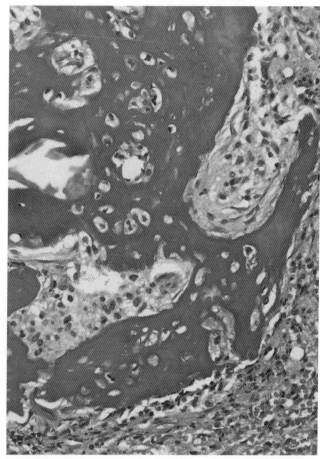

Figure 54–9. Bony sclerosis is commonly seen in mast cell disease, both radiographically and histologically, as shown in this photomicrograph.

Figure 54–8. These radiographs show the shoulder (*A*) and pelvis (*B*) of a patient with mastocytosis. Some of the focal lesions are sclerotic; others are lytic, with surrounding sclerosis.

CHAPTER 55

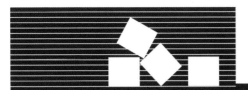

Langerhans' Cell Histiocytosis (Histiocytosis X)

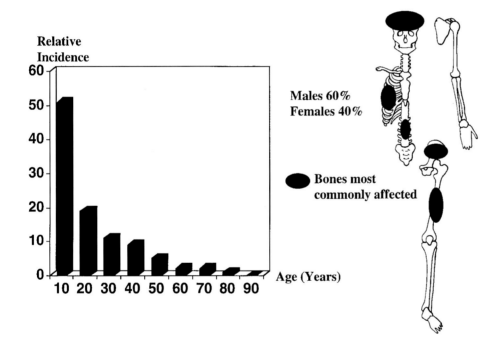

Males 60%
Females 40%

● Bones most
commonly affected

CLINICAL SIGNS

1. A mass may be palpable on physical examination.
2. Cutaneous seborrhea-like lesions may be identified, indicating skin involvement.
3. Hearing loss or decreased balance may indicate involvement of the mastoid region.
4. Marked tenderness in the region of the affected bone may be found on physical examination.

CLINICAL SYMPTOMS

1. Pain is the most frequent presenting complaint.
2. A swelling may also be noted in the region of the bone involved.
3. Only rarely will the lesion be discovered incidentally on radiographic examination.
4. Protean clinical symptoms are seen in multisystem disease, e.g., Hand-Schüller-Christian or Letterer-Siwe variants.

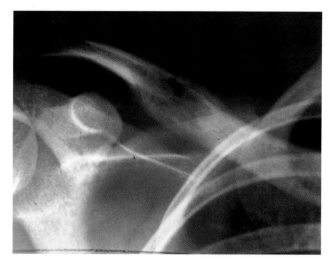

Figure 55–1. This radiograph shows an example of Langerhans' cell histiocytosis of the clavicle. The lesion is poorly marginated, and associated new bone formation is present. A similar appearance could be caused by Ewing's sarcoma or osteomyelitis.

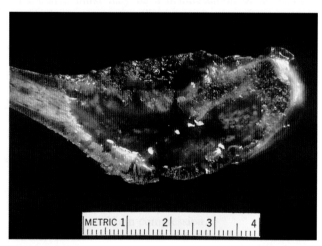

Figure 55–2. Another example of Langerhans' cell histiocytosis of the clavicle demonstrates the gross pathologic features of the condition. The lesional tissue may be quite loose and runny. Lesions that extend beyond the cortex, as shown here, may simulate the appearance of a malignant neoplasm radiographically.

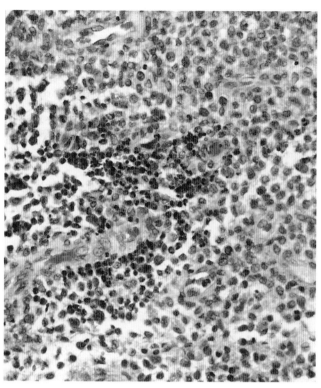

Figure 55–3. At low magnification, Langerhans' cell histiocytosis is a lesion composed of multiple cell types. Eosinophils may be prominent, as in this case, or sparse. In this lesion, the loose nature of the process is evident, and an eosinophilic "abscess" is present.

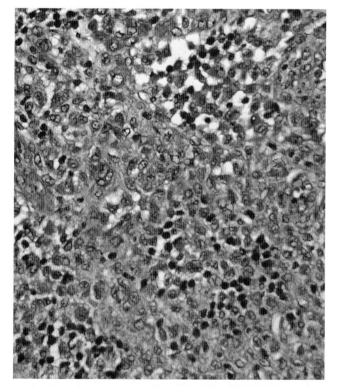

Figure 55–4. At higher magnification, the polymorphous nature of the process is evident. The Langerhans' cell–type histiocytes have abundant cytoplasm and a coffee bean–shaped nucleus. Lymphocytes, plasma cells, and polymorphonuclear leukocytes are scattered throughout the lesional tissue.

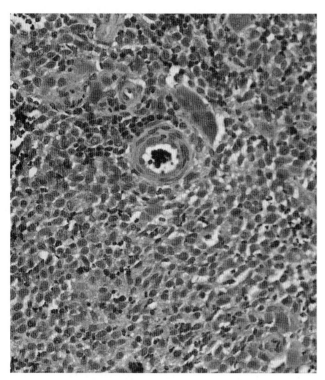

Figure 55–5. Multinucleated giant cells, as shown in this photomicrograph, may be seen in Langerhans' cell histiocytosis. Mitotic activity may be fairly brisk, but this feature does not appear to correlate with the clinical course of the disease.

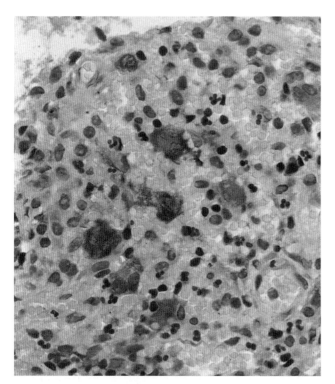

Figure 55–6. Immunohistochemical techniques may be helpful in substantiating the diagnosis of Langerhans' cell histiocytosis. The polymorphous nature of the infiltrate frequently raises consideration of the differential diagnosis of chronic osteomyelitis. In such cases, immunostains for S-100 protein and CDI$_a$ may be helpful in identifying the characteristic Langerhans' cells of Langerhans' cell histiocytosis.

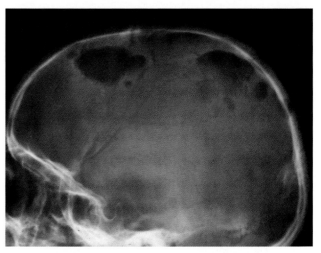

Figure 55–7. This radiograph shows multiple calvarial lesions, most of which are serpiginous with sharp margination. This is one of the radiographic appearances of Langerhans' cell histiocytosis.

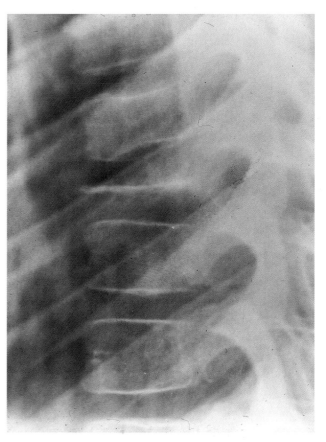

Figure 55–8. Uniform compression of a thoracic vertebra is shown in this radiograph. This condition, termed "vertebra plana," is another presentation of Langerhans' cell histiocytosis.

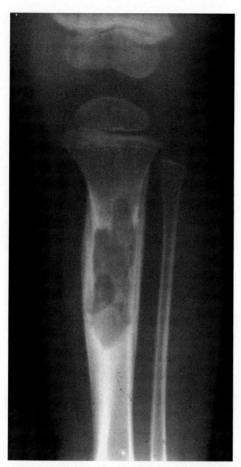

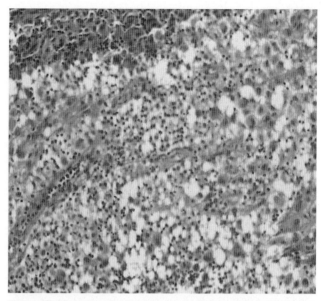

Figure 55–10. At low magnification, lesional tissue in Langerhans' cell histiocytosis often has a loose, edematous appearance, as in this case of an L4 vertebral lesion.

Figure 55–9. This radiograph demonstrates the typical appearance of Langerhans' cell histiocytosis involving the tibial diaphysis. The medullary lesion has a serpiginous margin that is well defined. The "hole within a hole" appearance and the thick, solid periosteal new bone formation are also characteristic.

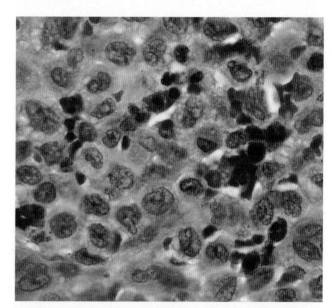

Figure 55–11. At high magnification, the cytologic features of the nuclei of the Langerhans' cells are identifiable. The nucleus is oval or bean-shaped and has a characteristic longitudinal groove if viewed en face.

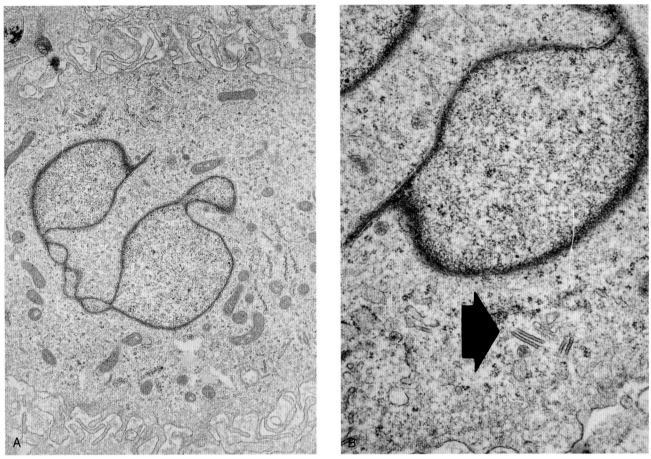

Figure 55–12. Ultrastructural investigation can help in identifying the characteristic features of Langerhans' cell histiocytosis. The lobulated nucleus is identifiable (*A*), but the feature that is diagnostic of the condition is the presence of the characteristic granules *(arrow) (B).*

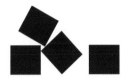

VASCULAR TUMORS

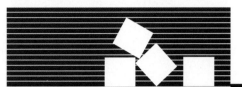

CHAPTER 56

Hemangioma

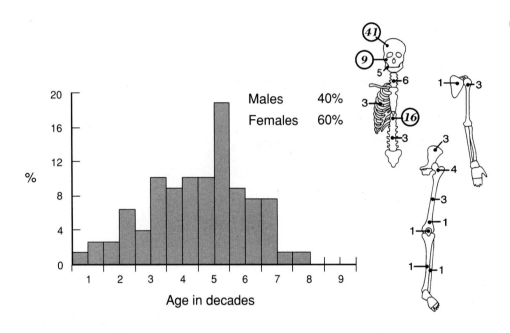

Males   40%
Females 60%

% — Age in decades

CLINICAL SIGNS

1. Local pain and swelling are frequently seen in cases involving the skull and ribs.
2. Vertebral lesions may result in a compression fracture and resultant neurologic signs.
3. Severe hemorrhage may be encountered at the time of surgery.

CLINICAL SYMPTOMS

1. The majority of hemangiomas are incidental findings on radiography.

2. Swelling is frequently noted and is related to expansion of the affected bone. This is particularly true of lesions involving the skull.
3. Local pain is a less common complaint.
4. Spinal lesions may produce spinal cord compression.

MAJOR RADIOGRAPHIC FEATURES

1. In the calvarium the features are as follows:
   a. The lesion is small and oval with sharp margins.
   b. The lesion has a sunburst or granular appearance.
   c. Fifteen per cent are multicentric.

2. In the spine the features are as follows:
   a. The lesion has a "corduroy" or honeycomb appearance.
   b. The lesion has a polka-dot appearance on computed tomography (CT) scan.
   c. The lesion may have a soft tissue mass or an associated pathologic fracture.
3. In the long bones there is no specific appearance.

RADIOGRAPHIC DIFFERENTIAL DIAGNOSIS

1. For calvarial lesions:
   a. Langherhans' cell histiocytosis.
   b. Epidermoid cyst.
2. For vertebral lesions:
   a. Paget's disease.
   b. Metastatic carcinoma.
3. For long bone lesions:
   a. Angiosarcoma.
   b. Other sarcomas.

MAJOR PATHOLOGIC FEATURES

Gross

1. Grossly, these lesions are soft, friable, red, and bloody.
2. Tumors may be more firm and fleshy if they are capillary in type.
3. Bony trabeculae coursing through the tumor may be grossly evident and are the counterpart of the "sunburst" seen radiographically in some cases.

Microscopic

1. At low magnification, these lesions may show large, cavernous vascular spaces or small capillary-type vascular spaces.
2. The vascular nature is evident at low magnification, with the vascular spaces being lined by a thin, attenuated endothelial lining.
3. At higher magnification, the endothelial cells are inconspicuous, as are their nuclei, which are small and dark.

PATHOLOGIC DIFFERENTIAL DIAGNOSIS

Benign lesions:

1. Disappearing bone disease.
2. Lymphangioma.

Malignant lesions:

1. Angiosarcoma.
2. Adamantinoma.

TREATMENT

Primary Modality: Observation is recommended for the usual lesion with an asymptomatic presentation. Curettage and grafting are used for the symptomatic lesion.

Other Possible Approaches: The symptomatic spinal lesion is treated with radiation therapy, with a dose of 3000 to 4000 rads. Surgical treatment with laminectomy is reserved for patients with spinal cord compression. Spinal angiography is helpful in these instances.

References

Asch MJ, Cohen AH, and Moore TC: Hepatic and splenic lymphangiomatosis with skeletal involvement: report of a case and review of the literature. Surgery 76:334–339, 1974.

Dorfman HD, Steiner GC, and Jeffe JL: Vascular tumors of bone. Hum Pathol 2:349–376, 1971.

Karlin CA, and Brower AC: Multiple primary hemangiomas of bone. AJR 129:162–164, 1977.

Keel SB, and Rosenberg AE: Hemorrhagic epithelioid and spindle cell hemangioma: a newly recognized, unique vascular tumor of bone. Cancer 85(9):1966–1972, 1999.

Kleer CG, Unni KK, and McLeod RA: Epithelioid hemangioendothelioma of bone. Am J Surg Pathol 20(11):1301–1311, 1996.

Tillman RM, Choong PF, Beabout JW, et al: Epithelioid hemangioendothelioma of bone. Orthopedics 20(2):177–180, 1997.

Unni KK, Ivins JC, Beabout JW, and Dahlin DC: Hemangioma, hemangiopericytoma, and hemangioendothelioma (angiosarcoma) of bone. Cancer 27:1403–1414, 1971.

Wenger DE, and Wold LE: Benign vascular lesions of bone: radiologic and pathologic features. Skeletal Radiol 29(2):63–74, 2000.

Wold LE, Swee RG, and Sim FH:. Vascular lesions of bone. Pathol Annu 20 Pt 2:101–137, 1985.

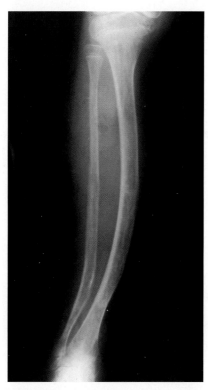

Figure 56–1. This radiograph shows an extensive hemangioma of the lower leg involving the soft tissues as well as the tibia and fibula. The bones contain lytic areas and are attenuated and bowed.

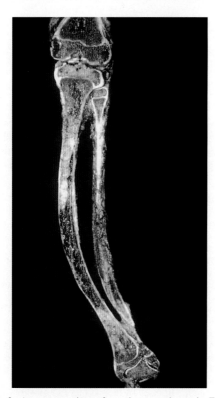

Figure 56–2. A gross specimen from the case shown in Figure 56–1 demonstrates the marked bowing of the tibia and fibula that was evident radiographically. Grossly, hemangiomas are red, hemorrhagic lesions that may bleed extensively at the time of biopsy.

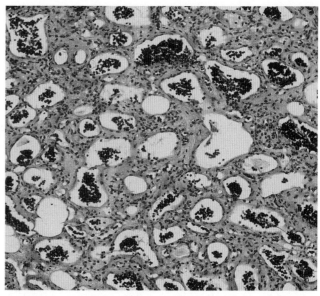

Figure 56–3. At low magnification, hemangiomas may show large, dilated vascular spaces, as seen in this case. Such lesions are termed "cavernous hemangiomas." In other cases, small, capillary-like spaces may predominate; these lesions are termed "capillary hemangiomas."

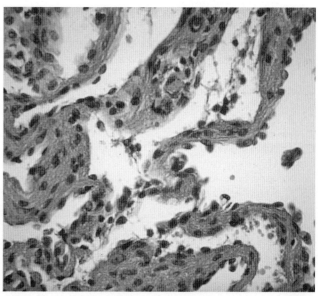

Figure 56–4. At high magnification, the endothelial cells lining the vascular spaces are inconspicuous. This feature helps to distinguish hemangiomas from low-grade angiosarcoma. The nuclei of the endothelial cells in a hemangioma are dark-staining and are flattened adjacent to the vascular lumina.

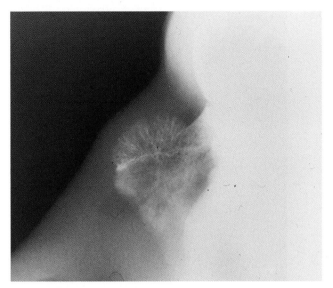

Figure 56–5. This radiograph illustrates the "sunburst" appearance of a hemangioma involving the nasal bones. This appearance is due to the presence of radiating spicules of bone in the lesion.

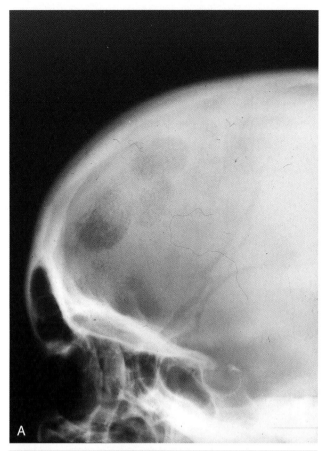

A

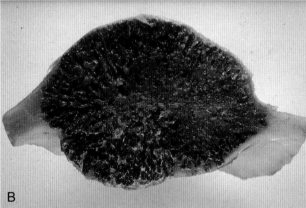

B

Figure 56–6. The calvarium is a common location for hemangiomas. *A,* This radiograph illustrates multicentric involvement showing three frontal bone lesions with sharp margination and a granular appearance. The gross appearance of such calvarial hemangiomas is shown in *B.* The radiating spicules of bone are visible traversing the lesion.

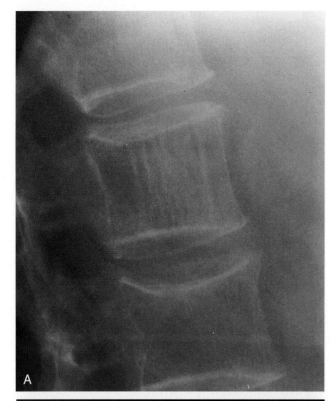

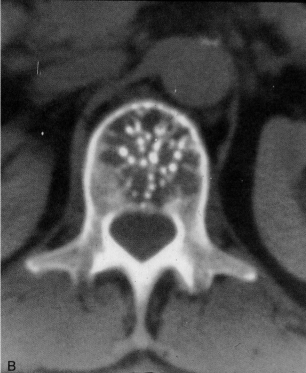

Figure 56–7. *A,* The coarse vertical trabecular appearance of a vertebral hemangioma results in the so-called corduroy vertebra. *B* shows the computed tomographic (CT) cross-sectional appearance of a similar vertebral hemangioma. In cross-section, the coarse trabeculae result in a polka-dot pattern.

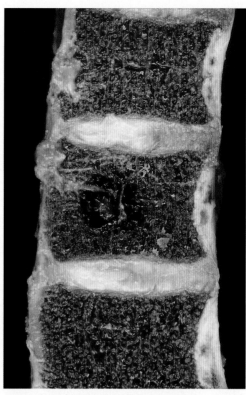

Figure 56–8. Grossly, hemangiomas of the vertebrae, shown in this photograph, are common findings during postmortem examination. Such lesions are small and generally clinically silent.

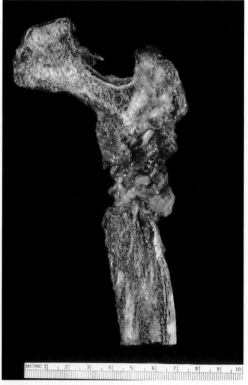

Figure 56–9. This gross specimen of the proximal femur exhibits the bony dissolution associated with phantom bone disease (massive osteolysis, Gorham's disease).

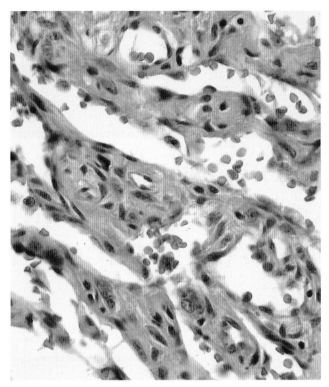

Figure 56–10. The histologic features of phantom bone disease are often indistinguishable from those of a hemangioma, as this femoral lesion demonstrates. The clinical history is often helpful in differentiating these two conditions.

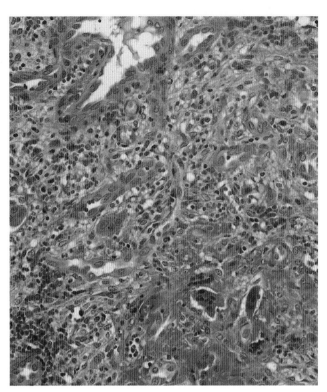

Figure 56–12. Some hemangiomas may appear histologically more solid, as in this example from the fibula. In addition, the endothelial cells of such tumors may become more plump, showing epithelioid cytologic features. Such tumors have been designated "epithelioid hemangiomas."

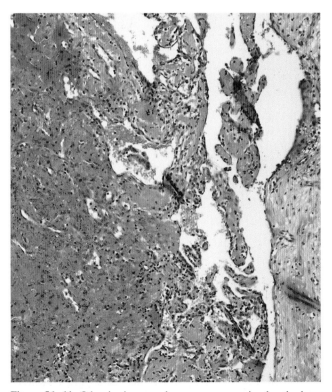

Figure 56–11. Other benign vascular processes may involve the bone and show a histologic pattern similar to that of a hemangioma. This photomicrograph shows an arteriovenous fistula with associated thrombus formation that resulted in a distal fibular defect.

CHAPTER 57

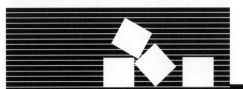

Hemangioendothelioma, Epithelioid Hemangioendothelioma, and Angiosarcoma

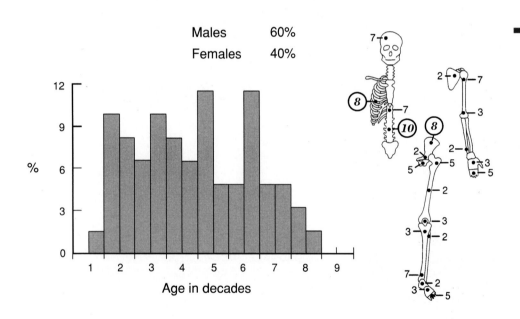

Males 60%
Females 40%

CLINICAL SIGNS

1. Local tenderness may be the only finding on physical examination.

CLINICAL SYMPTOMS

1. Pain is the usual clinical symptom.
2. Rarely, a mass may be noted if the lesion involves a superficial bone.

MAJOR RADIOGRAPHIC FEATURES

1. There is no specific radiographic appearance.
2. The most common pattern is that of a purely lytic lesion without periosteal reaction.
3. The radiographic appearance correlates with the histologic grade. High-grade lesions appear more permeative and destructive than do low-grade lesions.
4. Multifocal disease may be seen and, when present, frequently tends to cluster in one anatomic region.

RADIOGRAPHIC DIFFERENTIAL DIAGNOSIS

1. Osteosarcoma.
2. Fibrosarcoma.
3. Malignant fibrous histiocytoma.
4. Malignant lymphoma.
5. Metastatic carcinoma.
6. Hemangioma.

MAJOR PATHOLOGIC FEATURES

Gross

1. The lesional tissue is usually grossly red and bloody.
2. Tumors vary in consistency but are generally soft. Residual bony trabeculae may be present, particularly in low-grade lesions, giving the tumor a firmer consistency.
3. Necrotic tumor may be present but is most often seen in high-grade lesions.

Microscopic

1. The histologic features vary considerably in this group from low-grade tumors, which are obviously vasoformative, to high-grade, which may show areas of spindle cell proliferation without obvious vessel formation.
2. Low-grade tumors show plump endothelial cells lining vascular spaces. At higher magnification, the nuclei may appear histiocytoid or epithelioid. High-grade tumors show greater cytologic variation and mitotic activity and less histologic differentiation than their low-grade counterparts.
3. The radiographic appearance correlates with the histologic grade. High-grade lesions appear more permeative and destructive than do low-grade lesions.
4. Reticulin stains may be helpful in defining the vascular nature of the tumor by showing that the proliferating cells are clustered within a meshwork of reticulin fibers.
5. Immunohistochemical stains for endothelial and mesenchymal markers (e.g., Factor VIII–related antigen and vimentin) are variably positive.

PATHOLOGIC DIFFERENTIAL DIAGNOSIS

Benign lesions:

1. Hemangioma.
2. Disappearing bone disease.

Malignant lesions:

1. Metastatic carcinoma.
2. Fibrosarcoma.
3. Telangiectatic osteosarcoma.
4. Adamantinoma.

TREATMENT

Primary Modality: Treatment is dependent upon the grade of the lesion. Low-grade lesions that are unifocal may be treated with en bloc resection with a wide surgical margin. Low-grade multifocal lesions may be effectively treated with radiation therapy or amputation. High-grade lesions may be treated with either radiation therapy or ablative surgery, although some lesions are amenable to limb-saving resection.

Other Possible Approaches: Chemotherapy has been used with limited success in some cases of high-grade tumors.

References

Campanacci M, Boriani S, and Giunti A: Hemangioendothelioma of bone: a study of 29 cases. Cancer 46:804–814, 1980.

Dorfman HD, Steiner GC, and Jaffe HL: Vascular tumors of bone. Hum Pathol 2:349–376, 1971.

Garcia-Moral CA: Malignant hemangioendothelioma of bone: review of world literature and report of two cases. Clin Orthop 82:70–79, 1972.

Kleer CG, Unni KK, and McLeod RA: Epithelioid hemangioendothelioma of bone. Am J Surg Pathol 20(11):1301–1311, 1996.

Rosai J, Gold J, and Landy R: The histiocytoid hemangiomas: a unifying concept embracing several previously described entities of skin, soft tissue, large vessels, bone, and heart. Hum Pathol 10:707–730, 1979.

Tillman RM, Choong PF, Beabout JW, et al: Epithelioid hemangioendothelioma of bone. Orthopedics 20(2):177–180, 1997.

Unni KK, Ivins JC, Beabout JW, and Dahlin DC: Hemangioma, hemangiopericytoma, and hemangioendothelioma (angiosarcoma) of bone. Cancer 27:1403–1414, 1971.

Volpe R, and Mazabraud A: Hemangioendothelioma (angiosarcoma) of bone: a distinct pathologic entity with an unpredictable course. Cancer 49:727–736, 1982.

Weiss SW, and Enzinger FM: Epithelioid hemangioendothelioma: a vascular tumor often mistaken for a carcinoma. Cancer 50:970–981, 1982.

Wold LE, Unni KK, Beabout JW, et al: Hemangioendothelial sarcoma of bone. Am J Surg Pathol 6:59–70, 1982.

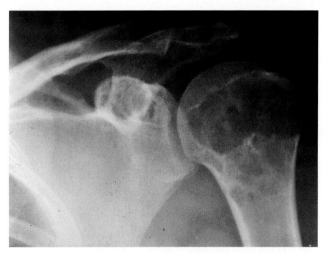

Figure 57–1. This radiograph of the shoulder shows a multicentric, purely lytic process involving the clavicle, scapula, and humerus. The presence of multiple lesions, generally purely lytic in character, in the same anatomic region suggests a diagnosis of angiosarcoma.

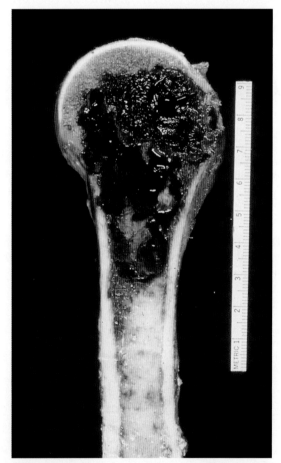

Figure 57–2. The gross specimen in this case of multicentric angiosarcoma correlates well with its radiographic appearance. These tumors generally are red and hemorrhagic. Although the tumor has not extended into the adjacent soft tissue, cortical erosion is evident.

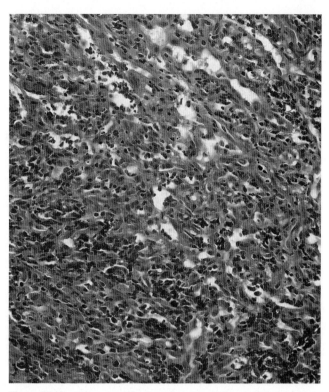

Figure 57–3. At low magnification, these tumors are variable in appearance. In general, however, their vasoformative nature is evident. Most commonly, the vascular spaces are small, as demonstrated in this lesion from the humerus.

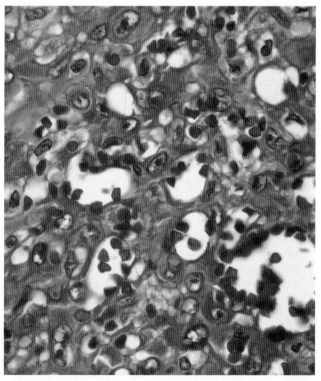

Figure 57–4. At high magnification, the cytologic atypia of these lesions varies from case to case. As this photomicrograph shows, the nuclei are plump, hyperchromatic, and variable in shape. They bulge into the vascular lumina, and tufting may occasionally be seen.

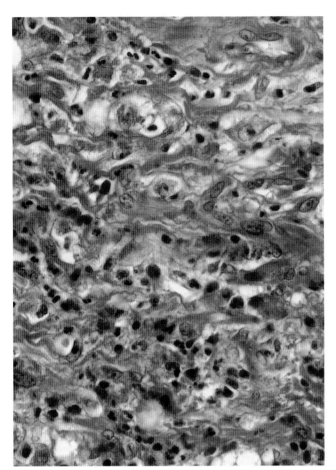

Figure 57–16. Eosinophils are commonly found in benign and malignant vascular tumors. This example of a high-grade angiosarcoma has numerous eosinophils in a region of the tumor that shows little vasoformative morphology.

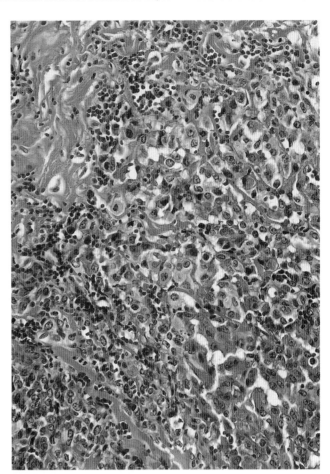

Figure 57–17. High-grade angiosarcomas may show little vasoformation and may even have "epitheliod" cytologic features, as in this tumor of the ilium.

CHAPTER 58

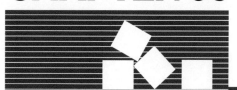

Hemangiopericytoma

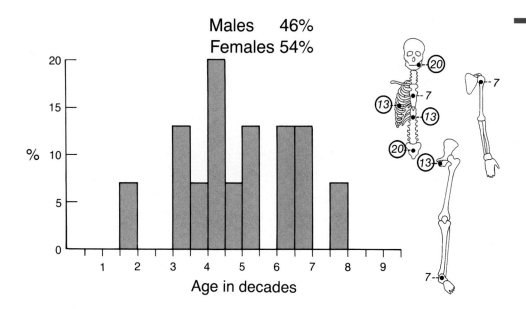

Males 46%
Females 54%

% (y-axis: 0, 5, 10, 15, 20)

Age in decades (x-axis: 1–9)

CLINICAL SIGNS

1. A mass lesion is palpable on physical examination.
2. The mass most commonly is tender to palpation.

CLINICAL SYMPTOMS

1. Local pain is present.
2. Swelling is noted in the region of the tumor.

MAJOR RADIOGRAPHIC FEATURES

1. This rare primary tumor of bone generally has a nonspecific radiographic appearance.
2. More than two thirds are purely lytic.
3. Most have a malignant appearance, and their radiographic appearance roughly correlates with the histologic grade of the tumor.
4. A honeycomb appearance occasionally is seen.

RADIOGRAPHIC DIFFERENTIAL DIAGNOSIS

1. Any lytic primary bone tumor.
2. Lytic metastatic tumors of bone.

MAJOR PATHOLOGIC FEATURES

Gross

1. The tumor is usually firm.
2. The lesional tissue is most often red and bloody.

Microscopic

1. At low magnification, this tumor is composed of round to oval cells.
2. The tumor is hypercellular.
3. Numerous thin-walled blood vessels course through the tumor.
4. The blood vessels are branched and "staghorn" in shape.
5. At higher magnification, the degree of cytologic atypia is variable.
6. Mitotic activity in the tumor is also variable.
7. No matrix is produced by the tumor cells.

PATHOLOGIC DIFFERENTIAL DIAGNOSIS

Benign lesions:

1. Glomus tumor.
2. Capillary hemangioma.

Malignant lesions:

1. Mesenchymal chondrosarcoma.
2. Small cell osteosarcoma.

3. Metastatic hemangiopericytoma (particularly common with hemangiopericytomas of the meninges).

TREATMENT

Primary Modality: En bloc resection with a wide margin and skeletal reconstruction if feasible. Amputation may be necessary to achieve an adequately wide margin.

Other Possible Approaches: Radiotherapy for surgically inaccessible lesions. Multiple drug chemotherapy protocols used in an adjuvant setting may be employed.

References

Dunlop J: Primary haemangiopericytoma of bone: report of two cases. J Bone Joint Surg (Br) 55:854–857, 1973.
Tang JS, Gold RH, Mirra JM, and Eckardt J: Hemangiopericytoma of bone. Cancer 62(4):848–859, 1988.
Vang PS, and Falk E: Haemangiopericytoma of bone. Review of the literature and report of a case. Acta Orthop Scand 51(6):903–907, 1980.
Wold LW, Unni KK, Cooper KL, et al: Hemangiopericytoma of bone. Am J Surg Pathol 6:53–58, 1982.

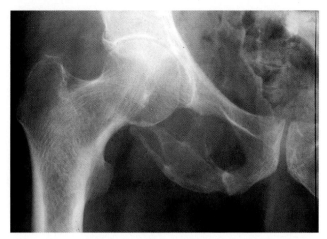

Figure 58–1. This radiograph shows a purely lytic hemangiopericytoma of the ischium. The lesion exhibits features of a malignant lesion but is otherwise nonspecific.

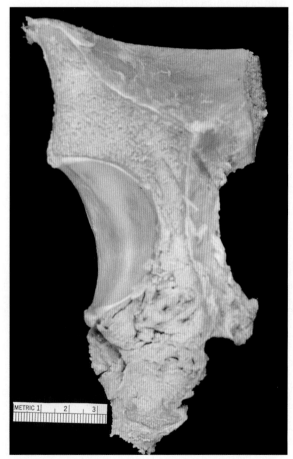

Figure 58–2. Grossly, the ischial hemangiopericytoma is relatively nondescript. The lesional tissue is firm and fibrous. Such tissue may be reddish and bloody.

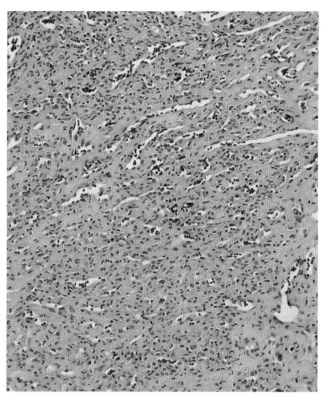

Figure 58–3. This low-power photomicrograph shows a relatively hypocellular tumor composed of void cells arranged around vascular spaces. This tumor of the thoracic vertebra in a 38-year-old man exhibits histologic features of a "benign" hemangiopericytoma.

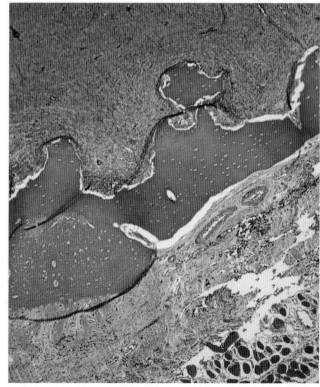

Figure 58–4. At low magnification, more aggressive hemangiopericytomas may show cortical erosion, as is evident in this lesion involving a rib.

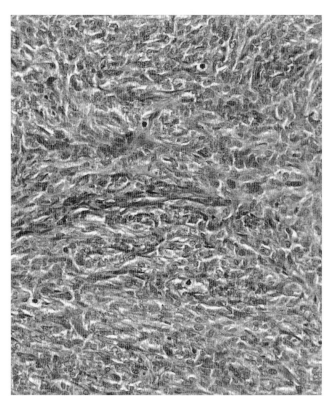

Figure 58–5. Frankly malignant hemangiopericytomas show greater cellular pleomorphism and atypia, as can be seen in this photomicrograph of a primary osseous tumor that also shows moderate mitotic activity.

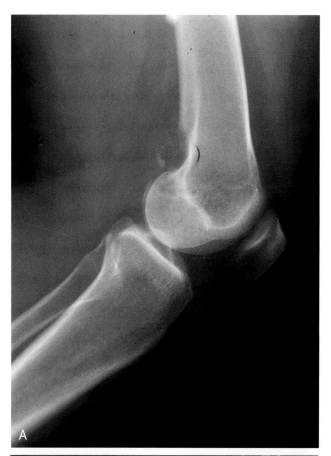

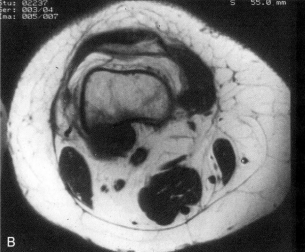

Figure 58–7. A radiograph (*A*) and an axial magnetic resonance imaging (MRI) scan (*B*) of a hemangiopericytoma of the posterior lower femur show destruction of the cortex and extension into the soft tissues. The appearance favors malignancy. The lesion is seen best on MRI.

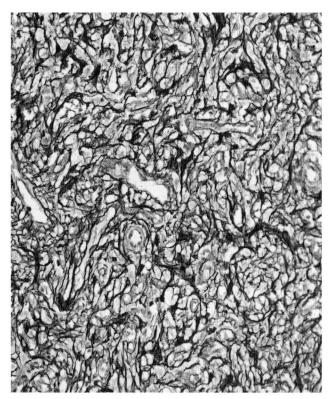

Figure 58–6. A reticulin stain, such as seen here, may accentuate the vascular nature of these tumors. The fine reticulin meshwork that surrounds each cell is helpful in identifying the lesion as a hemangiopericytoma.

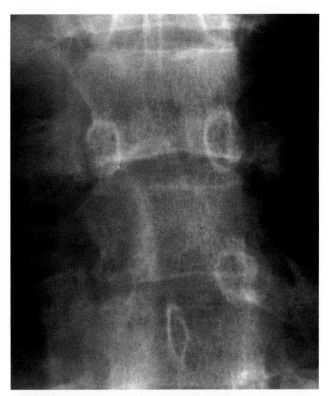

Figure 58–8. Hemangiopericytomas of the meninges show a propensity to osseous metastases, as can be seen in this radiograph of the thoracic spine. Note the lytic destruction of the left pedicle and adjacent vertebral body.

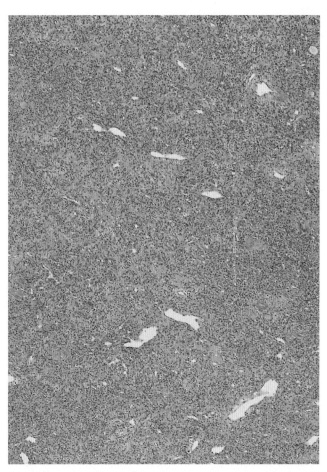

Figure 58–10. The low-power hemangiopericytomatous pattern illustrated in this case of an ischial tumor can also be seen in mesenchymal chondrosarcoma, small cell osteosarcoma, and Ewing's sarcoma. Careful search for matrix in the tumor and immunohistochemical evaluation of the tumor will by exclusion lead to a diagnosis of hemangiopericytoma.

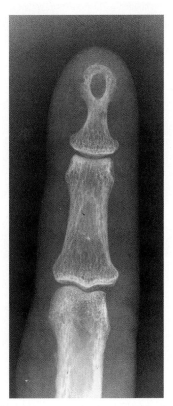

Figure 58–9. Glomus tumors are benign examples of pericytic tumors. These lesions are most commonly identified in the distal phalanx radiographically. Note the well-circumscribed lytic defect of the distal phalangeal tuft in this case.

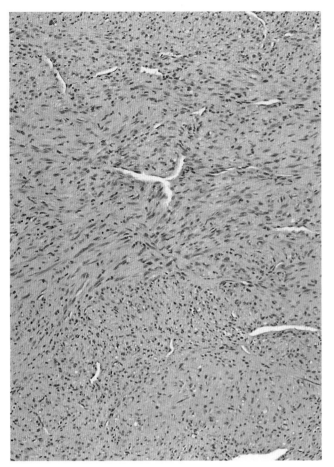

Figure 58–11. A hemangiopericytomatous pattern is commonly seen in cases of congenital fibromatosis, as in this photomicrograph of a skull lesion from a young patient.

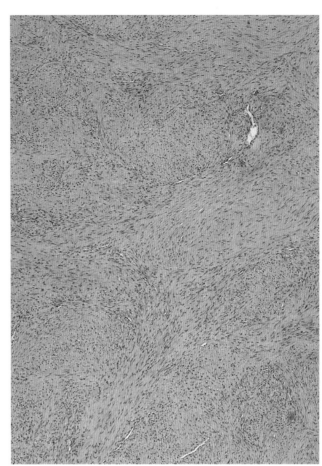

Figure 58–12. A vaguely lobulated pattern is often present in congenital fibromatosis, as in this photomicrograph. Hemangiopericytomas are more uniform in their histologic appearance.

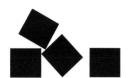

F

TUMORS OF
UNKNOWN ORIGIN

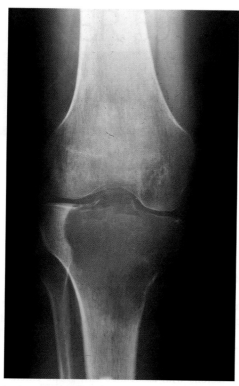

Figure 59–1. This anteroposterior radiograph of the knee shows a large, purely lytic, eccentric lesion involving the proximal tibia. The lesion extends to the end of the bone, and there is expansion of the bone and associated cortical destruction. The features are typical of giant cell tumor.

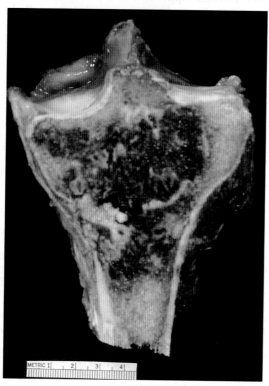

Figure 59–2. The gross pathologic appearance of the lesion correlates well with its radiographic appearance in Figure 59–1. The tumor varies in color from brown to yellow and extends to the articular surface.

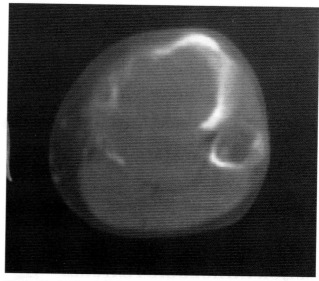

Figure 59–3. The computed tomographic (CT) scan in this case also shows the lesion to be purely lytic, a feature that helps support a diagnosis of giant cell tumor. Cortical destruction and soft tissue extension, evidence of aggressive behavior, are commonly seen in giant cell tumor.

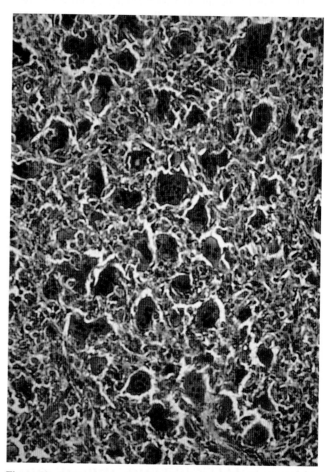

Figure 59–4. At low magnification, giant cell tumor consists of a "sea" of mononuclear cells within which multinucleated giant cells are scattered in a uniform manner.

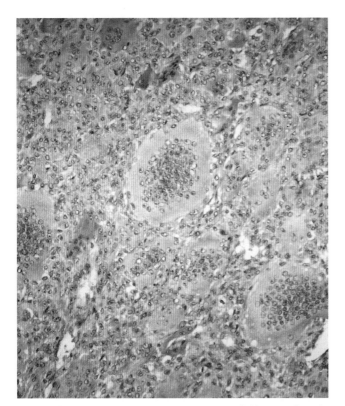

Figure 59–5. Although the histologic appearance of this tumor from the proximal humerus is typical of giant cell tumor, the aggressive radiographic features exhibited by the lesion suggested the possibility of telangiectatic osteosarcoma.

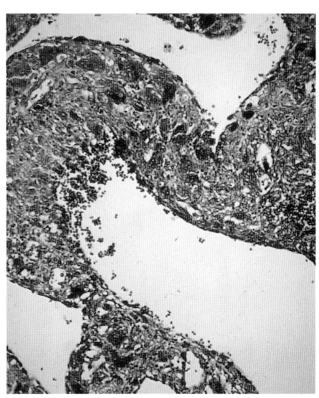

Figure 59–7. Secondary aneurysmal bone cyst may complicate giant cell tumor. In cases such as this, identification of the underlying giant cell tumor may be difficult.

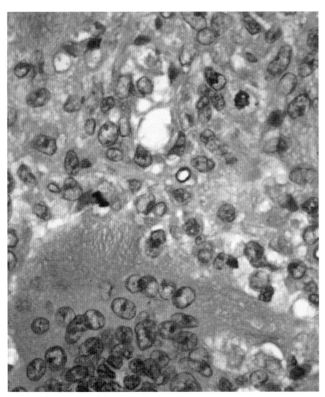

Figure 59–6. At high magnification, the nuclei of the mononuclear stromal cells are similar to those of the multinucleated giant cells. This feature is evident in this tumor from the proximal humerus. Mitotic activity may be brisk in giant cell tumors.

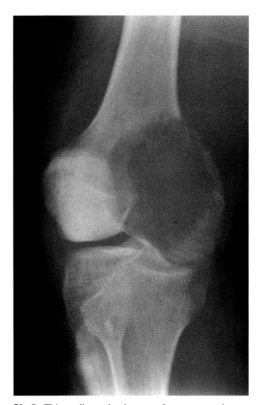

Figure 59–8. This radiograph shows a large, eccentric, aggressive-appearing giant cell tumor of the distal femur. The purely lytic nature of the lesion, its extension to the articular surface, and its eccentric location favor a diagnosis of giant cell tumor.

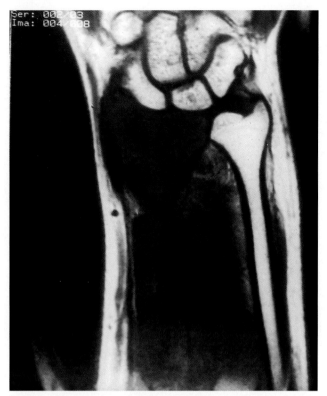

Figure 59–9. This magnetic resonance (MR) image of a giant cell tumor of the distal radius demonstrates the utility of this imaging modality, particularly for tumors in peripheral locations. The distal radius is a common site for giant cell tumor.

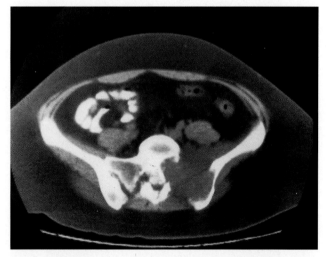

Figure 59–10. As with chordoma, CT scans are helpful in detecting giant cell tumors of the sacrum. These tumors (such as the one shown in this radiograph) may cause extensive destruction of the bone, and the soft tissue involvement generally is better appreciated with CT.

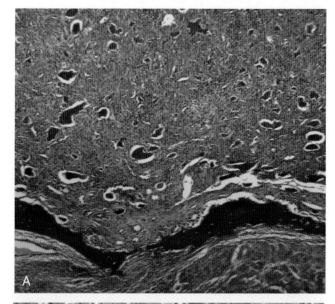

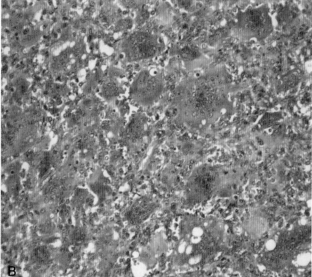

Figure 59–11. A rim of reactive tumor (*A*) frequently surrounds soft tissue recurrences of giant cell tumor. The recurrences—whether osseous, soft tissue, or pulmonary metastases—show the same histologic features as the primary tumor (*B*).

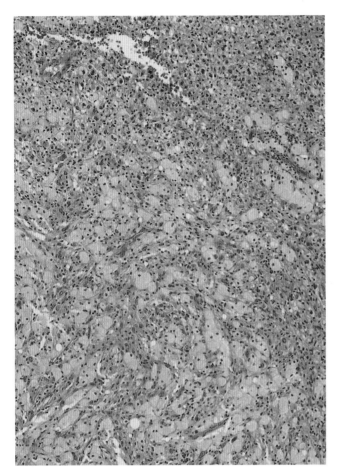

Figure 59–12. Degeneration is common within giant cell tumor. Xanthomatous change is illustrated in this photomicrograph of a distal femoral tumor.

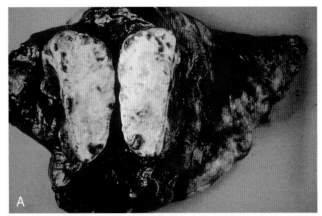

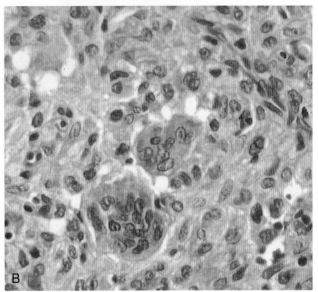

Figure 59–13. The pulmonary metastases, gross pathologic features, (*A*) that rarely complicate the clinical course of treated giant cell tumor exhibit the same cytologic similarity between mononuclear and multinucleated cells, as shown in this photomicrograph (*B*).

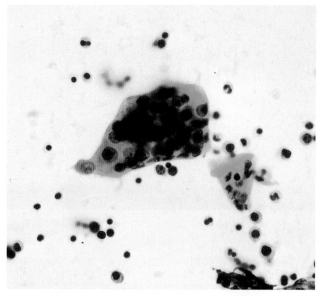

Figure 59–14. Aspiration biopsy of giant cell tumors generally shows numerous multinucleated giant cells, as seen in this aspirate of a sacral lesion.

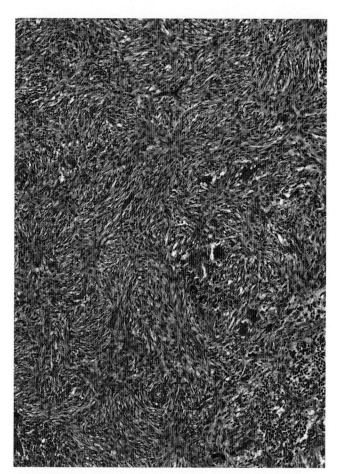

Figure 59–16. Although giant cell tumor typically does not contain spindle cells, some tumors show a fibrous histiocytoma-like pattern, as in this case of a giant cell tumor of the proximal fibula.

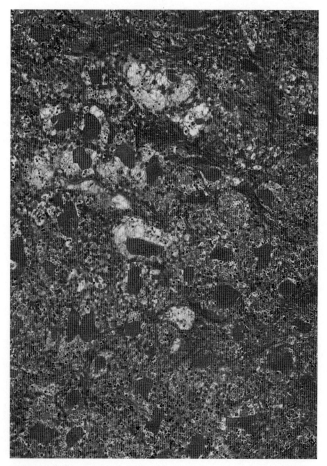

Figure 59–15. Giant cell tumors may become infarcted, as in this tumor from the proximal humerus. "Ghost" tumor cells and giant cells may be seen in such cases.

CHAPTER 60

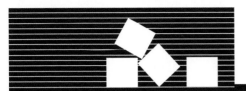

Malignancy in Giant Cell Tumor (Malignant Giant Cell Tumor)

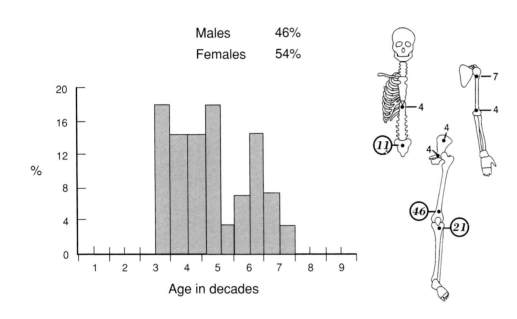

Males   46%
Females   54%

%

Age in decades

CLINICAL SIGNS

1. A tender mass lesion in the region of a previously treated giant cell tumor is commonly present on physical examination.
2. Cutaneous changes from prior radiation therapy are commonly found.

CLINICAL SYMPTOMS

1. Pain is the most common symptom.
2. Nearly all patients give a history of a previous giant cell tumor having been treated more than ten years (on average) before the recent onset of pain.

3. Seventy-five per cent of patients have received prior radiation therapy as part of treatment for the giant cell tumor.
4. Only rarely is an abrupt change in the symptoms related to the development of a "malignant giant cell tumor" in a patient who has not received prior radiation therapy.

MAJOR RADIOGRAPHIC FEATURES

1. A de novo malignant giant cell tumor has the same radiographic appearance as a benign giant cell tumor, and the two cannot be distinguished.
2. A secondary malignant giant cell tumor is usually seen

363

many years (average of 10 to 13 years) after treatment that included radiation therapy.
3. Serial changes that occur more than three years after the original treatment are highly suspect for secondary malignant giant cell tumor.

RADIOGRAPHIC DIFFERENTIAL DIAGNOSIS

1. Benign giant cell tumor.
2. Recurrent giant cell tumor.
3. Osteomyelitis.

MAJOR PATHOLOGIC FEATURES

Gross

1. The tumor expands the end of the bone and generally has broken through the cortex.
2. Zones of necrosis are identifiable; however, necrosis can be seen in benign giant cell tumors as well.
3. Extension into the surrounding soft tissue is generally present.
4. Hemorrhagic foci may also be identified.

Microscopic

1. At low magnification, the tumor is hypercellular and generally is composed of spindle cells.
2. Matrix production may be, but generally is not, present.
3. The arrangement of the spindle cells may be in a "herringbone," storiform, or haphazard pattern.
4. At higher magnification, the spindle cells show marked pleomorphism and nuclear atypia characterized by variation in size, shape, and staining qualities.
5. In general, mitotic activity is brisk.
6. Most commonly, no residual benign giant cell tumor is identifiable in the lesion. On rare occasions, however, zones of otherwise typical giant cell tumor may be identified adjacent to the high-grade sarcoma.

PATHOLOGIC DIFFERENTIAL DIAGNOSIS

Benign lesions:

1. Giant cell tumor.
2. Metaphyseal fibrous defect (fibroma).

Malignant lesions:

1. Osteosarcoma.
2. Fibrosarcoma.
3. Malignant fibrous histiocytoma.

TREATMENT

Primary Modality: Preoperative chemotherapy and wide surgical resection. Aggressive behavior and extensive involvement often mandate amputation to achieve an adequate margin.

Other Possible Approaches: Chemotherapy, radiation therapy for surgically inaccessible lesions, and thoracotomy for metastatic pulmonary disease.

References

Hutter RVP, Worcester JN Jr, Francis KC, et al: Benign and malignant giant cell tumors of bone: a clinicopathological analysis of the natural history of the disease. Cancer *15*:653–690, 1962.

Meis JM, Dorfman HD, Nathanson SD, et al: Primary malignant giant cell tumor of bone: "dedifferentiated" giant cell tumor. Mod Pathol *2*:541–546, 1995.

Nascimento AG, Huvos AG, and Marcove RC: Primary malignant giant cell tumor of bone: a study of eight cases and review of the literature. Cancer *44*:1393–1402, 1979.

Ortiz-Cruz EJ, Quinn RH, Fanburg JC, et al: Late development of a malignant fibrous histiocytoma at the site of a giant cell tumor. Clin Orthop *318*:199–204, 1995.

Rock MG, Sim FH, Unni KK, et al: Secondary malignant giant-cell tumor of bone. Clinicopathological assessment of nineteen patients. J Bone Joint Surg Am *68(7)*:1073–1079, 1986.

Sanerkin NG: Malignancy, aggressiveness, and recurrence in giant cell tumor of bone. Cancer *46*:1641–1649, 1980.

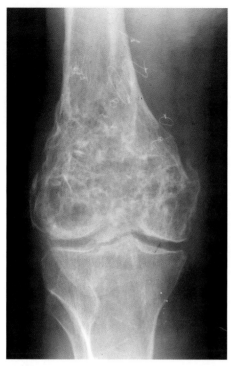

Figure 60–1. This radiograph shows a sarcoma arising from the site of a prior benign giant cell tumor. The development of the sarcoma is often obscured by the distortion caused by the previous tumor. In many cases, serial studies are essential to make the diagnosis with confidence.

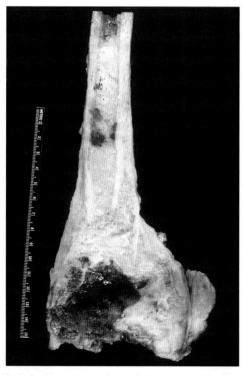

Figure 60–2. In this gross specimen of the tumor seen in Figure 60–1, the distal femur has been replaced by a firm fibrous tumor, which has destroyed the medial cortex of the femur. This sarcoma, which showed the histologic pattern of growth of a fibrosarcoma, occurred in a patient who had received radiation therapy for a giant cell tumor 12 years previously.

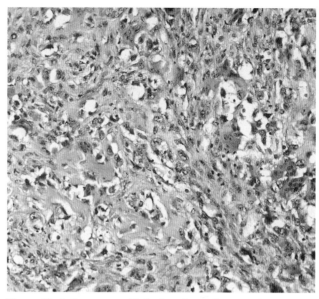

Figure 60–3. In contrast with benign giant cell tumors, in which the mononuclear cells contain nuclei similar to those in the multinucleated giant cells, malignancies arising in giant cell tumors show marked nuclear pleomorphism, as this photomicrograph illustrates.

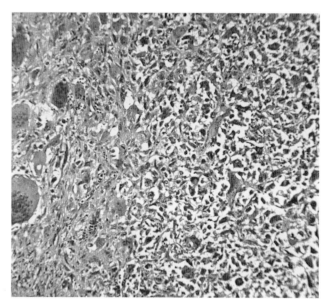

Figure 60–4. Although malignancy is rarely identified de novo in giant cell tumors, when such cases are encountered, both a benign giant cell tumor component and a sarcoma should be histologically identifiable. This photomicrograph shows a distal femoral tumor from a 28-year-old man that radiographically was classic for a benign giant cell tumor. Histologically, the lesion shows a pattern typical of benign giant cell tumor as well as a sarcomatous component.

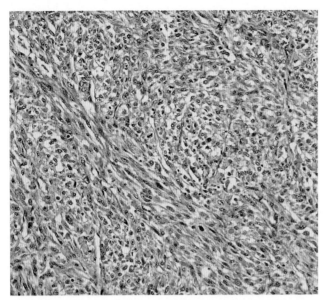

Figure 60–5. Malignancies that arise in the region of a prior giant cell tumor almost uniformly consist of spindle-shaped cells. This tumor shows some features of a malignant fibrous histiocytoma. Osseous and chondroid matrix production may also be evident in these tumors.

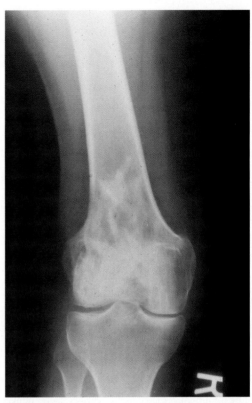

Figure 60–7. This radiograph demonstrates the appearance of a distal femur 16 years after curettage, grafting, and radiation therapy for a benign giant cell tumor.

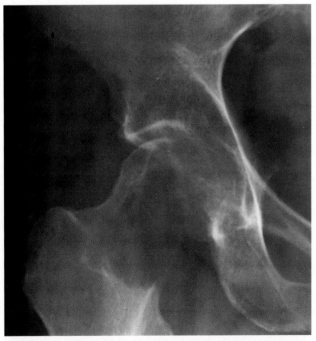

Figure 60–6. This radiograph shows a de novo malignant giant cell tumor of the proximal femur, characterized by an aggressive appearance and lytic destruction extending to the bone end. Benign giant cell tumors may also cause this type of change.

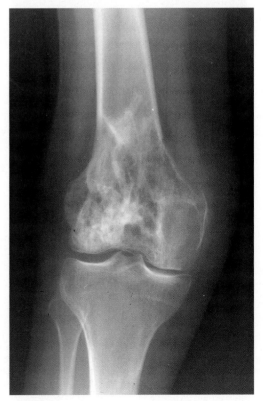

Figure 60–8. In this view, taken five months after the radiograph shown in Figure 60–7, the appearance of the lesion has changed. Lytic destruction due to secondary fibrosarcoma has developed.

CHAPTER 61

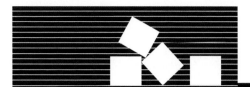

Adamantinoma

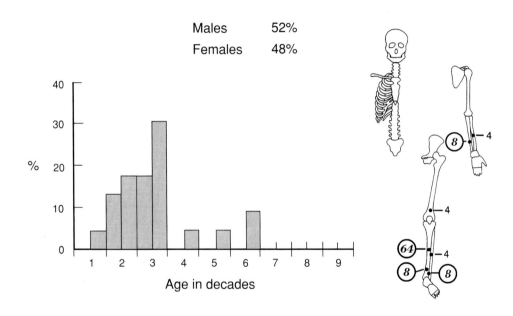

Males   52%
Females   48%

CLINICAL SIGNS

1. A mass lesion is the only usual finding on physical examination.

CLINICAL SYMPTOMS

1. Pain is the most common initial symptom.
2. A mass lesion is rarely the initial symptom.
3. The duration of symptoms may be several months to many years.

MAJOR RADIOGRAPHIC FEATURES

1. The lesion occurs in the diaphysis of the tibia.
2. Eccentric lucencies are connected by sclerosis.
3. A dominant central lesion is present.

4. Expansion of the affected bone is common.
5. Multicentricity of the lesion may be present.
6. The fibula may be affected as well.

RADIOGRAPHIC DIFFERENTIAL DIAGNOSIS

1. Osteofibrous dysplasia.
2. Fibrous dysplasia.
3. Fibroma.

MAJOR PATHOLOGIC FEATURES
Gross

1. These tumors tend to be well circumscribed at their periphery and arranged in a lobulated fashion.

2. The tumor is generally gray or white.
3. The consistency varies from firm and fibrous to soft.
4. Cystic spaces containing blood or straw-colored fluid may be encountered.

Microscopic

1. The tumors may show a myriad of histologic patterns; however, they share an epithelioid low-power pattern.
2. The most common pattern is that of epithelioid islands of cells with peripheral columnar cells showing nuclear palisading.
3. Toward the center of the epithelioid islands, the cells are arranged in a looser pattern with spindling (stellate reticulum–like appearance).
4. Hypocellular fibrous connective tissue occupies the space between the epithelioid islands, and disorganized bone may be seen in these regions, resulting in a pattern that mimics osteofibrous dysplasia.
5. The epithelioid islands may show squamous cytologic features and even keratin production.
6. A vascular pattern with the spaces merging into the epithelial islands is common.
7. The tumor may be purely spindle-celled, mimicking fibrosarcoma; however, a cortical location and a lack of cytologic atypia should suggest a diagnosis of adamantinoma.

PATHOLOGIC DIFFERENTIAL DIAGNOSIS

Benign lesions:

1. Osteofibrous dysplasia.
2. Fibrous dysplasia.

Malignant lesions:

1. Metastatic carcinoma.
2. Angiosarcoma.

TREATMENT

Primary Modality: En bloc removal with a wide surgical margin is done. Reconstruction of the bone can be achieved with an intercalary allograft or vascularized fibular graft. Amputation may be necessary for large or recurrent lesions.

Other Possible Approaches: Simple excision with a marginal margin is discouraged because of a high recurrence rate. Therapeutic lymph node dissection has occasionally been necessary for metastatic disease.

References

Campanacci M, Giunti A, Bertoni F, et al: Adamantinoma of the long bones: the experience at the Istituto Ortopedico Rizzoli. Am J Surg Pathol 5:533–542, 1981.
Keeney GL, Unni KK, Beabout JW, and Pritchard DJ: Adamantinoma of long bones. A clinicopathologic study of 85 cases. Cancer 64(3):730–737, 1989.
Knapp RH, Wick MR, Scheithauer BW, and Unni KK: Adamantinoma of bone: an electron microscopic and immunohistochemical study. Virchows Arch (Pathol Anat) 398:75–86, 1982.
Rock MG, Beabout JW, Unni KK, and Sim FH: Adamantinoma. Orthopedics 6:472–477, 1983.
Rosai J, and Pinkus GS: Immunohistochemical demonstration of epithelial differentiation in adamantinoma of the tibia. Am J Surg Pathol 6:427–434, 1982.
Weiss SW, and Dorfman HD: Adamantinoma of long bones: an analysis of nine new cases with emphasis on metastasizing lesions and fibrous dysplasia–like changes. Hum Pathol 8:141–153, 1977.

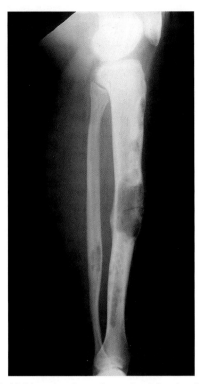

Figure 61–1. Multicentric adamantinoma involving the tibia and fibula is shown in this radiograph of the lower extremity. Multiple lytic areas with surrounding sclerosis are present. Note the dominant central expansile lesion.

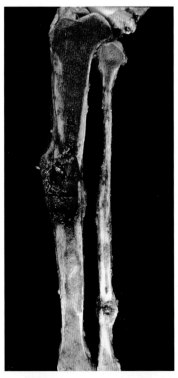

Figure 61–2. The bisected gross specimen in this case reveals the involvement of both the tibia and the fibula, as shown in Figure 61–1. Such multicentric disease is not uncommon; indeed, this gross appearance is virtually diagnostic. The multicentric nature of the disease may explain recurrences in cases treated with marginal excision.

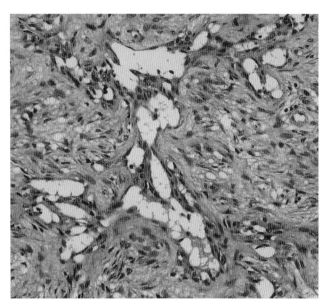

Figure 61–3. The low-power pattern of adamantinoma is that of a lesion composed of islands of epithelioid cells lying within a hypocellular fibrous connective tissue. At the periphery of these islands is a palisading of the nuclei. Toward the center of the islands, the cells have a looser arrangement and a more stellate appearance (so-called stellate reticulum).

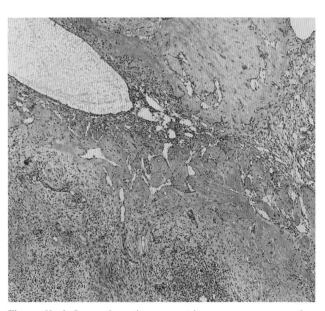

Figure 61–4. Some adamantinomas contain more open spaces; when these are blood-filled, the appearance may mimic that of a vascular neoplasm.

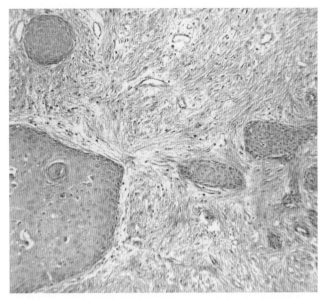

Figure 61–5. Squamous differentiation, as shown in this case, may be so prominent as to mimic the appearance of a squamous cell carcinoma. Other tumors may appear glandular and therefore look like metastatic adenocarcinoma.

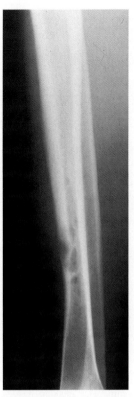

Figure 61–7. Multiple small cortical lucencies are apparent in this example of an adamantinoma involving the tibia. The lucencies are connected by sclerotic regions.

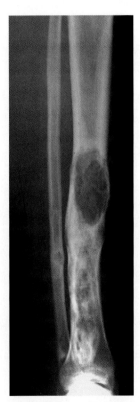

Figure 61–6. The typical appearance of a multicentric adamantinoma involving the tibia and fibula is shown in this radiograph. The dominant lesion involves the diaphysis of the tibia and is centrally located.

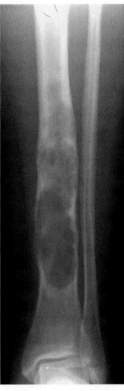

Figure 61–8. Adamantinomas are slow-growing lesions and, as such, may result in significant expansion of the affected bone prior to diagnosis of the lesion. This example shows diaphyseal expansion of the tibia with a sclerotic margin, another feature indicating slow growth.

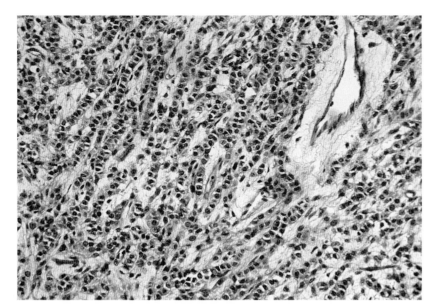

Figure 61–9. At times, the arrangement of the epithelioid cells may give rise to a single-file pattern, mimicking poorly differentiated adenocarcinoma. This tumor had been present in the tibia for 50 years.

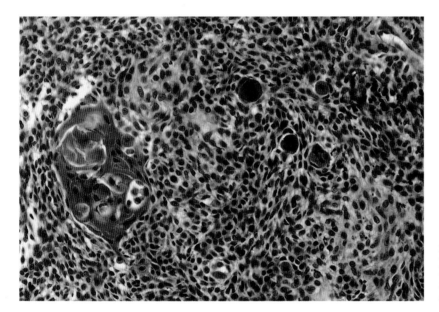

Figure 61–10. Squamous differentiation may be so prominent that squamous pearl formation occurs. Such cases may have a deceptively bland cytologic appearance and suggest the diagnosis of squamous cell carcinoma arising in chronic osteomyelitis.

CHAPTER 62

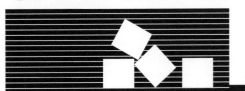

Chordoma

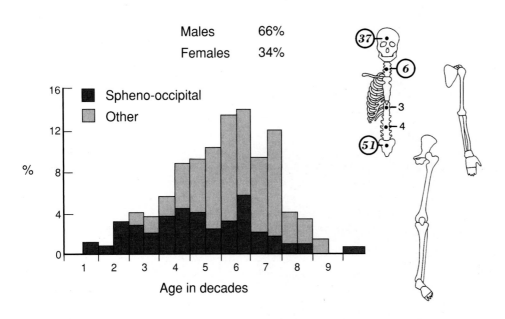

Males   66%
Females   34%

CLINICAL SIGNS

1. Sacral tumors generally extend anteriorly and thus produce a presacral mass appreciable on rectal examination.
2. Spheno-occipital tumors cause cranial nerve VI palsy but may also result in cranial nerve VII and VIII abnormalities. Downward growth may produce a nasopharyngeal mass lesion.
3. Vertebral chordomas give rise to nerve root compression or spinal cord compression signs, but those in the cervical region may also result in symptoms suggestive of a chronic retropharyngeal abscess.

CLINICAL SYMPTOMS

1. Symptoms and duration are variable and depend upon tumor location (sacral, spheno-occipital, or vertebral); however, they are usually of long duration.

2. Sacral tumors nearly always are associated with pain in the sacral or coccygeal region. Constipation may be experienced.
3. Spheno-occipital tumors generally cause symptoms related to involvement of cranial nerves. Of these, cranial nerves VI, VII, and VIII are the most frequently involved.
4. Vertebral chordomas may cause symptoms owing to nerve root or spinal cord compression.

MAJOR RADIOGRAPHIC FEATURES

1. The lesion is in the sacrum or clivus.
2. Midline destruction is seen. (Regardless of location—sacral, clival, or vertebral—all chordomas are midline lesions.)
3. Poor margination and an associated soft tissue mass are commonly present.

4. Fifty per cent of all chordomas are seen to be calcified on radiography.
5. Computed tomography (CT) and magnetic resonance imaging (MRI) are the best modalities to delineate the extent of the lesion.

RADIOGRAPHIC DIFFERENTIAL DIAGNOSIS

1. Metastatic carcinoma.
2. Myeloma.
3. Giant cell tumor.
4. Neurogenic tumor.

MAJOR PATHOLOGIC FEATURES

Gross

1. Chordomas generally are soft, grayish tumors that have a gelatinous consistency grossly.
2. The tumor tends to be well circumscribed and may even show gross lobulation.
3. In both the sacral and the spheno-occipital regions, the tumor tends to elevate the periosteum of the affected bone, extending into the presacral and cranial cavities, respectively.

Microscopic

1. At low magnification, chordomas characteristically are arranged in a lobulated fashion, with fibrous septa separating the lobules.
2. The tumor generally is arranged in chords or strands of cells.
3. Between the chords of cells is abundant intercellular mucoid matrix.
4. At higher magnification, the cells have abundant eosinophilic vacuolated cytoplasm (physaliferous cells). The boundaries between cells in the strands are indistinct, resulting in a syncytial quality.
5. In the spheno-occipital region, some tumors have a histologic appearance very similar to that of chondrosarcoma (chondroid chordoma).

PATHOLOGIC DIFFERENTIAL DIAGNOSIS

Benign lesions:

1. Chondromyxoid fibroma.

Malignant lesions:

1. Metastatic carcinoma.
2. Chordosarcoma.

TREATMENT

Primary Modality: En bloc resection with a marginal or wide margin is performed; sacrificing involved nerve roots provides the best chance for cure. Sacral lesions below the third sacral vertebra can be removed with a posterior approach; lesions above this level are approached both anteriorly and posteriorly.

Other Possible Approaches: Adjuvant radiation therapy is utilized for narrow or contaminated margins and surgically inaccessible lesions. Radiation therapy is particularly helpful for tumors in the spheno-occipital region.

References

Bjornsson J, Wold LE, Ebersold MJ, and Laws ER: Chordoma of the mobile spine. Cancer 71:735–740, 1993.

Chambers PW, and Schwinn CP: Chordoma: a clinicopathologic study of metastasis. Am J Clin Pathol 72:765–776, 1979.

Eriksson B, Gunterberg B, and Kindblom LG: Chordoma: a clinicopathologic and prognostic study of a Swedish national series. Acta Orthop Scand 52:49–58, 1981.

Kaiser TE, Pritchard DJ, and Unni KK: Clinicopathologic study of sacrococcygeal chordoma. Cancer 53:2574–2578, 1984.

Meis JM, Raymond AK, Evans JL, et al: "Dedifferentiated" chordoma. Am J Surg Pathol 11:516–525, 1987.

Mindell ER: Current concepts review: chordoma. J Bone Joint Surg (Am) 63:501–505, 1981.

Mitchell A, Scheithauer BW, Unni KK, et al: Chordoma and chondroid neoplasms of the spheno-occiput. An immunohistochemical study of 41 cases with prognostic and nosologic implications. Cancer 72(10):2943–2949, 1993.

Rosenthal DI, Scott JA, Mankin JH, et al: Sacro-coccygeal chordoma: magnetic resonance imaging and computed tomography. AJR Am J Roentgenol 145:143–147, 1983.

Volpe R, and Mazabraud A: A clinicopathologic review of 25 cases of chordoma (a pleomorphic and metastasizing neoplasm). Am J Surg Pathol 7:161–170, 1983.

Wold LE, and Laws ER Jr: Cranial chordomas in children and young adults. J Neurosurg 59:1043–1047, 1983.

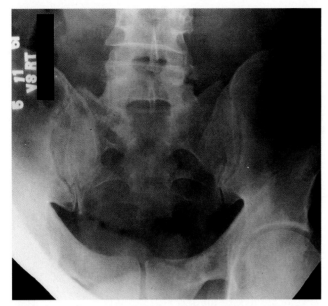

Figure 62–1. This radiograph illustrates how difficult it may be to demonstrate a chordoma in the sacrum with a routine anteroposterior view.

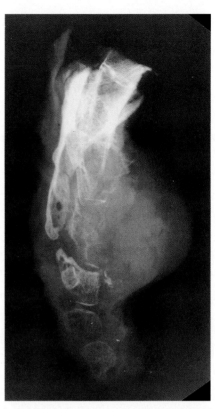

Figure 62–3. The specimen radiogram exhibits the same features seen in the gross specimen. Lateral radiographs of the pelvis may help visualize a sacral chordoma, as do computed tomography (CT) and magnetic resonance imaging (MRI).

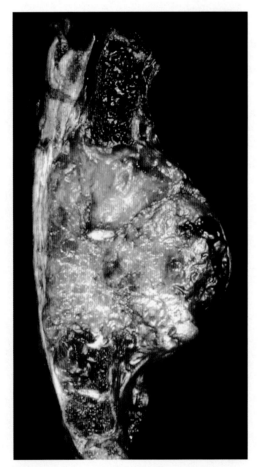

Figure 62–2. The gross pathologic features in this case (also shown in Fig. 62–1) demonstrate destruction of a significant portion of the sacrum and extension of the tumor into the presacral space.

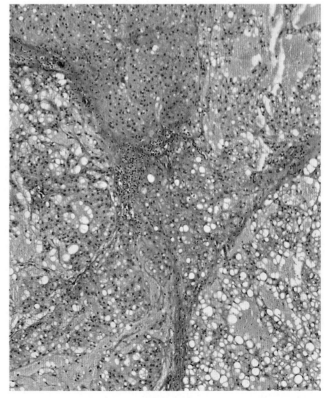

Figure 62–4. At low magnification, chordomas are characteristically lobulated tumors, as this photomicrograph shows.

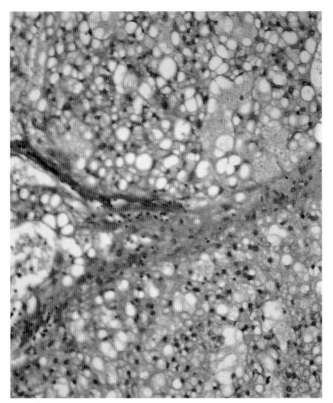

Figure 62–5. Within the lobules, the tumor is mildly cellular, and numerous cytoplasmic vacuoles are identifiable even at medium magnification. Chording of the cells is a feature that varies from tumor to tumor and need not be prominent.

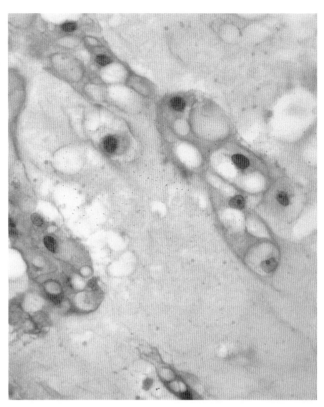

Figure 62–7. Chording of the cells, as seen in this photomicrograph, is a feature that can result in a histologic pattern similar to that of a mucinous adenocarcinoma.

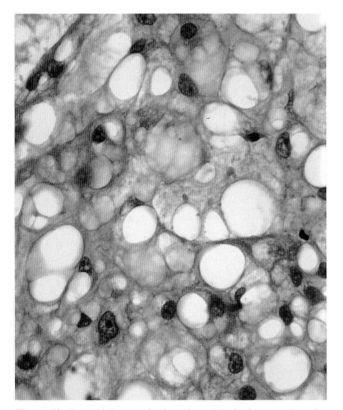

Figure 62–6. At high magnification, the cytologic features show that the cells have abundant vacuolated cytoplasm. Such cells have been termed "physaliferous."

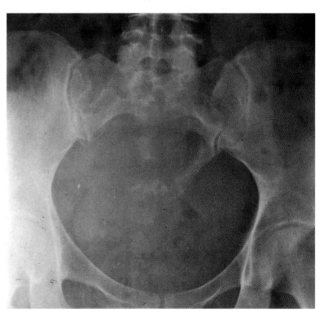

Figure 62–8. This radiograph shows a chordoma presenting as a large, poorly marginated, midline, destructive tumor of the sacrum. An area of central calcification is present.

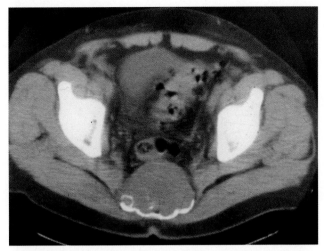

Figure 62–9. This CT scan shows the typical features of a sacral chordoma, with bony destruction and anterior extension of the lesion.

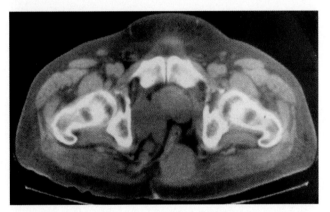

Figure 62–10. Multiple soft tissue nodules of recurrent chordoma are identifiable in this CT scan. These tumors have a propensity for such recurrences, and CT or MRI usually is needed to detect them.

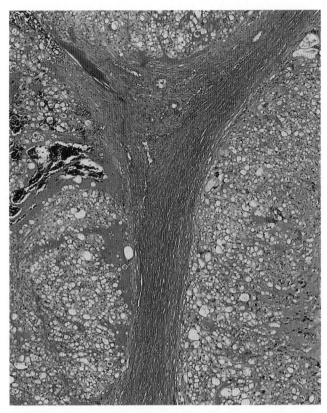

Figure 62–11. The lobulated pattern of growth of a chordoma is evident in this sacral tumor. Soft tissue extensions of the tumor maintain this pattern.

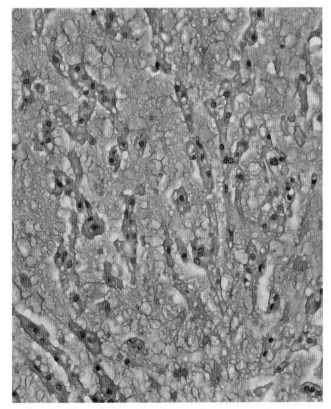

Figure 62–12. Chording and the physaliferous quality of the cytoplasm are evident in this photomicrograph.

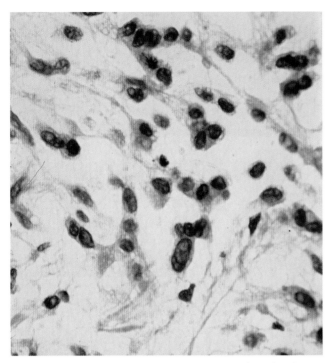

Figure 62–13. Chording is also evident in this tumor involving the seventh thoracic vertebra. Although some mesenchymal and even epithelial tumors may exhibit a similar pattern of chorded growth, the diagnosis of chordoma is valid only for midline tumors.

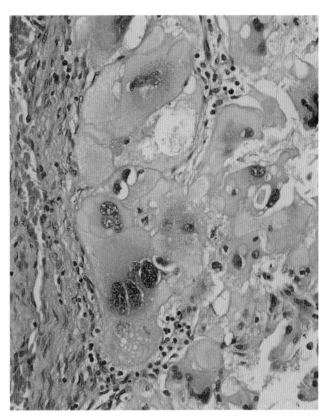

Figure 62–15. Marked cytologic pleomorphism may be seen in sacral chordomas, as illustrated in this photomicrograph. Such atypia is most commonly seen after radiation therapy or with recurrence of a tumor.

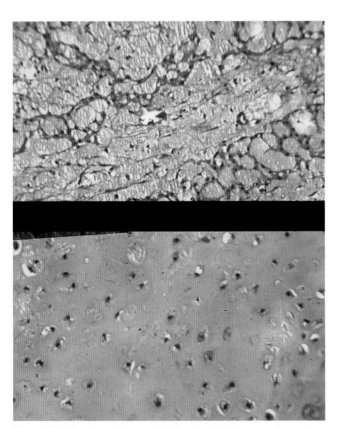

Figure 62–14. In the spheno-occipital region, some tumors show a mixture of chondroid and chordoid features histologically. Such tumors have been termed "chondroid chordomas."

CHAPTER 63

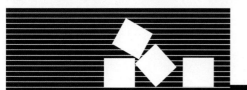

Ewing's Sarcoma

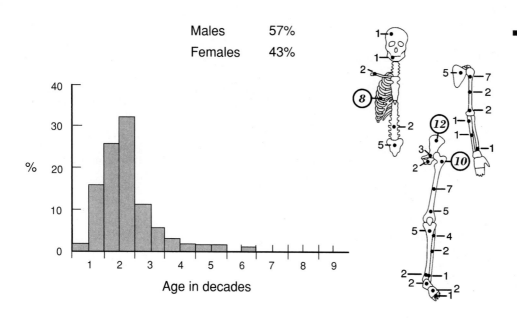

Males   57%
Females   43%

CLINICAL SIGNS

1. A palpable, tender mass lesion is found.
2. Fever and an increased erythrocyte sedimentation rate may be seen.
3. Anemia and leukocytosis may also be present.

CLINICAL SYMPTOMS

1. Local pain is the first symptom in 50 per cent of patients. Although it may be intermittent at first, pain tends to increase in severity over time.
2. Swelling is commonly present at the time of diagnosis but is rarely the first symptom.
3. Fever and other constitutional symptoms suggestive of an infection may be present.

MAJOR RADIOGRAPHIC FEATURES

1. The tumor most commonly presents as an extensive diaphyseal lesion.
2. The lesion has a permeative pattern of growth and is poorly marginated.
3. The lesion may be lytic or sclerotic, or it may have regions of both lysis and sclerosis evident radiographically.
4. Characteristically, there is prominent periosteal new bone formation.
5. A soft tissue mass most commonly accompanies the osseous lesion.
6. An isotope bone scan, computed tomography (CT), and magnetic resonance imaging (MRI) are helpful in defining the lesion.

RADIOGRAPHIC DIFFERENTIAL DIAGNOSIS

1. Malignant lymphoma.
2. Osteosarcoma.
3. Osteomyelitis.
4. Langerhans' cell histiocytosis.

MAJOR PATHOLOGIC FEATURES

Gross

1. The tumor is characteristically gray-white.
2. The tumor is moist and glistening.
3. The tumor may be almost liquid and can mimic the appearance of pus.

Microscopic

1. The low-power appearance is that of a "small round cell tumor" with little intercellular stroma.
2. Between the areas of highly cellular tumor, fibrous strands that compartmentalize the tumor may be identified.
3. At high magnification, the cells are uniform and round to oval.
4. The nuclei are round to oval and have a delicate, finely dispersed chromatin pattern.
5. Nucleoli, if present, are inconspicuous.
6. Mitotic figures are not abundant.
7. The majority of tumors have glycogen identifiable in the cytoplasm (periodic acid–Schiff–positive and diastase-sensitive).
8. The tumor is reticulin-poor and does not show evidence of matrix production.

PATHOLOGIC DIFFERENTIAL DIAGNOSIS

Benign lesions:

1. Chronic osteomyelitis.

Malignant lesions:

1. Malignant lymphoma.
2. Mesenchymal chondrosarcoma.
3. Small cell osteosarcoma.
4. Metastatic neuroblastoma.

TREATMENT

Primary Modality: radiation therapy to control the primary lesion. An effort is made to avoid irradiating an actively growing physis. Combination chemotherapy to control occult systemic disease is used in conjunction with the radiotherapy.

Other Possible Approaches: preoperative chemotherapy followed by resection with or without postoperative radiation therapy. Increased emphasis is being placed on the addition of surgical treatment to the overall management of Ewing's tumor.

References

Bacci G, Picci P, Gitelis S, et al: The treatment of localized Ewing's sarcoma: the experience at the Istituto Ortopedico Rizzoli in 163 cases treated with and without adjuvant chemotherapy. Cancer 49:1561–1570, 1982.

Devoe K, and Weidner N: Immunohistochemistry of small round-cell tumors. Semin Diagn Pathol 17(3):216–224, 2000.

Eggli KD, Quiogue T, and Moser RP Jr: Ewing's sarcoma. Radiol Clin North Am 31(2):325–337, 1993.

Kissane JM, Askin FB, Fokulkes M, et al: Ewing's sarcoma of bone: clinicopathologic aspects of 303 cases from the Intergroup Ewing's Sarcoma Study. Hum Pathol 14:773–779, 1983.

Mendenhall CM, Marcus RB Jr, Enneking WF, et al: The prognostic significance of soft tissue extension in Ewing's sarcoma. Cancer 51:913–917, 1983.

Nascimento AG, Unni KK, Pritchard DJ, et al: A clinicopathologic study of 20 cases of large-cell (atypical) Ewing's sarcoma of bone. Am J Surg Pathol 4:29–36, 1980.

Rosen G, Caparros B, Nirenberg A, et al: Ewing's sarcoma: ten-year experience with adjuvant chemotherapy. Cancer 47:2204–2213, 1981.

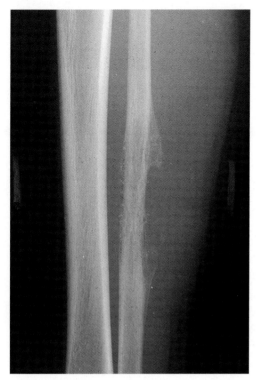

Figure 63–1. This radiograph of Ewing's sarcoma shows the characteristic lytic appearance of such tumors. A diaphyseal location, as in this case involving the fibula, is most common. The periosteum is generally elevated in such cases, resulting in Codman's triangle and an associated soft tissue mass.

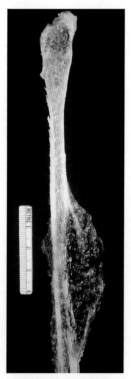

Figure 63–2. The gross pathologic features of this fibular Ewing's sarcoma correlate well with the radiographic features shown in Figure 63–1. The lesional tissue is frequently soft and hemorrhagic, as in this case. A small incisional biopsy may yield a loose gray-white tissue that mimics the gross features of an osteomyelitis.

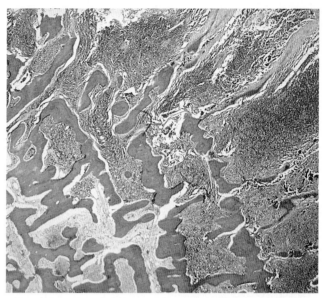

Figure 63–3. At low magnification, Ewing's sarcoma is a highly cellular tumor composed of small round cells. The periosteum is elevated by this cellular proliferation, resulting in a layering of periosteal new bone that may appear as an "onion skin" radiographically. The reactive new bone is shown in this photomicrograph.

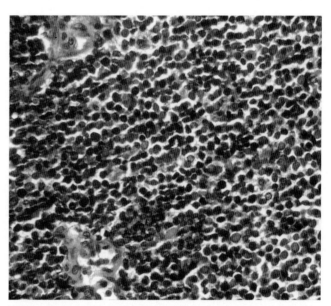

Figure 63–4. At higher magnification, Ewing's sarcoma is composed of small round cells; frequently, however, two cell types are identifiable. The nuclei of the most prominent type are round with a regular chromatin pattern; if nucleoli are present, they are indistinct. The second cell type contains a dark, hyperchromatic nucleus and is thought to represent a degenerative change.

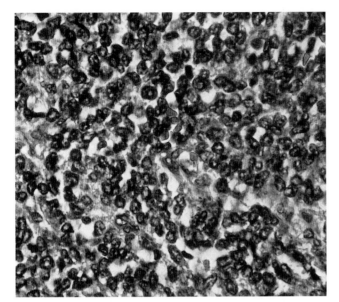

Figure 63–5. Ewing's sarcoma is homogeneous at high magnification, and no matrix is identifiable within the tumor. In contrast, small cell osteosarcoma should have identifiable osteoid within the tumor.

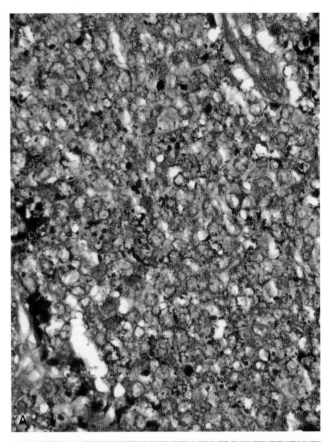

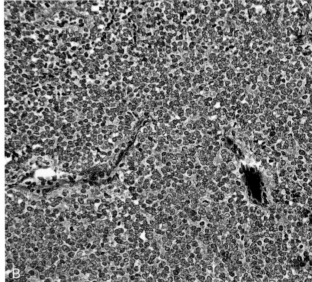

Figure 63–6. Two special stains, the periodic acid–Schiff (PAS) stain and the reticulin stain, are helpful in confirming the diagnosis of Ewing's sarcoma. Ewing's sarcoma is generally, but not uniformly, PAS-positive (*A*) and reticulin-poor (*B*).

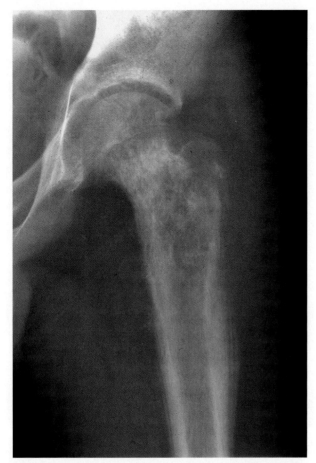

Figure 63–7. This radiograph shows Ewing's sarcoma of the proximal femur. The lesion is long and poorly marginated. The multilaminae, or "onion skin," periosteal reaction is evident.

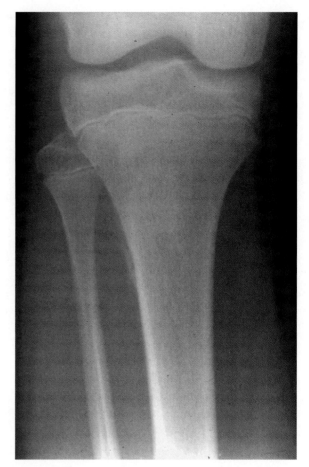

Figure 63–9. This plane radiograph shows only new bone formation associated with Ewing's sarcoma of the proximal tibia.

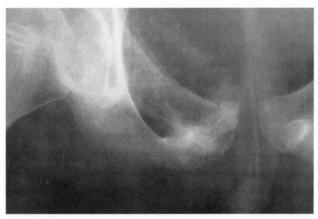

Figure 63–8. This Ewing's sarcoma of the pubic ramus shows irregular lysis, spiculated new bone, and an associated soft tissue mass. These features are frequently seen with this tumor.

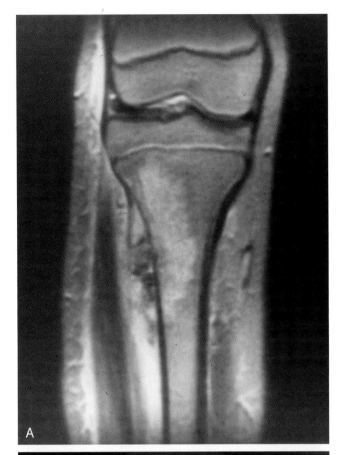

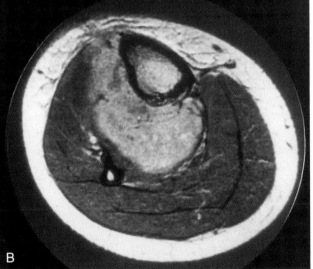

Figure 63–10. Although the plane radiographic features are unimpressive (see Fig. 63–9), coronal magnetic resonance imaging (MRI) shows a fairly large intramedullary tumor with cortical destruction and elevation of the periosteum (*A*). Axial MRI of the same tumor shows a large soft tissue mass typical of this tumor (*B*). This case demonstrates the utility of computed tomography (CT) and MRI in the evaluation of cases that are inconspicuous on plane radiographic evaluation.

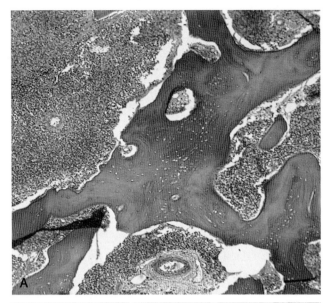

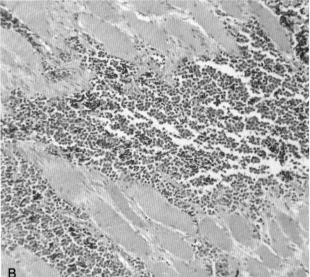

Figure 63–11. These photomicrographs illustrate the permeative nature of the pattern of growth of Ewing's sarcoma, whether it is in bone (*A*) or involves the soft tissues adjacent to the affected bone (*B*).

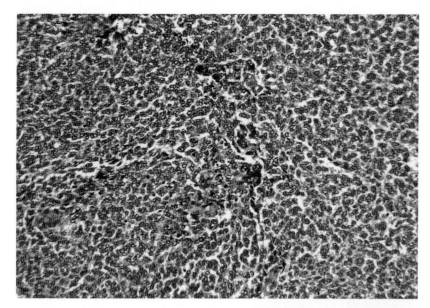

Figure 63–12. The cytologic features of Ewing's sarcoma are homogeneous, as this photomicrograph shows. Foci of necrosis may be present.

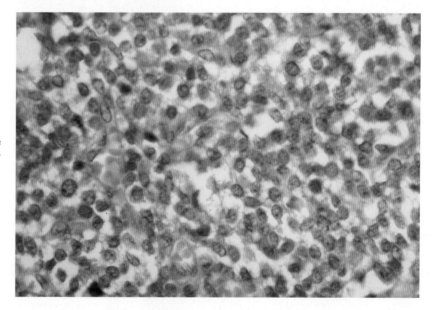

Figure 63–13. At high magnification, the nuclei are uniform and show a finely granular chromatin pattern.

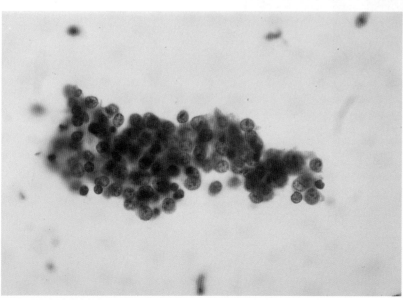

Figure 63–14. Fine-needle aspiration of Ewing's sarcoma yields small, uniform cells, which may be found in clusters but are generally noncohesive in smear preparations. Although diagnosis of the primary tumor with this technique is possible, its main utility is in confirming metastatic disease, as in this case of a transthoracic needle aspirate in a patient with a primary tumor in the ilium.

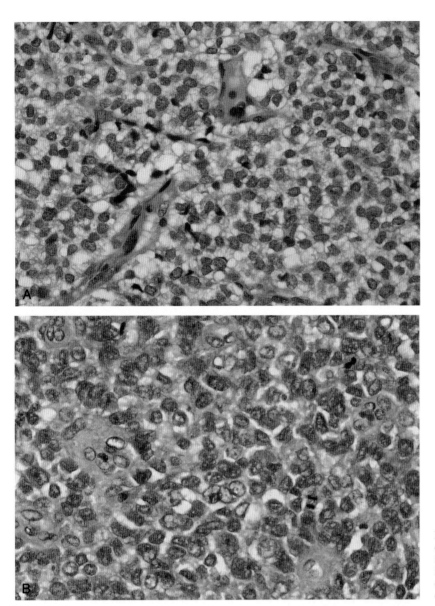

Figure 63–15. *A*, The photomicrograph shows the cytologic characteristics of typical Ewing's sarcoma in contrast to the "atypical" Ewing's sarcoma shown in *B*. Atypical Ewing's sarcoma demonstrates greater cytologic pleomorphism than the uniform small cell cytology of typical Ewing's sarcoma.

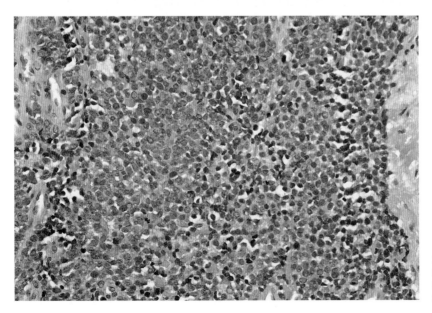

Figure 63–16. Ewing's sarcoma of the small bones is associated with a better prognosis than Ewing's sarcoma in other locations. The tumor shown in this photomicrograph involved a carpal bone.

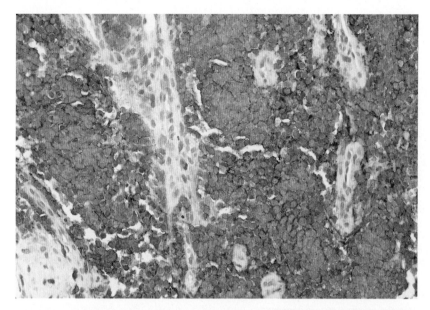

Figure 63–17. Immunohistochemical stains for lymphoid markers and CD99 (MIC2) can be helpful in distinguishing Ewing's sarcoma from lymphoma and other "small round cell tumors." This Ewing's sarcoma of the small bones of the hand shows strong CD99 positivity.

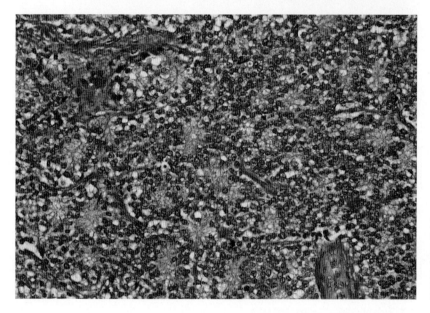

Figure 63–18. Ewing's sarcoma shows a spectrum of histologic patterns ranging from a sheet-like proliferation of small cells to the pattern of primitive neuroectodermal tumor (PNET) illustrated in this photomicrograph. Tumors that show the typical pattern of Ewing's sarcoma may show a PNET histologic pattern with recurrence.

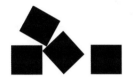

SECONDARY
SARCOMAS

CHAPTER 64

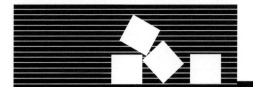

Paget's Sarcoma

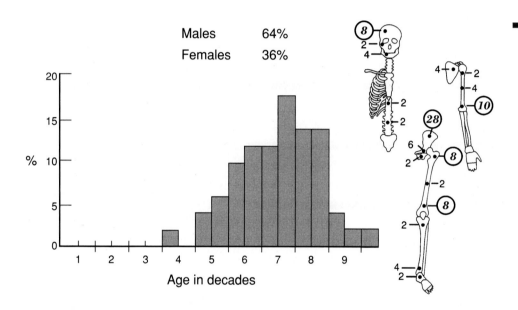

Males 64%
Females 36%

CLINICAL SIGNS

1. A painful mass lesion is felt in the region of the affected bone.
2. Symptoms are rapidly progressive.

CLINICAL SYMPTOMS

1. Pain is felt in the affected region. An increase in pain in one bone in a patient with Paget's disease should arouse suspicion of the development of a sarcoma.
2. Swelling may be due to soft tissue extension of the tumor.

MAJOR RADIOGRAPHIC FEATURES

1. Most tumors are purely lytic, although sclerotic and mixed lesions do occur.

2. The bone of origin usually shows changes of Paget's disease.
3. The tumor extends into the surrounding soft tissue.
4. There is a pattern of "geographic" bone destruction.
5. Computed tomography (CT) or magnetic resonance imaging (MRI) may be useful for detection when a soft tissue component is present. Compared with uncomplicated Paget's disease with respect to location, these sarcomas have a predilection for the humerus and only rarely arise in the spine.

RADIOGRAPHIC DIFFERENTIAL DIAGNOSIS

1. Paget's disease with marked lysis.
2. Florid Paget's disease extending into soft tissues.

MAJOR PATHOLOGIC FEATURES

Gross

1. A destructive lesion involves the bone and extends into the soft tissues.
2. The soft, fleshy tumor generally is whitish to brown.

Microscopic

1. At low magnification, the tumor is highly cellular.
2. The tumor generally is composed of spindle cells.
3. At higher magnification, the spindle cells show significant pleomorphism and cytologic atypia.
4. The specific diagnosis may be that of osteosarcoma, fibrosarcoma, or malignant fibrous histiocytoma.

PATHOLOGIC DIFFERENTIAL DIAGNOSIS

Benign lesions:

1. Lytic phase of Paget's disease (radiographic, primarily).
2. Fracture callus.
3. Myositis ossificans (heterotopic ossification).

Malignant lesions:

1. Malignant lymphoma.
2. Osteosarcoma.
3. Fibrosarcoma.
4. Malignant fibrous histiocytoma.

TREATMENT

Primary Modality: Usually, the tumor's aggressive behavior, with extensive local involvement, requires amputation to achieve an adequately wide surgical margin.

Other Possible Approaches: Preoperative chemotherapy and limb-saving resection may be chosen if surgical staging suggests that an adequately wide margin can be achieved. Radiation therapy is used for surgically inaccessible lesions, and an aggressive approach with thoracotomy is employed for pulmonary metastases.

References

Boutin RD, Spitz DJ, Newman JS, et al: Complications in Paget disease at MR imaging. Radiology 209(3):641–651, 1998.

Donath J, Szilagyi M, Fornet B, et al: Pseudosarcoma in Paget's disease. Eur J Radiol 10(10):1664–1668, 2000.

Haibach H, Farrell C, and Dittrich FJ: Neoplasms arising in Paget's disease of bone: a study of 82 cases. Am J Clin Pathol 83:594–600, 1985.

Lamovec J, Rener M, and Spiler M: Pseudosarcoma in Paget's disease of bone. Ann Diagn Pathol 3(2):99–103, 1999

Wick MR, Siegal GP, McLeod RA, et al: Sarcomas of bone complicating osteitis deformans (Paget's disease): fifty years' experience. Am J Surg Pathol 5:47–59, 1981.

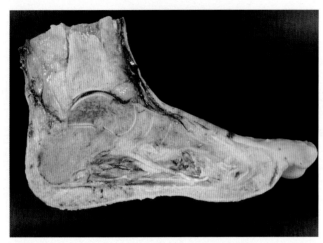

Figure 64–1. This gross specimen shows a case of Paget's sarcoma involving the distal tibia. The patient initially had suffered a pathologic fracture of the distal tibia and had been treated conservatively for the fracture, as the underlying malignancy was radiographically subtle. The tumor has broken through the cortex and extended into the soft tissues of the foot.

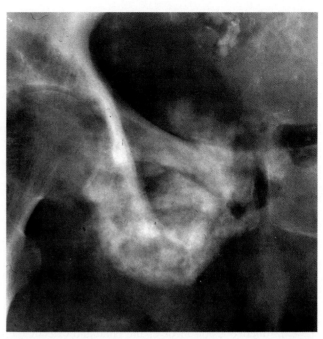

Figure 64–3. A blastic Paget sarcoma, arising in the ischium and pubis in a region of pre-existing Paget's disease, is shown in this radiograph. The soft tissue component of the tumor contains bony mineralization indicative of an osteosarcoma.

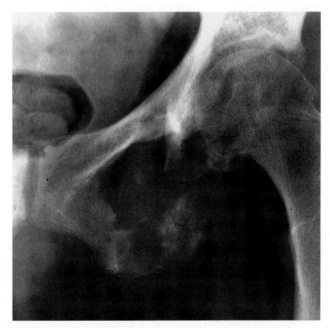

Figure 64–2. This radiograph shows a lytic Paget sarcoma arising in the ischium with pre-existing Paget's disease and causing considerable bone destruction.

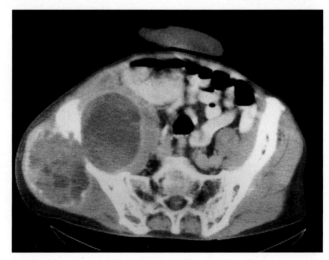

Figure 64–4. This computed tomographic (CT) scan shows Paget's sarcoma of the pelvis with a large soft tissue component surrounding the iliac bone. Both innominate bones show evidence of Paget's disease as well.

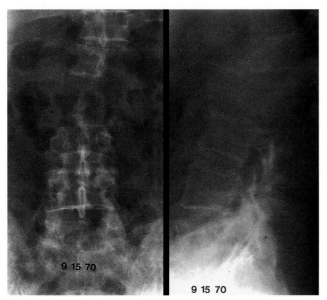

Figure 64–5. This radiograph reveals extensive lysis of a vertebra due to uncomplicated Paget's disease. The radiographic appearance is that of a malignancy; however, the spine is a rare site for this complication of Paget's disease.

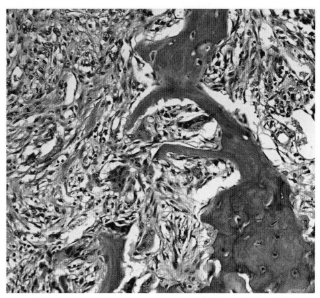

Figure 64–7. Some sarcomas that complicate Paget's disease do not demonstrate matrix production. This photomicrograph shows such a case. These lesions may be classified as fibrosarcomas or as malignant fibrous histiocytomas, depending upon other features evident in the tumor.

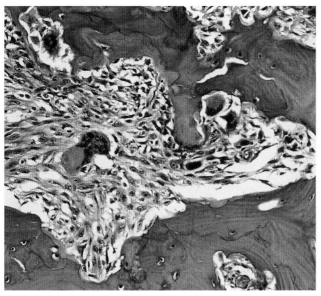

Figure 64–6. Paget's sarcomas may show a variety of histologic patterns. As this photomicrograph illustrates, osteosarcoma is the most common.

CHAPTER 65

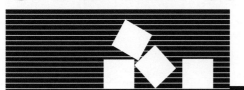

Postradiation Sarcoma

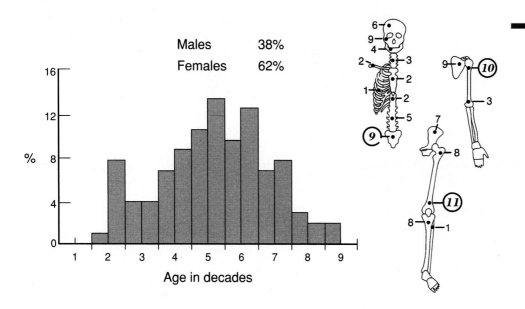

Males   38%
Females   62%

% (y-axis: 0, 4, 8, 12, 16)

Age in decades (x-axis: 1 through 9)

CLINICAL SIGNS

1. A tender mass lesion is found on physical examination.
2. Skin changes compatible with prior radiation therapy may be present.

CLINICAL SYMPTOMS

1. Pain is felt in the region of prior radiation therapy.
2. The interval between radiation therapy and diagnosis of sarcoma has varied from 2.75 to 55 years in cases treated at the Mayo Clinic, with an average interval of 15.1 years.
3. A swelling may be noted by the patient.

MAJOR RADIOGRAPHIC FEATURES

1. The tumor may arise from normal bone or in an area of a pre-existing lesion within the radiation portal.
2. The underlying bone often is altered by radiation, surgery, the pre-existing abnormality, or some combination of these.
3. The underlying changes in the affected bone may obscure the lesion early in the course of the disease.
4. The latent period ranges from 2.75 to 55 years, with an average of 15.1 years.
5. Postradiation sarcomas are radiographically similar to conventional tumors.

6. A soft tissue mass, cortical destruction, and extra-osseous bone production are indicative of sarcoma.

RADIOGRAPHIC DIFFERENTIAL DIAGNOSIS

1. Metastatic disease.
2. Radiation-induced change without sarcoma.
3. Osteoporosis.
4. Insufficiency stress fracture.

MAJOR PATHOLOGIC FEATURES

Gross

1. These tumors tend to be soft and fleshy.
2. The tumor has most commonly extended beyond the confines of the affected bone and has an associated soft tissue mass.
3. Foci of hemorrhage and necrosis may be identifiable.
4. Matrix production in the form of osteoid or even cartilage may be seen, and calcification may be present on a degenerative basis.

Microscopic

1. At low magnification, the pattern varies from tumor to tumor. Of postradiation sarcomas compiled by the Mayo Clinic, the majority (approximately 50%) showed osteoid production and were classified as osteosarcomas.
2. Spindle cell tumors lacking osteoid matrix production were the second largest group, accounting for 42 per cent of the total, with the majority of these being classified as fibrosarcomas and the remainder as malignant fibrous histiocytomas.
3. At higher magnification, the cytologic characteristics are those of a pleomorphic high-grade sarcoma. The nuclei vary in size, shape, and nuclear staining characteristics.

PATHOLOGIC DIFFERENTIAL DIAGNOSIS

Benign lesions:

1. Reactive spindle cell proliferation in the region of prior irradiation.
2. Fracture callus at a site of pathologic fracture after radiation therapy.

Malignant lesions:

1. Osteosarcoma.
2. Fibrosarcoma.
3. Malignant fibrous histiocytoma.

TREATMENT

Primary Modality: preoperative chemotherapy and limb-saving resection if a wide surgical margin can be achieved. Reconstruction is individualized and depends upon the location of the tumor. Amputation will be necessary if surgical staging indicates that an adequately wide margin cannot be achieved to preserve the neurovascular structures.

Other Possible Approaches: radiation therapy for lesions in inaccessible sites, thoracotomy for pulmonary metastases, or chemotherapy protocols similar to those used for osteosarcoma.

References

Brady LW: Radiation-induced sarcomas of bone. Skeletal Radiol 4(2):72–78, 1979.
Ergun H, and Howland WJ: Postradiation atrophy of mature bone. CRC Crit Rev Diagn Imaging 12(3):225–243, 1980.
Frassica FJ, Frassica DA, Wold LE, et al: Postradiation sarcoma of bone. Orthopedics 16(1):105–106, 109, 1993.
Frassica FJ, Sim FH, Frassica DA, and Wold LE: Survival and management considerations in postirradiation osteosarcoma and Paget's osteosarcoma. Clin Orthop (270):120–127, 1991.
Unni KK, and Dahlin DC: Premalignant tumors and conditions of bone. Am J Surg Pathol 3(1):47–60, 1979.
Weatherby RP, Dahlin DC, and Ivins JC: Postradiation sarcoma of bone: review of 78 Mayo Clinic cases. Mayo Clin Proc 56:294–306, 1981.

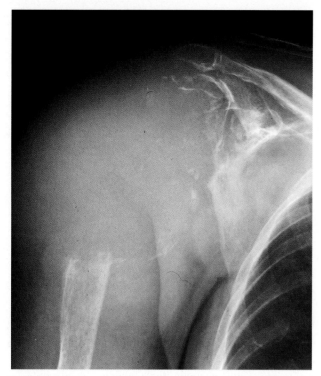

Figure 65–1. This radiograph shows a postradiation sarcoma of the proximal humerus, with nearly complete destruction of the bone and an associated soft tissue mass. The tumor arose eight years after radiation therapy for carcinoma of the breast. Radiation-induced changes are present in the remaining humerus and the scapula.

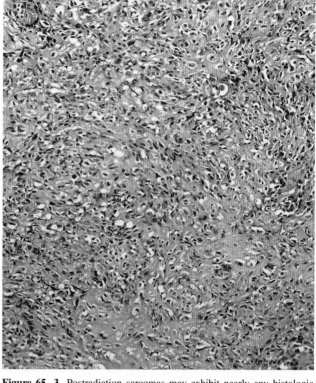

Figure 65–3. Postradiation sarcomas may exhibit nearly any histologic pattern of growth and differentiation. This tumor, which arose in the distal femur of a young woman who had received radiation therapy for a hemangioendothelial sarcoma, shows bony matrix production.

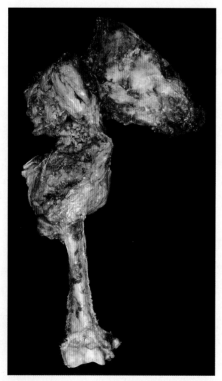

Figure 65–2. The gross specimen from the forequarter amputation performed in the case shown in Figure 65–1 shows the total destruction of the proximal humerus. Hemorrhagic necrosis and soft tissue extension are commonly seen in postradiation sarcomas of this size.

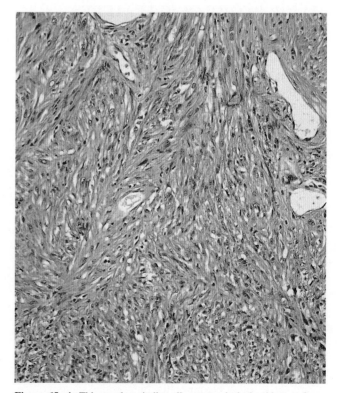

Figure 65–4. This purely spindle cell sarcoma lacked evidence of matrix production and was classified as a postradiation fibrosarcoma. The tumor arose in the humerus 55 years after radiation therapy.

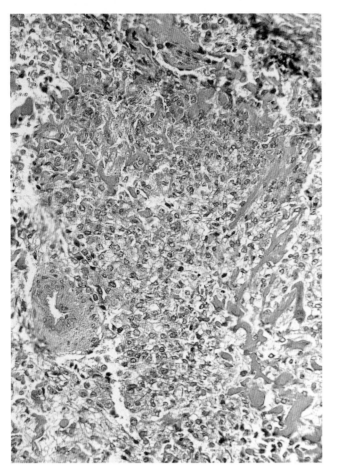

Figure 65–5. This photomicrograph shows a postradiation osteosarcoma that arose after treatment for histiocytosis X of the mandible.

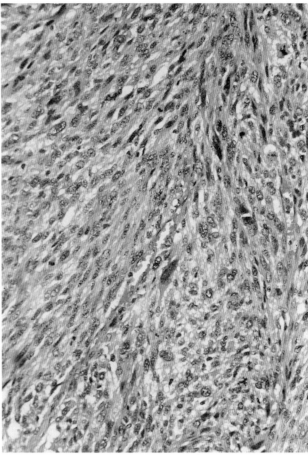

Figure 65–6. The proximal humerus frequently lies within the radiation field for patients receiving adjuvant radiation therapy for metastatic breast carcinoma. This fibrosarcoma arose in the proximal humerus in such a clinical setting.

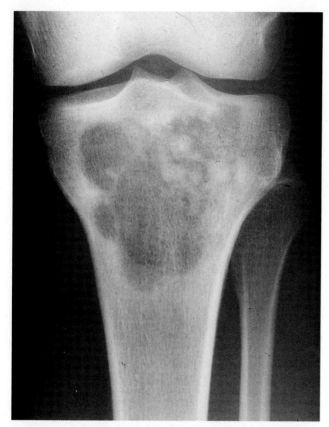

Figure 65–7. This radiograph shows a postradiation osteosarcoma of the proximal tibia. The large malignant-appearing tumor shows areas of ossification.

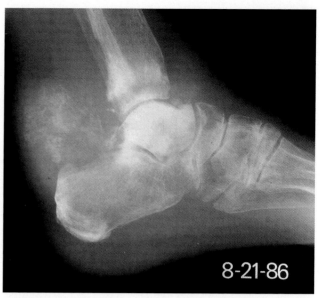

8-21-86

Figure 65–9. This example of a postradiation sarcoma developed multi-focally in the foot and ankle of a radium watch–dial painter.

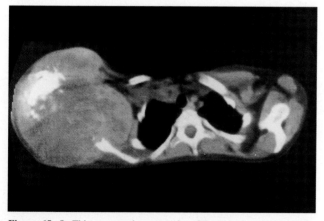

Figure 65–8. This computed tomography (CT) scan shows a postradiation sarcoma of the proximal humerus. The ossified malignancy also demonstrates a huge necrotic soft tissue component.

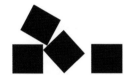

TUMOR-LIKE CONDITIONS

CHAPTER 66

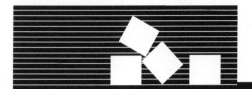

Neurilemmoma

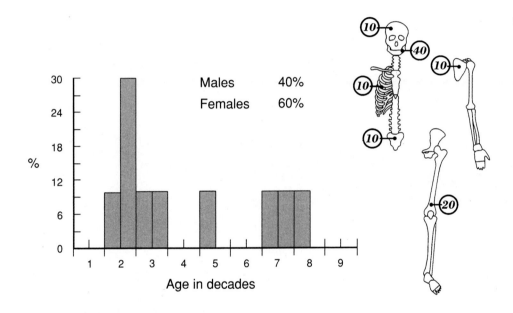

Males   40%
Females   60%

CLINICAL SIGNS

1. There are generally no specific findings on physical examination.
2. A small mass lesion may be found if the lesion involves a superficial bone, e.g., the mandible.
3. Stigmata of neurofibromatosis may be present in some cases.

CLINICAL SYMPTOMS

1. Many neurilemmomas are asymptomatic.
2. A minority of lesions produce pain.
3. A minority of lesions produce a swelling that is noticed by the patient

MAJOR RADIOGRAPHIC FEATURES

1. The lesion has a benign appearance, with sharp margins and a sclerotic rim.
2. Intraosseous tumors usually arise near the end of the bone and within the shaft.
3. Erosion of the bone by a tumor arising in nerves contiguous to bone is the most common presentation.

RADIOGRAPHIC DIFFERENTIAL DIAGNOSIS

1. Fibroma.
2. Fibrous dysplasia.
3. Chondromyxoid fibroma.
4. Neurofibroma.

MAJOR PATHOLOGIC FEATURES

Gross

1. The lesion is generally well circumscribed.
2. The tissue is firm but may show regions of myxoid and cystic change.
3. The tissue is yellow to brown.
4. The lesion's relationship to a nerve or its canal may be appreciated.

Microscopic

1. At low magnification, the lesion is hypocellular and composed of spindle cells.
2. Between the spindle cells is a loose, myxoid-appearing matrix.
3. Focally, the nuclei of the spindle cells may be clustered in a linear fashion (Verocay bodies).
4. At higher magnification, the nuclei are generally small and hyperchromic. However, they may become irregular in size, shape, and staining characteristics—features that are ascribed to degeneration.
5. No mitotic figures are identified.

PATHOLOGIC DIFFERENTIAL DIAGNOSIS

Benign lesions:

1. Myxoma.

Malignant lesions:

1. Fibrosarcoma.
2. Malignant fibrous histiocytoma, myxoid variant.

TREATMENT

Primary Modality: Conservative surgical excision with a marginal margin is used.

Other Possible Approaches: These lesions, which may become very large when they arise in the sacrum, can be "shelled out," preserving sacral nerve roots.

References

De la Monte SM, Dorfman HD, Chandra R, and Malawer M: Intraosseous schwannoma: histologic features, ultrastructure, and review of the literature. Hum Pathol 15(6):551–558, 1984.
Fawcett KJ, and Dahlin DC: Neurilemmoma of bone. Am J Clin Pathol 147:759–766, 1967.
Gordon EJ: Solitary intraosseous neurilemmoma of the tibia: review of intraosseous neurilemmoma and neurofibroma. Clin Orthop 117:271–282, 1976.
Vicas E, Bourdua S, and Charest F: Le neurilemmome du sacrum: presentation d'un cas. Union Med Can 103:1057–1060, 1974.

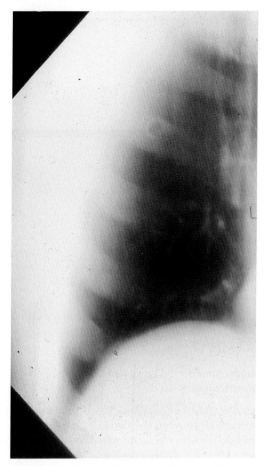

Figure 66–1. This radiograph shows a small oval neurilemmoma of the anterior rib. The sharp margination, sclerotic rim, and cortical expansion indicate a benign process.

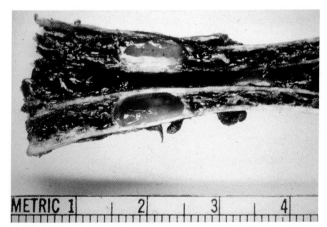

Figure 66–2. This resected rib (also seen in Fig. 66–1) shows cystic degenerative changes. Such changes frequently occur in neurilemmomas but may also be found in fibrous dysplasia involving the rib.

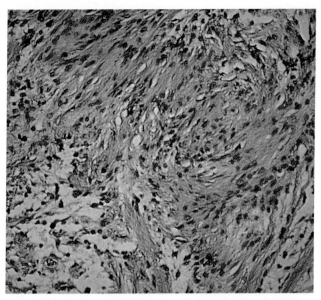

Figure 66–3. This photomicrograph of a mandibular neurilemmoma shows the admixture of spindle and round cells commonly seen in this lesion. Frequently, lipid-laden histiocytes are so prominent as to be grossly evident as yellowish areas in the tumor.

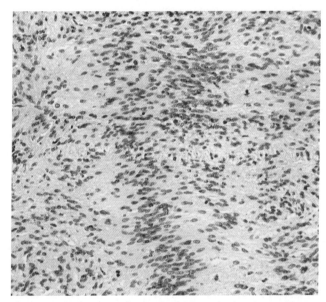

Figure 66–4. This photomicrograph of a femoral tumor from a 16-year-old girl shows the classic palisading of the nuclei of the spindle cells evident in neurilemmomas of peripheral nerves.

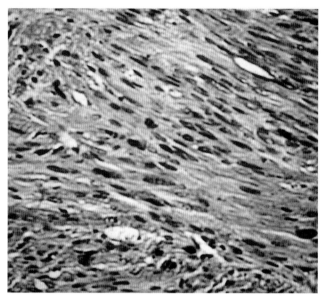

Figure 66-5. At high magnification, cytologic atypia may be seen in neurilemmomas, as in this mandibular lesion. Mitotic activity should essentially be absent in neurilemmomas; this feature helps to distinguish such lesions with "degenerative atypia" from sarcomas.

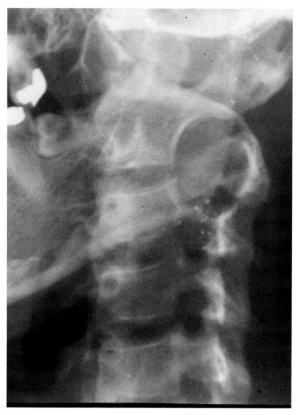

Figure 66-7. This neurilemmoma of the cervical nerve root has resulted in marked erosion and expansion of the C2-C3 intervertebral foramen.

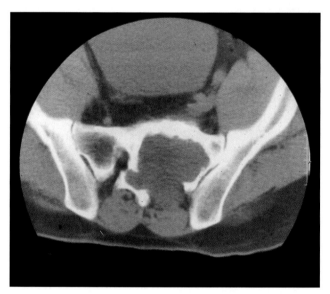

Figure 66-6. This computed tomography (CT) scan shows a neurilemmoma of the sacrum. The slowly enlarging tumor has eroded and destroyed bone around the left sacral foramen.

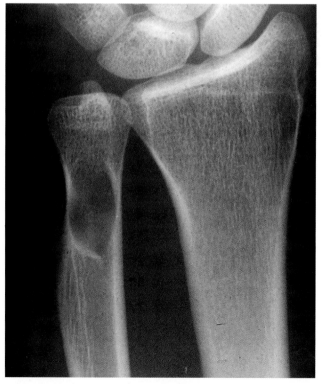

Figure 66-8. An intraosseous neurilemmoma of the distal ulna is shown in this radiograph. Very sharp margination is evident, as is the sclerotic rim; these are indications of a benign process.

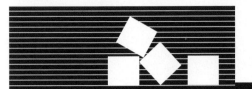

CHAPTER 67

Aneurysmal Bone Cyst

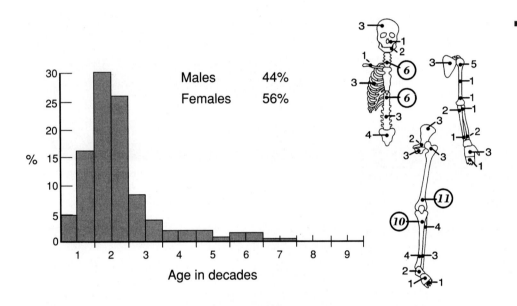

Males   44%
Females   56%

CLINICAL SIGNS

1. Swelling may be evident on physical examination.
2. Aneurysmal bone cyst frequently involves the vertebra—usually the posterior elements—and as such may cause signs and symptoms of cord compression or compression of emerging nerves.

CLINICAL SYMPTOMS

1. Pain is the most common symptom at presentation; it is usually of short duration.
2. Swelling may be noticed, and the size of the lesion tends to increase until therapy is instituted.

MAJOR RADIOGRAPHIC FEATURES

1. "Ballooned" or "aneurysmal" cystic expansion of the affected bone is evident.
2. No significant matrix mineralization is seen.
3. The lesion affects the metaphysis in long bones and the dorsal elements in vertebral locations.
4. Sclerotic rim and periosteal new bone formation are common.
5. The tumor may have an aggressive appearance, simulating that of a sarcoma.

RADIOGRAPHIC DIFFERENTIAL DIAGNOSIS

1. Unicameral bone cyst (simple cyst).
2. Giant cell tumor.

3. Sarcoma, particularly osteosarcoma, telangiectatic type.
4. Osteoblastoma when in the vertebra.

MAJOR PATHOLOGIC FEATURES

Gross

1. The lesional tissue is hemorrhagic, consisting of un-clotted blood and more "fleshy," solid aggregates of tissue.
2. Blood may fill the region of the tumor as the overlying bone is unroofed, but it does not spurt in a pulsatile fashion from the lesion. At the periphery of the lesion, an eggshell-thin layer of new periosteal bone is characteristically present.

Microscopic

1. At low magnification, cavernous spaces that may be filled with blood are identified.
2. The walls of the spaces contain spindled fibroblastic cells, multinucleated giant cells, and thin strands of bone.
3. At high magnification, the spaces are seen to lack an endothelial lining.

PATHOLOGIC DIFFERENTIAL DIAGNOSIS

Benign lesions:

1. Giant cell tumor.
2. Giant cell reparative granuloma (giant cell reaction).
3. Simple bone cyst.

Malignant lesions:

1. Telangiectatic osteosarcoma.

TREATMENT

Primary Modality: excision, curettage, and bone grafting. When the lesion is in an expendable bone such as the fibula or a rib, resection with a marginal or wide margin is preferred. In a patient who is asymptomatic, persistence of a cyst in a portion of a grafted lesion that has not been expanding on serial roentgenograms may be managed by close observation.

Other Possible Approaches: surgical adjuvant treatment with cryosurgery or chemical cautery. Injection of steroids in the lesion is also being explored. Radiation therapy is not recommended because of the potential for malignant transformation.

References

Dahlin DC, and McLeod RA: Aneurysmal bone cyst and other non-neoplastic conditions. Skeletal Radiol 8:243–250, 1982.

Gipple JR, Pritchard DJ, and Unni KK: Solid aneurysmal bone cyst. Orthopedics 15(12):1433–1436, 1992.

Levy WM, Miller AS, Bonakdarpour A, and Aegerter W: Aneurysmal bone cyst secondary to other osseous lesions: report of 57 cases. Am J Clin Pathol 63:1–8, 1975.

Ruiter DJ, vanRijssel TG, and ven der Velde EA: Aneurysmal bone cysts: a clinicopathological study of 105 cases. Cancer 39:2231–2239, 1977.

Vergel De Dios AM, Bond JR, Shives TC, et al: Aneurysmal bone cyst: a clinicopathologic study of 238 cases. Cancer 69(12):2921–2931, 1992.

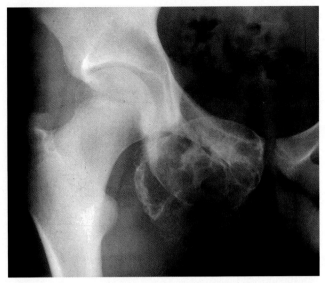

Figure 67–1. This radiograph of the pelvis shows a large aneurysmal bone cyst of the ischium and pubis, with marked expansion of the affected bones. No matrix mineralization is present, and the lesion is surrounded by a thin shell of bone.

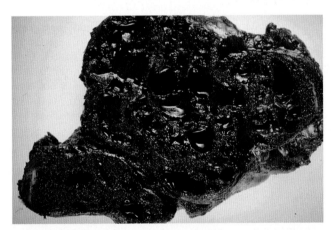

Figure 67–2. The gross specimen from the lesion seen in Figure 67–1 shows the typical features of aneurysmal bone cyst. The lesion is hemorrhagic and cystic. Numerous septa are identified; they may be somewhat gritty, as bone may be present in them.

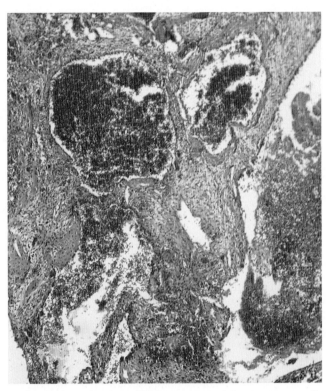

Figure 67–3. At low magnification, aneurysmal bone cysts generally contain numerous blood-filled spaces, as illustrated in this photomicrograph.

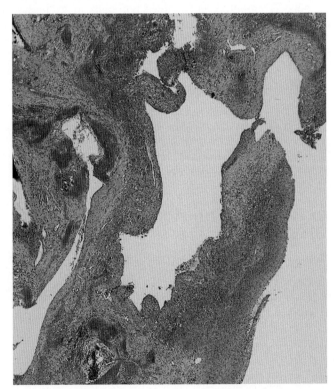

Figure 67–4. When the lesion is curetted, the spaces may collapse, as this photomicrograph shows. Blood may not be prominent because it may be lost during processing of the specimen. When the curetted specimen is collapsed, the presence of benign multinucleated giant cells within the lesion may result in a histologic pattern superficially mimicking that of giant cell tumor.

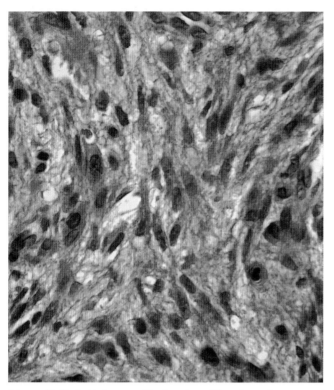

Figure 67–5. At higher magnification, the solid portions of aneurysmal bone cyst show a loose arrangement of the spindle cells. Mitotic activity may be brisk, this being the histologic counterpart of the clinical fact that the lesion may grow rapidly.

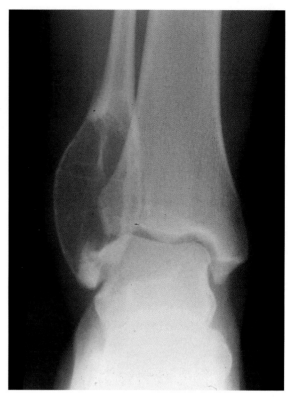

Figure 67–7. This aneurysmal bone cyst of the lower fibula shows marked expansion of the metaphysis. The overall appearance is that of a benign process.

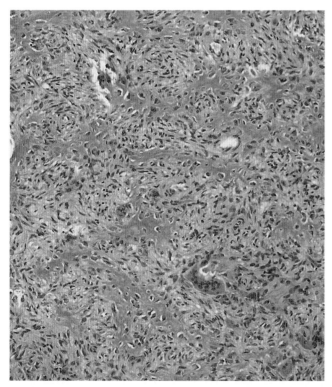

Figure 67–6. The solid portion of this aneurysmal bone cyst of the tibia shows bone production. This, combined with the aggressive radiographic appearance that may be present and the brisk mitotic activity generally seen in such lesions, may lead to a mistaken diagnosis of osteosarcoma.

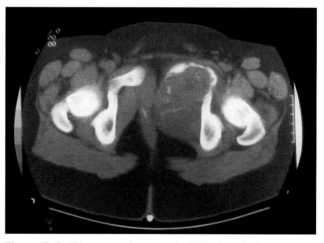

Figure 67–8. This computed tomography (CT) view of a large aneurysmal bone cyst of the pelvis shows an inhomogeneous soft tissue component associated with the lesion. Such an appearance may suggest a diagnosis of sarcoma.

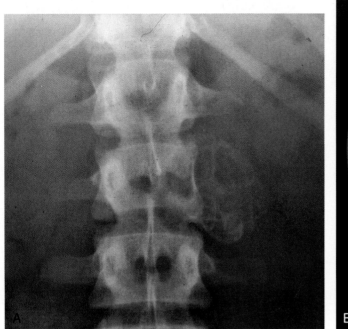
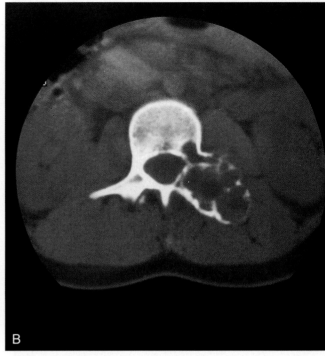

Figure 67–9. This radiograph (*A*) and CT scan (*B*) demonstrate an aneurysmal bone cyst involving the L2 vertebra. When the vertebrae are involved, it is generally the posterior or dorsal elements that are affected; the radiographic appearance is that of an expansile, lytic defect.

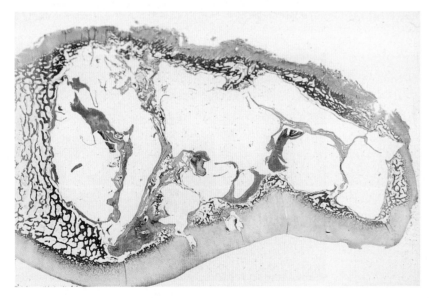

Figure 67–10. Multiple septa are present in an aneurysmal bone cyst, as shown in this low-power photomicrograph in which the fibrous septa are seen traversing the cystic space.

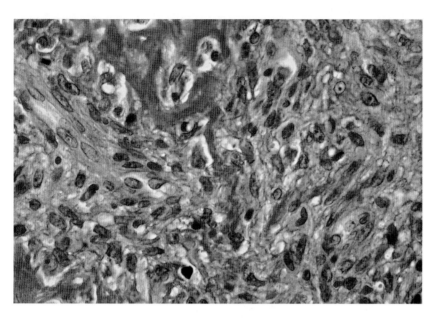

Figure 67–11. The fibrous bone present in the septa of the lesion may suggest the possibility that the lesion is an osteosarcoma. However, the loose arrangement of the lesion, its vascular appearance, and the presence of bone may also mimic the appearance of osteoblastoma.

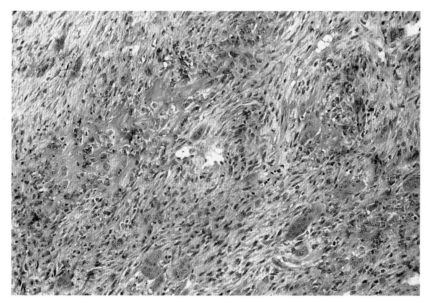

Figure 67–12. The loose pattern of arrangement shown in this low-power photomicrograph indicates that the lesion is proliferative in nature and not neoplastic.

CHAPTER 68

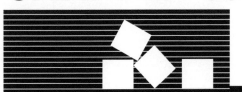

Unicameral Bone Cyst (Simple Cyst)

CLINICAL SIGNS

1. The majority of these lesions are incidental radiographic "abnormalities."
2. A painful mass occasionally may be identified on physical examination.

CLINICAL SYMPTOMS

1. The majority of tumors are asymptomatic.
2. The onset of pain is abrupt (associated with pathologic fracture).
3. Rarely, swelling in the region of the lesion may be noticed.

MAJOR RADIOGRAPHIC FEATURES

1. Cysts usually occur in the upper humerus or upper femur.
2. They frequently abut the epiphyseal plate.
3. They are often large and elongated.
4. Expansion is usually present but does not exceed the width of the epiphyseal plate.
5. There is sharp margination, often with trabeculation.
6. Pathologic fracture occurs and may result in healing or bone fragment settling to the dependent part of the lesion, indicative of fluid.

RADIOGRAPHIC DIFFERENTIAL DIAGNOSIS

1. Aneurysmal bone cyst.
2. Fibrous dysplasia.

MAJOR PATHOLOGIC FEATURES

Gross

1. The cystic cavity usually contains a straw-colored fluid.
2. If there has been bleeding into the cyst, pathologic fracture, or a previous attempt to insert a needle into the lesion, the fluid may be blood-tinged or frankly bloody.
3. Occasionally, partial or complete septation of the cyst may be seen.

Microscopic

1. At low magnification, the lining of the cyst appears as a thin rim of fibrous connective tissue.
2. Thicker areas of the cyst wall contain multinucleated giant cells.
3. Amorphous eosinophilic debris (probably fibrin) frequently is identified in the hypocellular fibrous connective tissue. This may undergo calcification, resulting in an appearance simulating that of cementum.
4. At higher magnification, no cytologic atypia is appreciated.

PATHOLOGIC DIFFERENTIAL DIAGNOSIS

Benign lesions:

1. Aneurysmal bone cyst.
2. Giant cell tumor.

Malignant lesions:

1. Osteosarcoma. Rarely, this has been mistakenly treated as a simple cyst. Radiographic features should aid in avoiding this mistake.

TREATMENT

Primary Modality: Treatment consists of dual-needle aspiration of the cyst and injection of methylprednisolone. Multiple steroid injections may be necessary to promote healing of the cyst.

Other Possible Approaches: In patients with loss of structural integrity in a weight-bearing bone associated with a large cyst, curettage and grafting are indicated.

References

Bauer TW, and Dorfman HD: Intraosseous ganglion: a clinicopathologic study of 11 cases. Am J Surg Pathol 6:207–213, 1982.

Boseker EH, Bickel WH, and Dahlin DC: A clinicopathologic study of simple unicameral bone cysts. Surg Gynecol Obstet 127:550–560, 1968.

Capanna R, Campanacci DA, and Manfrini M: Unicameral and aneurysmal bone cysts. Orthop Clin North Am 27(3):605–614, 1996.

Capanna R, Dal Monte A, Gitelis S, and Campanacci M: The natural history of unicameral bone cyst after steroid injection. Clin Orthop 166:204–211, 1982.

Lokiec F, and Wientroub S: Simple bone cyst: etiology, classification, pathology, and treatment modalities. J Pediatr Orthop B 7(4):262–273, 1998.

Schajowicz F, Sainz MC, and Slullitel JA: Juxta-articular bone cysts (intra-osseous ganglia): a clinicopathological study of eighty-eight cases. J Bone Joint Surg (Br) 61:107–116, 1979.

Wilkins RM: Unicameral bone cysts. J Am Acad Orthop Surg 8(4):217–224, 2000.

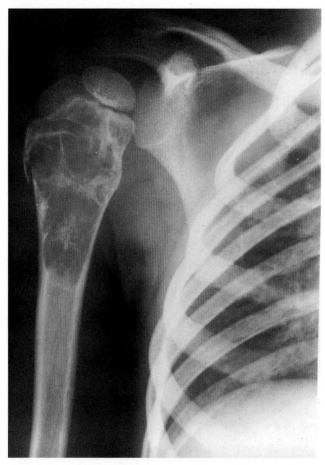

Figure 68–1. This radiograph shows a unicameral bone cyst abutting against the physis of the upper humerus. The lesion has resulted in mild expansion of the bone and shows sharp margination. A pathologic fracture is present, and trabeculation is evident.

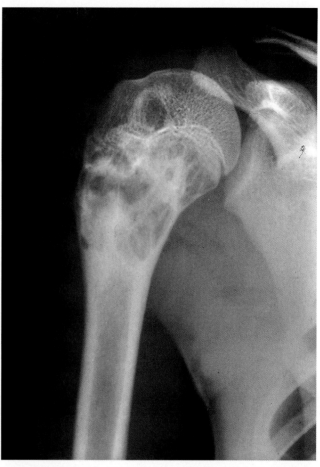

Figure 68–3. Considerable healing of this unicameral bone cyst of the proximal humerus has occurred after a pathologic fracture sustained eight months earlier.

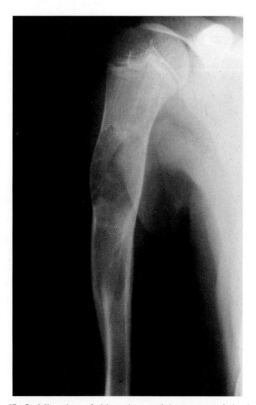

Figure 68–2. Migration of this unicameral bone cyst of the humerus has resulted in a diaphyseal location for the lesion.

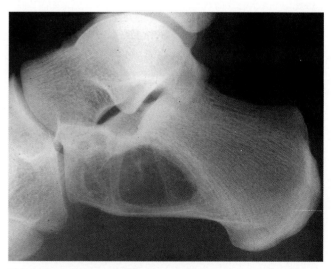

Figure 68–4. This radiograph shows a simple cyst of the calcaneus.

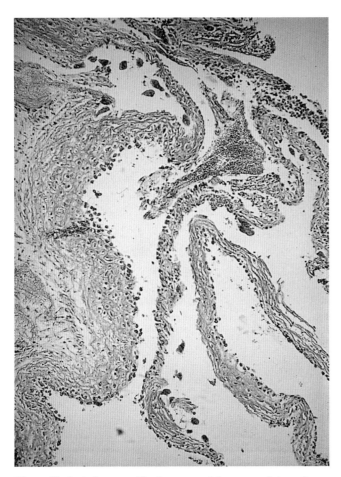

Figure 68–5. At low magnification, curetted fragments of tissue from a simple cyst may demonstrate septa similar to those seen in aneurysmal bone cyst. Usually, they show only a thin lining on the bone.

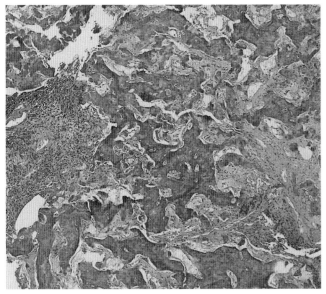

Figure 68–6. Reactive bone may be identified adjacent to simple cysts.

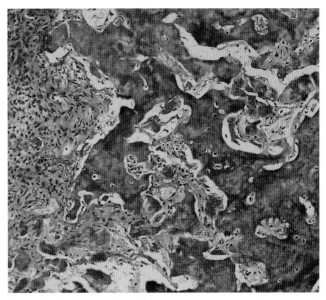

Figure 68–7. Some regions of the wall may contain multinucleated giant cells and have histologic features identical with those of aneurysmal bone cyst.

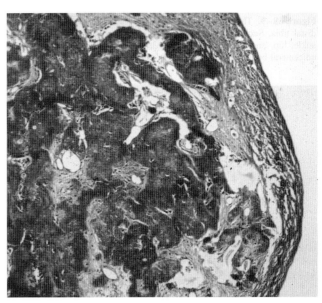

Figure 68–8. Eosinophilic aggregates of calcified fibrinous debris may be identified in the wall of the cyst. The histologic features of such debris may resemble cementum.

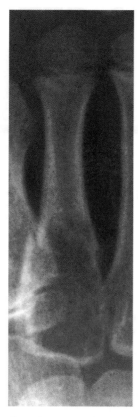

Figure 69–1. This radiograph shows a giant cell reaction of the proximal second metacarpal. There is cortical expansion and thinning by this purely lytic process.

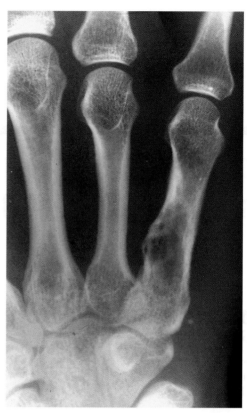

Figure 69–3. In this purely lytic giant cell reaction of the proximal metacarpal, the lesion is well marginated and shows cortical expansion and thinning.

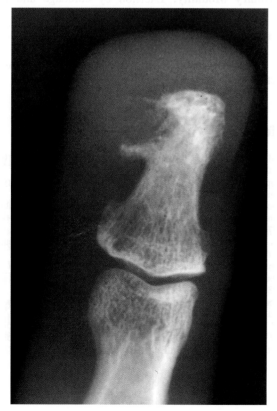

Figure 69–2. A giant cell reaction of the distal phalanx is shown in this radiograph. The lesion arose eccentrically and has extended into the soft tissues.

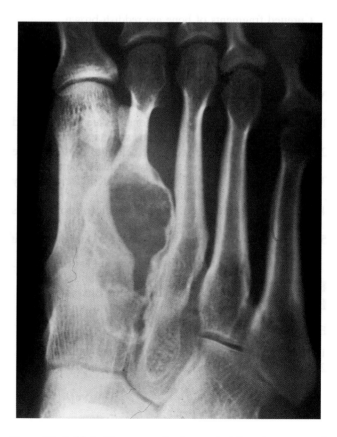

Figure 69–4. Marked bony expansion has resulted from the presence of this large, lytic giant cell reaction of the proximal second metatarsal.

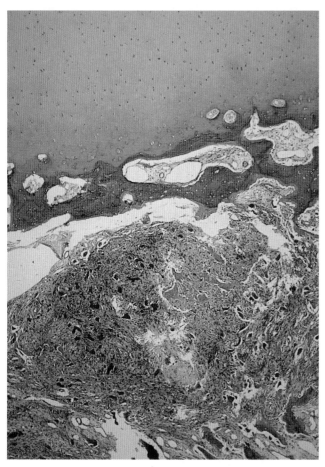

Figure 69–5. This photomicrograph shows a giant cell reaction extending to the end of a small bone in the hand. At low magnification, giant cells may be seen to slightly cluster in these lesions.

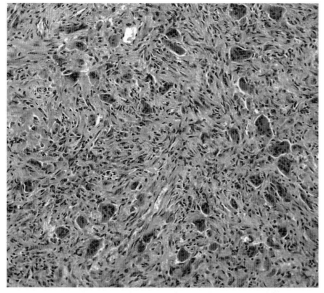

Figure 69–6. Giant cell reactions show a distinctly spindled mononuclear stromal component, as in this photomicrograph. This is in contrast with benign giant cell tumors, in which the mononuclear stromal component is round to oval.

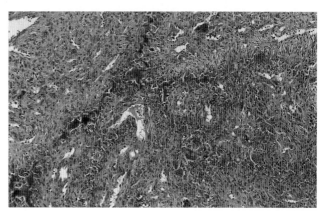

Figure 69–7. The stromal component of giant cell reactions is generally more collagenous than that of giant cell tumors. Osteoid may be seen in the stroma as well.

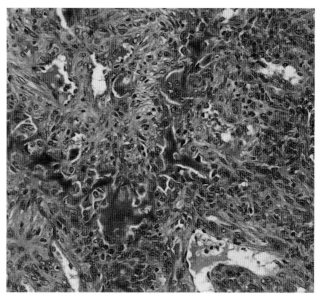

Figure 69–8. Giant cell reactions, like this lesion involving the fifth metacarpal, have histologic features similar to those of the solid variant of aneurysmal bone cyst.

CHAPTER 70

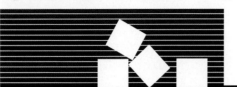

Fibroma (Metaphyseal Fibrous Defect)

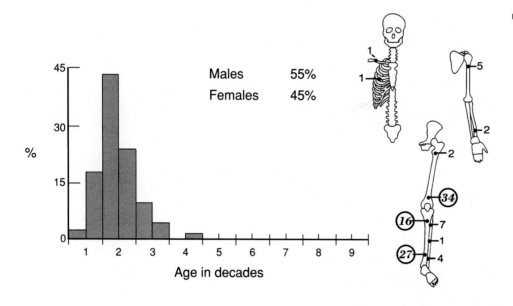

Males 55%
Females 45%

% (y-axis)

Age in decades (x-axis)

CLINICAL SIGNS

1. Physical examination is usually unrevealing in these cases.
2. A slight swelling may be present if the affected bone is near the skin, e.g., the distal tibia.

CLINICAL SYMPTOMS

1. These lesions are usually asymptomatic and are discovered on radiographic examination for an unrelated condition.
2. Local pain of short duration may be present.
3. Pathologic fracture may be the first clinical symp-tom.

MAJOR RADIOGRAPHIC FEATURES

1. The location of the lesion is metaphyseal.
2. The lesion is expansile and sharply marginated and is located in the cortex.
3. The lesion appears multilocular and has a scalloped margin.
4. The long axis of the lesion generally parallels that of the affected bone, and a sclerotic rim surrounds it.
5. Multiple lesions may be present.

RADIOGRAPHIC DIFFERENTIAL DIAGNOSIS

1. Chondromyxoid fibroma.
2. Fibrous dysplasia.

MAJOR PATHOLOGIC FEATURES

Gross

1. The cortex may be attenuated in the area of the lesion but remains intact unless pathologic fracture has occurred.
2. The lesion is well demarcated from the surrounding bone.
3. Curetted fragments are fibrous and vary from yellow to brown, depending upon the proportion of fibrous tissue to lipid-laden or hemosiderin-laden histiocytes present in the lesion.

Microscopic

1. At low magnification, the pattern is variable from region to region. Zones of spindle cells are arranged in a storiform pattern and interspersed with other foci containing more abundant histiocytic cells.
2. Giant cells are scattered throughout the lesion in irregular clusters. (In general, these cells contain fewer nuclei than the giant cells of giant cell tumor.)
3. Clusters of lipophages are scattered irregularly throughout the lesion.
4. Clusters of hemosiderin-laden macrophages are similarly dispersed.
5. At higher magnification, the nuclei of the spindled cells and histiocytes are regular. Mitotic figures may be present.
6. When pathologic fracture occurs, there may be associated reactive new bone formation.

PATHOLOGIC DIFFERENTIAL DIAGNOSIS

Benign lesions:

1. Giant cell tumor.
2. Benign fibrous histiocytoma.
3. Giant cell tumor of tendon-sheath type.
4. Pigmented villonodular synovitis.

Malignant lesions:

1. Malignant fibrous histiocytoma.
2. Osteosarcoma (if pathologic fracture and reactive new bone are misinterpreted).

TREATMENT

Primary Modality: If the diagnosis is certain and the lesion does not threaten the strength of the bone, observation alone is indicated.

Other Possible Approaches: Large lesions occupying more than 50 per cent of the bone diameter pose the risk of fracture. Curettage and bone grafting are curative. Pathologic fractures should be allowed to heal prior to surgical intervention.

References

Arata MA, Peterson HA, and Dahlin DC: Pathological fractures through non-ossifying fibromas. Review of the Mayo Clinic experience. J Bone Joint Surg (Am) 63:980–988, 1981.

Ritschl P, Hajek PC, and Pechmann U: Fibrous metaphyseal defects. Magnetic resonance imaging appearances. Skeletal Radiol 18:253–259, 1989.

Steiner GC: Fibrous cortical defect and nonossifying fibroma of bone: a study of the ultrastructure. Arch Pathol 97:205–210, 1974.

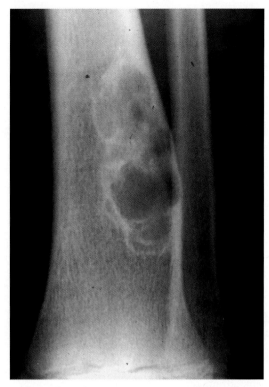

Figure 70–1. Metaphyseal fibrous defects, or fibromas, characteristically have a sharp peripheral margin and a sclerotic rim. These features are well demonstrated in this lesion of the distal diametaphyseal region of the tibia. The affected bone may be expanded, as in this case, and the lesion characteristically has a scalloped margin.

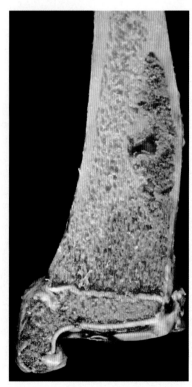

Figure 70–2. The gross pathologic features in this case correlate closely with the radiographic features shown in Figure 70–1. The patient had an incidental fibroma identified at the time of diagnosis of a distal femoral osteosarcoma, for which an above-the-knee amputation was performed.

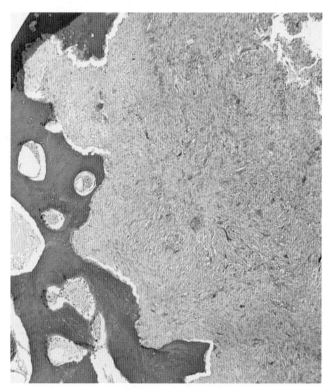

Figure 70–3. At low magnification, the well-circumscribed nature of a metaphyseal fibrous defect is evident at the periphery of the lesion. This photomicrograph shows the edge of a fibular lesion.

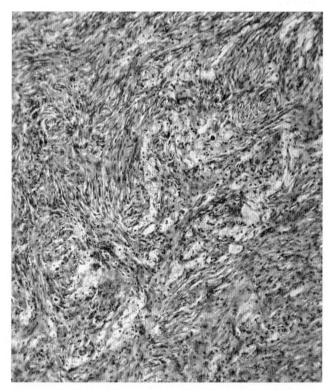

Figure 70–4. The histologic features of a fibroma vary from region to region within the lesion. The cells vary from spindled to round; some show phagocytic activity resulting in hemosiderin-laden or lipid-laden cytoplasm, as illustrated in this photomicrograph.

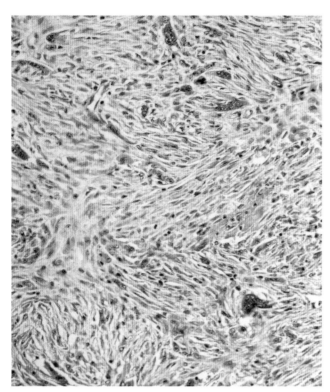

Figure 70–5. The pattern of cell arrangement at low magnification is frequently storiform, as shown in this field from a proximal tibial lesion.

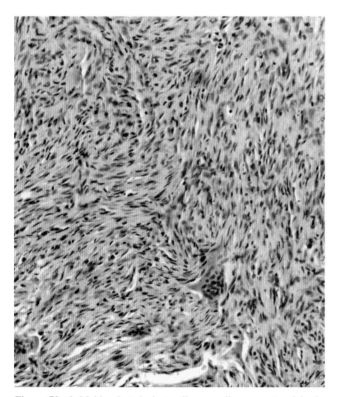

Figure 70–6. Multinucleated giant cells generally are scattered in the lesion; however, they may cluster slightly. This feature may suggest the histologic diagnosis of giant cell tumor; however, the location, radiographic features, ages, and spindled nature of the stromal cells are all characteristics that militate against such a diagnosis.

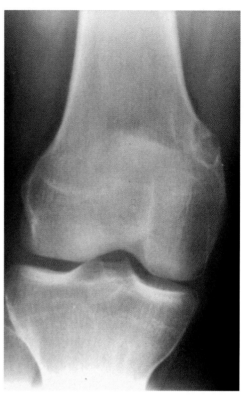

Figure 70–7. This radiograph reveals a small metaphyseal fibroma with a sharp sclerotic margin and slight expansion involving the distal femur. Such a lesion can be confidently identified on the basis of the radiographic features, and surgical intervention is unnecessary.

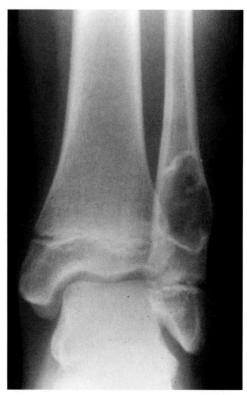

Figure 70–8. This fibroma of the distal fibula also shows the sharp margination and peripheral sclerosis characteristic of this group of lesions.

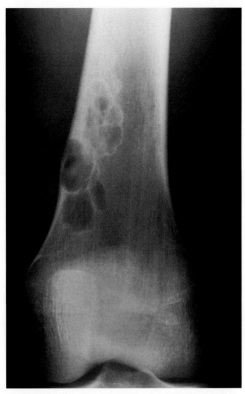

Figure 70–9. This radiograph illustrates the multilocular appearance of a fibroma involving the distal femur.

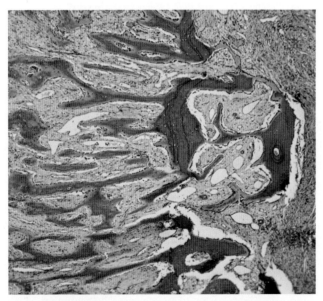

Figure 70–10. If pathologic fracture has occurred through a fibroma, a prominent periosteal reaction may be present. Although the orderly arrangement of the reaction at low magnification is a clue to its benign nature, disregarding this feature may result in a mistaken diagnosis of malignancy based upon the mitotic activity and production of osteoid that are evident at high magnification.

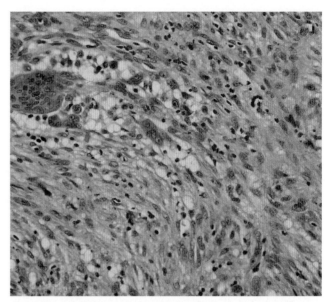

Figure 70–11. Fibroma and benign fibrous histiocytoma share histologic features; both lesions show phagocytic activity and a storiform pattern of growth. The diagnosis of benign fibrous histiocytoma is only viable in a clinical setting in which fibroma is rare. This fibroma shows the characteristic histologic features of these two lesions.

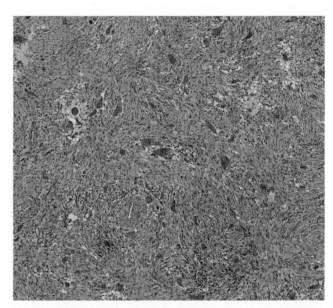

Figure 70–12. Numerous multinucleated giant cells may be present in a fibroma, as in this case involving the proximal tibia.

CHAPTER 71

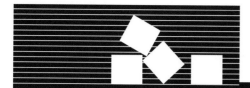

Avulsive Cortical Irregularity (Fibrous Cortical Defect, Periosteal Desmoid)

CLINICAL SIGNS

1. There are no findings on physical examination.

CLINICAL SYMPTOMS

1. These lesions are invariably silent clinically.
2. They are discovered as incidental radiographic findings, often following some trauma.

MAJOR RADIOGRAPHIC FEATURES

1. The lesion is characteristically located along medial posterior supracondylar ridges 1 to 2 cm above the epiphyseal plate, best seen in external rotation.
2. There is cortical fuzziness, irregularity, or spiculation.
3. There may be a small cortical defect.
4. There is no soft tissue mass.
5. The lesion is usually found in boys (3:1), and one third are bilateral.

RADIOGRAPHIC DIFFERENTIAL DIAGNOSIS

1. Osteosarcoma.

MAJOR PATHOLOGIC FEATURES

Gross

1. In general, these lesions are identified radiographically; biopsy is not necessary.
2. If biopsy is performed, the lesional tissue is found to be nondescript, fibrous, and soft.

Microscopic

1. At low magnification, the lesion is composed of spindle cells.
2. Lesional tissue is hypocellular, and abundant collagen is produced by the spindle cell component of the lesion.
3. At higher magnification, the fibroblasts show no cytologic atypia.
4. Mitotic figures are not identified.

PATHOLOGIC DIFFERENTIAL DIAGNOSIS

Benign lesions:

1. Fibroma.
2. Fibromatosis.

Malignant lesions:

1. Fibrosarcoma, well differentiated.

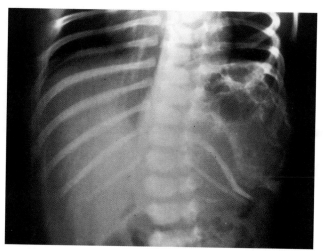

Figure 72–1. This radiograph shows a large mesenchymal hamartoma of the wall of the left lower side of the chest. The lesion is irregularly calcified and shows partial destruction of the seventh through tenth ribs.

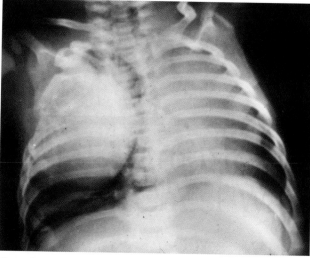

Figure 72–3. The size of such hamartomatous lesions is variable. This radiograph shows a very large lesion involving the right upper part of the chest; it contains a small amount of calcification in the upper portion of the soft tissue mass.

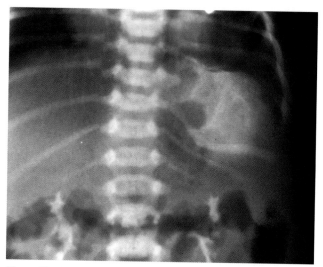

Figure 72–2. This radiograph illustrates the features of a mesenchymal hamartoma of the eighth through tenth ribs on the left side.

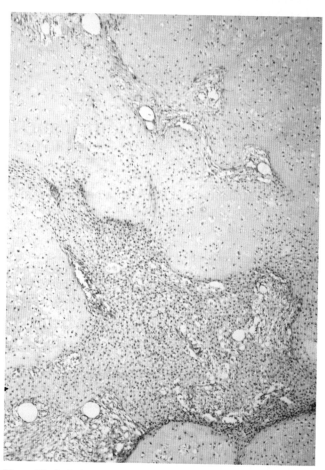

Figure 72–4. At low magnification, the mesenchymal hamartoma of the chest wall shows a variable histology. Chondroid regions are separated by more cellular regions, as in this photomicrograph.

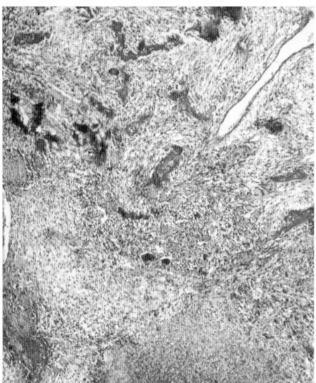

Figure 72–5. Although the solid portions of the lesion may demonstrate a worrisome spindle cell proliferation, mature bony trabeculae appear to arise from the spindle cell portion of the lesion, as this photomicrograph shows.

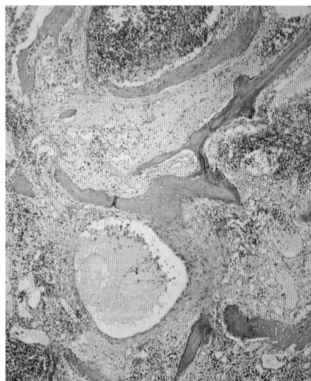

Figure 72–7. Aneurysmal bone cyst–like regions are commonly found in mesenchymomas of the chest wall. Such a region is shown in this photomicrograph.

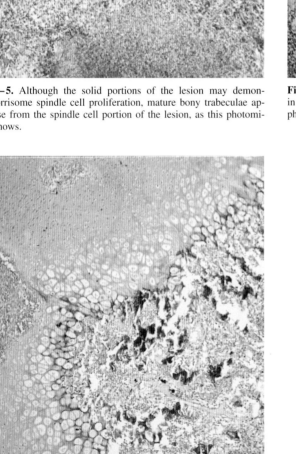

Figure 72–6. This photomicrograph illustrates the juxtaposition of normal cartilage and lesional cartilage in a mesenchymal hamartoma of the chest wall in a male newborn.

CHAPTER 73

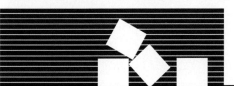

Osteomyelitis

CLINICAL SIGNS

1. Children are most commonly affected.
2. Pain is the most common sign; however, this may be minimal in infants.
3. Restricted range of motion and tenderness may be present.
4. In adults, osteomyelitis often complicates other conditions, e.g., chronic debilitating disease, drug addiction, and urinary tract infection.
5. A peripheral blood leukocytosis with a left shift in the differential is usually present; however, this is highly variable.
6. The erythrocyte sedimentation rate (ESR) is elevated.

CLINICAL SYMPTOMS

1. Fever may occur.
2. Local pain may be present (found most commonly around the knee in children because of involvement of the distal femur or proximal tibia).
3. Swelling in the region of the affected bone may be seen.

MAJOR RADIOGRAPHIC FEATURES

1. A permeative destructive pattern within the medullary cavity may be present.
2. A periosteal reaction may be present.
3. The radiographic identification of bony abnormality usually lags behind the clinical symptoms of the patient by seven to ten days.

RADIOGRAPHIC DIFFERENTIAL DIAGNOSIS

1. Osteoid osteoma.
2. Osteosarcoma.
3. Ewing's sarcoma.

MAJOR PATHOLOGIC FEATURES
Gross

1. Lesional tissue is often loose and "runny" and is surrounded by sclerotic bone.
2. Liquefactive change may be present.

Microscopic

1. An admixture of inflammatory cells may infiltrate the medullary space.
2. There may be loss of normal fatty or hematopoietic marrow.
3. Proliferation of loose edematous connective tissue may be seen within the medullary space.
4. Abscess formation may be present.
5. Necrotic bone (sequestrum) may be seen.
6. Approximately 95 per cent of cases of "uncomplicated" acute osteomyelitis are due to staphylococcal infection.

PATHOLOGIC DIFFERENTIAL DIAGNOSIS

1. Langerhans' cell histiocytosis (histiocytosis X).
2. Malignant lymphoma.
3. Myeloma.

TREATMENT

Medical

1. An accurate diagnosis is obtained by
   a. Aspiration of organisms for culture.
   b. Positive agglutination titers (e.g., *Brucella* and *Salmonella* infections).
2. Key comorbidity and risk factors—i.e., diabetes, intravenous (IV) drug use, human immunodeficiency virus (HIV) infection, and hemoglobinopathies—must be identified.

3. High-dose, organism-specific, parenteral antibiotic therapy is instituted.

Surgical

Treatment varies with the stage of infection, i.e., acute, subacute, or chronic.

1. Open drainage of acute infection is done.
2. Saucerization and excision of infected and dead bone, as well as debridement of tissues, are performed.
3. When necessary, local muscle flaps are used to provide coverage.

References

Hanssen AD, Rand JA, and Osmon DR: Treatment of the infected total knee arthroplasty with insertion of another prosthesis: the effect of antibiotic-impregnated bone cement. Clin Orthop 309:44–55, 1994.

Kraemer WJ, Saplys R, Waddell JP, and Martin J: Bone scan, gallium scan and total hip arthroplasty. J Arthoplasty 8:611–616, 1993.

Langerman RJ, et al: Osteomyelitis: diagnosing an often challenging infection. J Musculoskel Med 11:56–68, 1994.

Laughlin RT, Wright DG, Mader JT, and Calhoun JH: Osteomyelitis. Curr Opin Rheumatol 7:315–321, 1995.

Murray SD, and Kehl DK: Chronic recurrent multifocal osteomyelitis. J Bone Joint Surg (Am) 66: 1110–1112, 1984.

Patzakis MJ, et al: Symposium on current concepts in the management of osteomyelitis. Contemp Orthop 28:157–185, 1994.

Sonnen GM, and Henry NK: Pediatric bone and joint infections. Pediatr Clin North Am 43:933–947, 1996.

Sordahl OA, et al: Quantitative bone gallium scintigraphy in osteomyelitis. Skeletal Radiol 22:239–242, 1993.

Tuson CE, Hoffman EB, and Mann MD: Isotope bone scanning for acute osteomyelitis and septic arthritis in children. J Bone Joint Surg (Br) 76:306–310, 1994.

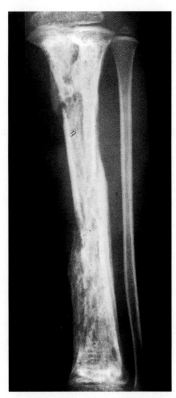

Figure 73–1. This radiograph illustrates bony destruction of a child's tibia caused by acute osteomyelitis. Such destruction may occur relatively rapidly. The tibia and femur are the most common sites of involvement in acute osteomyelitis.

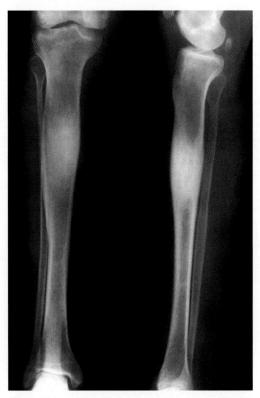

Figure 73–2. This radiograph shows another presentation pattern of acute osteomyelitis. Bony sclerosis, as in this case of osteomyelitis involving the femur, may simulate the radiographic appearance of an osteoid osteoma.

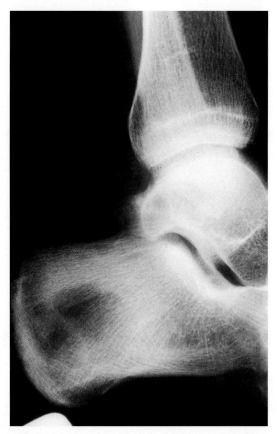

Figure 73–3. This radiograph reveals a relatively ill-defined lesion in the calcaneus that proved to be osteomyelitis on biopsy. Most cases of hematogenous osteomyelitis in the lower extremity involve the femur or tibia and those in the upper extremity involve the humerus preferentially.

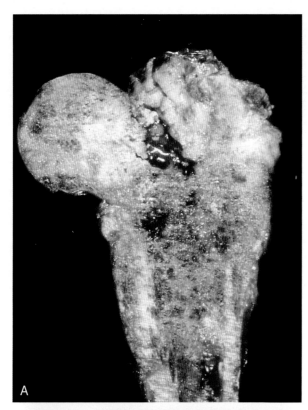

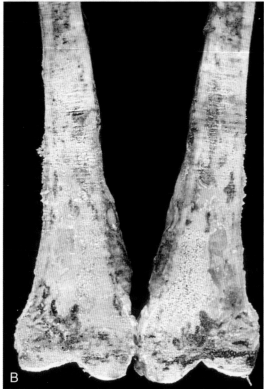

Figure 73–4. *A* and *B*, These two photographs of gross specimens show the marked bony destruction that may result from acute osteomyelitis. At the center of such regions of inflammatory reaction, fragments of dead bone (sequestra) may be present. Removal of the sequestra is necessary if the risk for reactivating osteomyelitis is to be minimized.

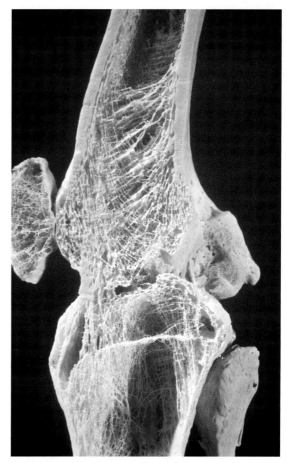

Figure 73–5. This photograph of a gross macerated specimen illustrates bony ankylosis across the knee joint in an adult patient who had long-standing osteomyelitis.

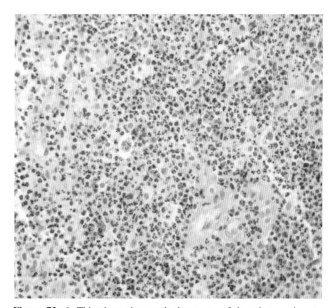

Figure 73–6. This photomicrograph shows one of the microscopic patterns of osteomyelitis. The inflammatory infiltrate in such cases may vary from being predominantly leukocytic to predominantly lymphocytic. Varying numbers of histiocytes are also commonly present.

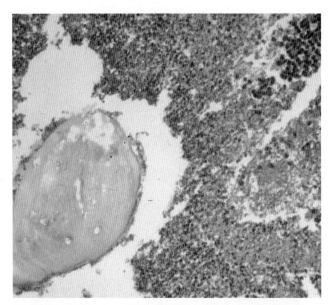

Figure 73–7. This photomicrograph illustrates osteomyelitis with an associated sequestrum. The dead bone is identified by the absence of viable osteocytes.

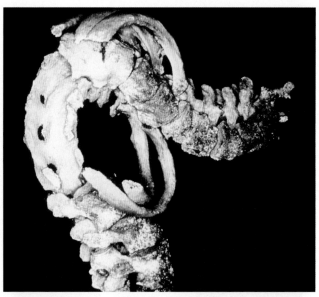

Figure 73–9. This photograph of a gross macerated specimen shows a spinal gibbus secondary to tuberculous osteomyelitis.

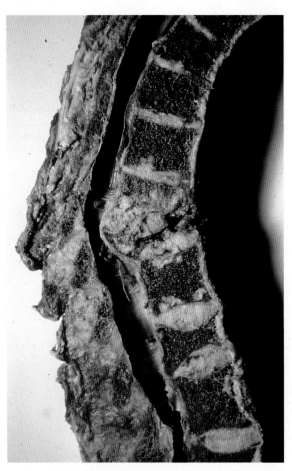

Figure 73–8. This photograph of a gross specimen illustrates a case of tuberculous osteomyelitis of the spine with bony destruction of a vertebral body. Tuberculous osteomyelitis may appear grossly "cheesy" because of granulomatous necrosis.

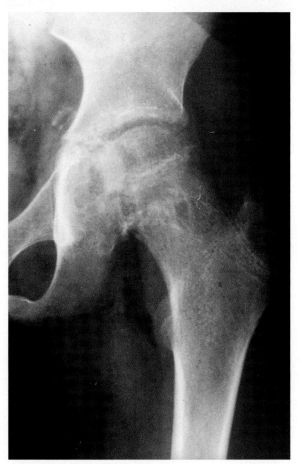

Figure 73–10. This radiograph illustrates bony destruction of the hip secondary to *Mycobacterium tuberculosis* infection.

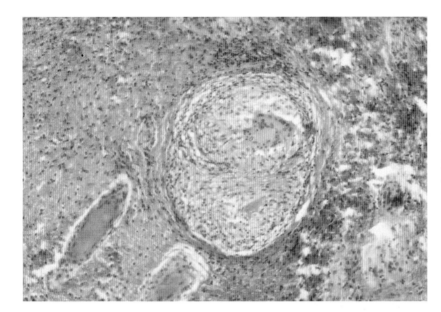

Figure 73–11. This photomicrograph reveals the granulomatous inflammation related to tuberculous osteomyelitis. Similar granulomatous reaction may be present in the synovium adjacent to the involved bone.

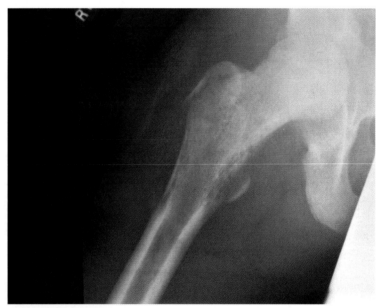

Figure 73–12. This radiograph demonstrates acute osteomyelitis of the proximal femur. The lesion shows a permeative radiographic pattern of destruction that is suggestive of a malignant tumor such as Ewing's sarcoma.

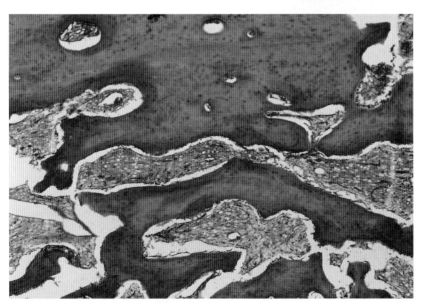

Figure 73–13. This photomicrograph shows a case of chronic osteomyelitis with marked bony sclerosis. The low-power appearance of the condition simulates that of a low-grade parosteal osteosarcoma.

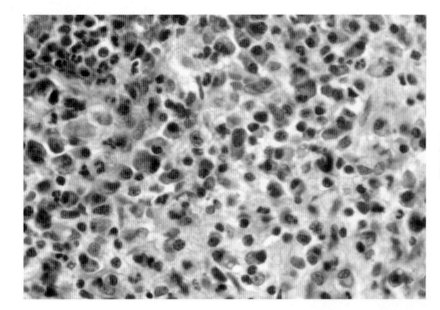

Figure 73–14. This photomicrograph illustrates a case of chronic osteomyelitis in which plasma cells predominate. Such cases can mimic myeloma in appearance.

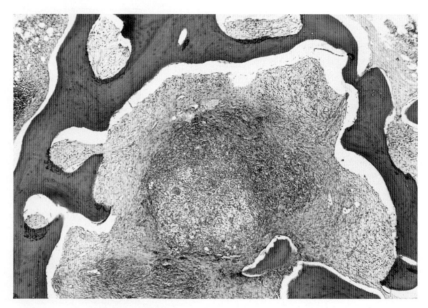

Figure 73–15. This low-power photomicrograph demonstrates the histologic appearance of Brodie's abscess. Such lesions typically simulate osteoid osteoma radiographically.

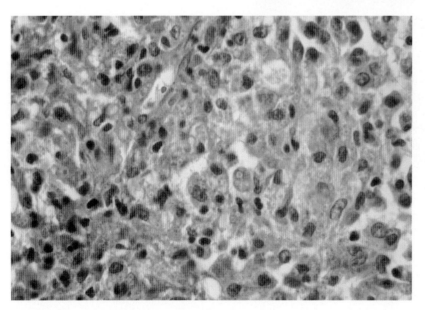

Figure 73–16. This photomicrograph shows the granulomatous response to *Histoplasma* infection in a patient with a prior history of Hodgkin's disease.

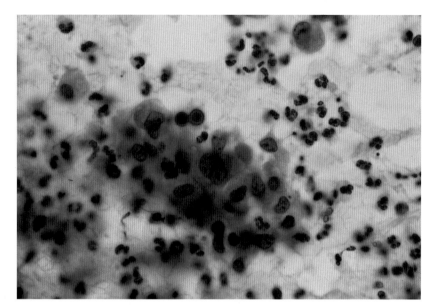

Figure 73–17. Fine-needle aspiration, with associated culture, can frequently help in diagnosing osteomyelitis. This case of blastomycotic osteomyelitis involved the ileum.

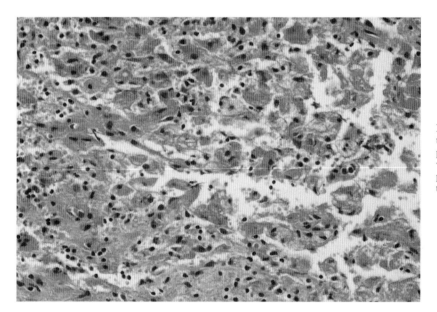

Figure 73–18. Whenever a diagnosis of xanthogranulomatous osteomyelitis is considered, the pathologist should also consider sinus histiocytosis with massive lymphadenopathy (SHML). SHML can present as bony disease, as in this case that involved the sacrum.

CHAPTER 74

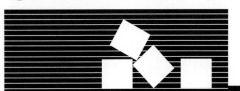

Avascular Necrosis

RISK FACTORS AND APPROXIMATE INCIDENCE

1. Corticosteroids are a risk factor in approximately 33 per cent of cases. (In these cases more than 50 per cent of patients have multiple lesions.)
2. Alcohol abuse is a risk factor in approximately 30 per cent of cases.
3. Trauma is a risk factor in approximately 5 per cent of cases.

CLINICAL SIGNS

1. Nearly 20 per cent of patients with prior subcapital fracture of the femoral neck will develop avascular necrosis of the femoral head.
2. Avascular necrosis is also associated with steroid therapy, alcoholism, Gaucher's disease, sickle cell disease, and caisson disease.
3. Any condition that interrupts the blood flow to the affected bone can result in avascular necrosis. Conditions such as systemic lupus erythematosus and related collagen vascular diseases may be associated with avascular necrosis.
4. Pathologic fracture may occur through the affected bone.

CLINICAL SYMPTOMS

1. There may be a sudden onset of pain in the affected joint.
2. The hip is most commonly involved (femoral head).

MAJOR RADIOGRAPHIC FEATURES

1. A change in the contour of the affected bone secondary to collapse of the infarcted area may be seen.
2. Increased density of the affected bone in the subchondral region may be present.
3. Approximately 50 per cent of patients have multiple joints involved.
4. Magnetic resonance imaging (MRI) is highly sensitive and specific when the clinical setting suggests a diagnosis of avascular necrosis.

RADIOGRAPHIC DIFFERENTIAL DIAGNOSIS

1. Osteoarthritis.
2. Chondroblastoma.
3. Malignant lymphoma.

MAJOR PATHOLOGIC FEATURES
Gross

1. The necrotic bone separates from the adjacent articular cartilage.
2. Hyperemia results in reddish discoloration of the bone just beyond the region of necrosis.
3. The necrotic bone is yellowish.
4. The necrotic bone may collapse into the remaining bone, flattening the contour of the articular surface.

Microscopic

1. The triangular sequestrum of dead bone retains the trabecular architecture of the native bone, but osteocytes are absent.
2. Fatty and hematopoietic marrow undergoes necrosis with the accumulation of lipid-laden histioctyes.
3. Fibrovascular connective tissue may proliferate in response to the ischemic injury at the periphery of the ischemic region.
4. Liquefactive necrosis may be present early in the course of the process.

PATHOLOGIC DIFFERENTIAL DIAGNOSIS

1. Storage disease.
2. Metabolic bone disease.
3. Acute osteomyelitis.

TREATMENT
Medical

1. The underlying disorder must be identified and treated.
2. Symptomatic measures for are given joint symptoms, e.g., nonsteroidal anti-inflammatory drugs (NSAIDs), physical therapy, ambulatory aids.

Surgical

Surgical treatment is individualized and varies with underlying disease.

1. Core decompression may be performed for early disease, i.e., stages I and II (remains controversial).
2. Nonvascularized or vascularized fibular bone graft may be undertaken for intermediate disease, i.e., stages II and III (remains controversial).
3. Total joint replacement may be indicated for advanced disease, i.e., stages IV and V.

References

Aglietti P, Buzzi JN, Buzzi R, Deschamps G. Idiopathic osteonecrosis of the knee. Aetiology, prognosis and treatment. J. Bone Joint Surg. Br. 65:588–597, 1983.

Catto, M. A histological study of avascular necrosis of the femoral head after trascervical fracture. J. Bone Joint Surg. Br. 47B:749–776, 1965.

Mont MA, Hungerford DS. Non-traumatic avascular necrosis of the femoral head. J. Bone Joint Surg. Am. 77:459–474, 1995.

Sissons HA, Nuovo MA, Steiner GC. Pathology of osteonecrosis of the femoral head. A review of experience at the Hospital for Joint Diseases, New York. Skeletal Radiol. 21:229–238, 1992.

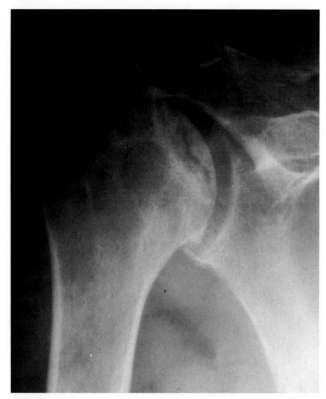

Figure 74–1. This radiograph of the proximal humerus shows a region of avascular necrosis in the humeral head. The subarticular bone shows a wedge-shaped region of radiopacity with the base adjacent to the articular cartilage.

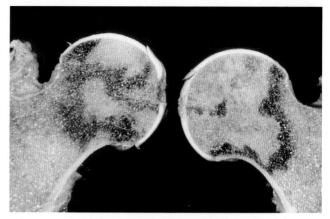

Figure 74–3. This photograph of a gross specimen of the femoral head illustrates a more recent example of avascular necrosis than that seen in Figure 74–2. The entire femoral head is infarcted, and the hyperemic region of bone at the edge of the infarct is easily identified.

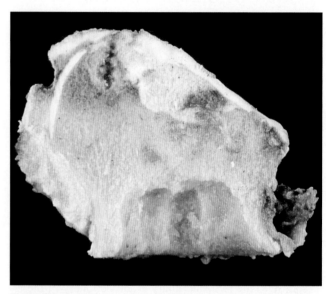

Figure 74–4. Altered mechanical properties of the articular cartilage secondary to avascular necrosis can lead to degenerative joint disease, as illustrated in this example in the femoral head. The underlying cause of the degenerative joint disease may be obscured by the marked degenerative changes.

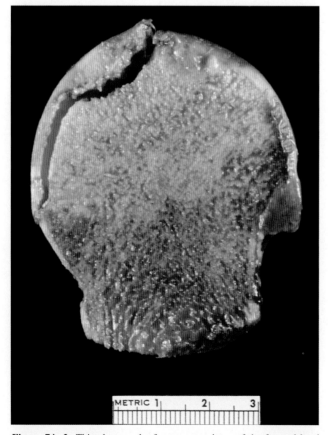

Figure 74–2. This photograph of a gross specimen of the femoral head illustrates an example of avascular necrosis. Note that the wedge-shaped region of yellowish discoloration corresponds to the area of infarction. The articular cartilage has been lifted from the underlying dead bone, resulting in alteration of the mechanical properties of the joint surface, which predisposes to degenerative joint disease.

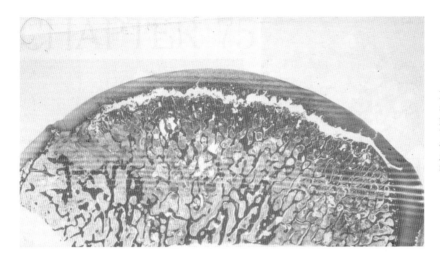

Figure 74–5. This low-power photomicrograph shows avascular necrosis in the femoral head of a patient with systemic lupus erythematosus. The wedge-shaped region identifiable radiographically is also appreciated in this specimen. Note that the region of infarction is also associated with loss of connection to the articular cartilage.

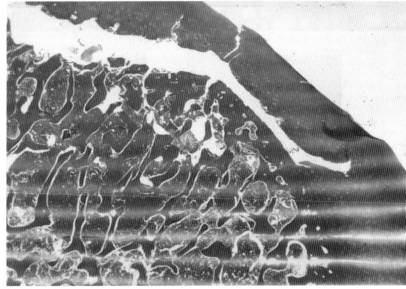

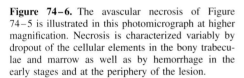

Figure 74–6. The avascular necrosis of Figure 74–5 is illustrated in this photomicrograph at higher magnification. Necrosis is characterized variably by dropout of the cellular elements in the bony trabeculae and marrow as well as by hemorrhage in the early stages and at the periphery of the lesion.

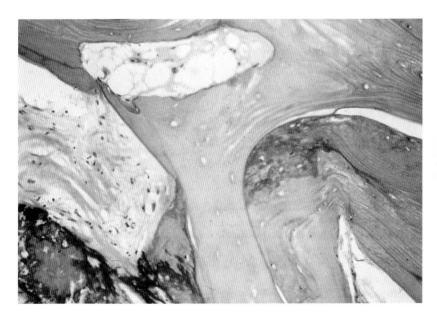

Figure 74–7. This photomicrograph illustrates the healing phase of avascular necrosis. Appositional new bone formation that uses the "scaffolding" of the pre-existing necrotic bone is evident.

6. Approximately one third of cases appear to arise from bone, one third arise from soft tissue, and one third involve both bone and soft tissue at the time of presentation.
7. When the first radiographic manifestation of the disease is in the soft tissues, then thinning and tapering of the circumference of the adjacent bone may subsequently be seen radiographically.

RADIOGRAPHIC DIFFERENTIAL DIAGNOSIS

1. Osseous hemangioma.
2. Idiopathic multicentric osteolysis.
3. Early osseous involvement may mimic a neoplasm of bone or a dysplastic condition such as fibrous dysplasia or neurofibromatosis.

MAJOR PATHOLOGIC FEATURES

1. Histologically, this condition is characterized by a proliferation of blood vessels and associated osteolysis. The vessels are usually thin-walled and capillary-like. Occasionally, they may show a more cavernous histologic appearance.
2. Reactive bone is not present in the region of the affected bone.
3. The affected bone is thinned and has been described as having a spongy consistency, evident grossly.
4. In areas where the bone has totally disappeared, there may be residual excess fibrous connective tissue.

PATHOLOGIC DIFFERENTIAL DIAGNOSIS

1. Hemangioma.
2. Lymphangioma.

TREATMENT

1. Supportive care is given, as most cases resolve spontaneously.
2. Surgical treatment involves wide resection of involved bone and soft tissue in surgically reconstructable areas (i.e., reconstruction of the hip, knee, shoulder with custom prosthetic implants).
3. Radiation therapy can be given for lesions that may be associated with significant morbidity (e.g., vertebral lesions). Moderate doses (e.g., 40 to 45 Gy) may be successful in eradicating the disease.

References

Assoun J, Richardi G, Railhac JJ, et al: CT and MRI of massive osteolysis of Gorham. J Comput Assist Tomogr 18(6):981–984, 1994.
Dominguez R, and Washowich TL: Gorham's disease or vanishing bone disease: plain film, CT, and MRI findings of two cases. Pediatr Radiol 24(5):316–318, 1994.
Dunbar SF, Rosenberg A, Mankin H, et al: Gorham's massive osteolysis: the role of radiation therapy and a review of the literature [review]. Int J Radiat Oncol Biol Physics 26(3):491–497, 1993.
Shives TC, Beabout JW, and Unni KK: Massive osteolysis. Clin Orthop (294):266–276, 1993.
Vinee P, Tanyu MO, Hauenstein KH, et al: CT and MRI of Gorham syndrome [review]. J Comput Assist Tomogr 18(6):985–859, 1994.

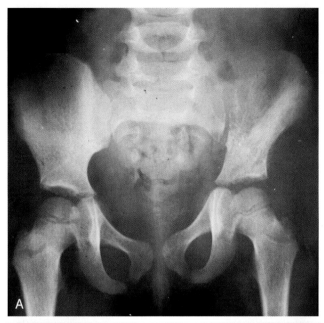

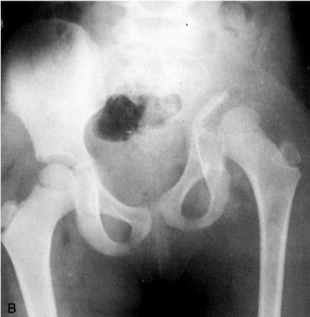

Figure 75–1. *A* and *B*, These two radiographs of the pelvis show the dramatic progression of bony dissolution over a period of two months in a patient with massive osteolysis.

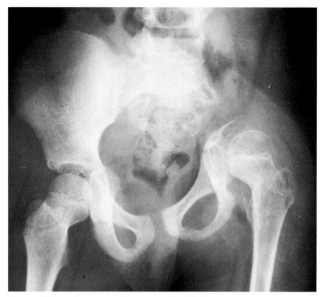

Figure 75–2. One year after the onset of symptoms, the pelvic bony dissolution has ceased and the affected bone begins to show healing with bony sclerosis.

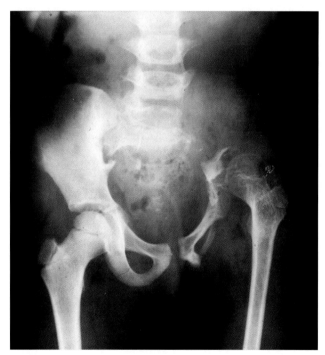

Figure 75–3. Three years after the onset of the disease illustrated in Figures 75–1 through 75–3, the process is stable. Bony deformity remains in the pelvis, but the bone has shown sclerotic changes related to healing.

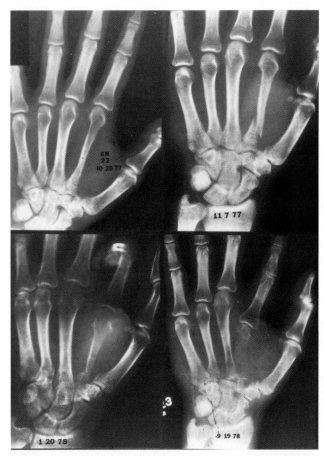

Figure 75–4. This series of radiographs illustrates massive osteolysis involving the metacarpal. Progressive bony dissolution with resultant tapering of the bone is characteristic of this process. Pathologic fracture may occur, as shown in this case.

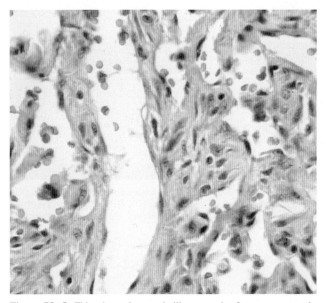

Figure 75–5. This photomicrograph illustrates the features commonly seen histologically in massive osteolysis. Hypervascularity or angiomatous changes may be present in the bone or soft tissues, as in this case.

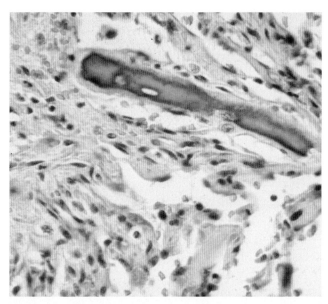

Figure 75–6. This photomicrograph shows the bland cytologic features of the endothelial cells lining the vessels of the bone in massive osteolysis. A thin bony trabecula is present. The vascular changes seen in some cases of massive osteolysis may suggest a diagnosis of hemangioma, or they may be relatively subtle.

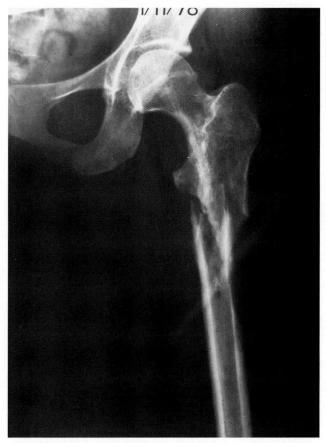

Figure 75–7. This radiograph illustrates massive osteolysis involving the proximal femur. There is an associated pathologic fracture through the diseased bone.

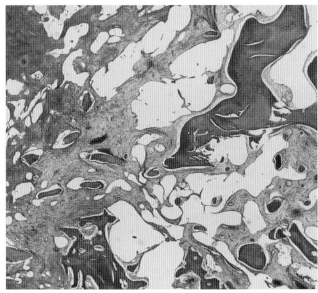

Figure 75–8. This photomicrograph reveals the hypervascular nature of diseased bone in massive osteolysis. Some cases show significantly less vascular transformation of the connective tissue than is evident in this case involving the femur.

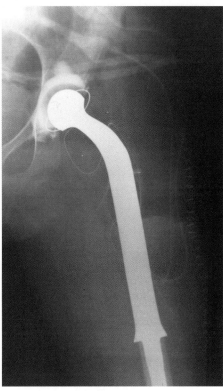

Figure 75–10. This radiograph illustrates the proximal femoral replacement used for reconstruction of the femur seen in Figures 75–7 and 75–9.

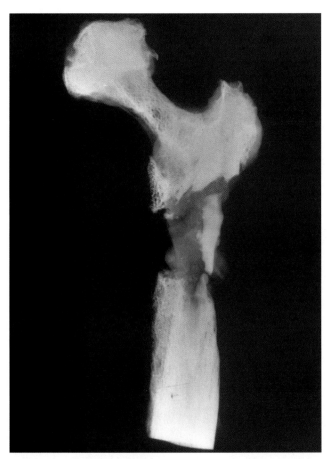

Figure 75–9. This radiograph shows the specimen taken after resection of the proximal femur illustrated in Figure 75–7. The pathologic fracture is also evident in the specimen radiograph.

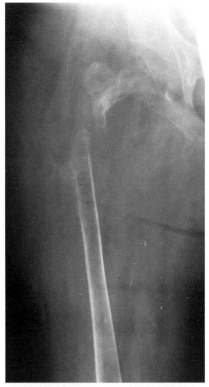

Figure 75–11. This radiograph shows massive osteolysis involving the right proximal femur. Pathologic fracture is present. Concentric narrowing of the femoral neck and the "sucked candy" appearance of the proximal end of the distal fragment are characteristic radiographic features of massive osteolysis.

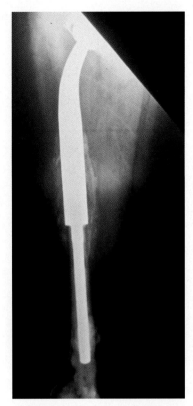

Figure 75–12. A custom prosthesis was used to reconstruct the defect remaining after resection of the proximal femoral lesion illustrated in Figure 75–11.

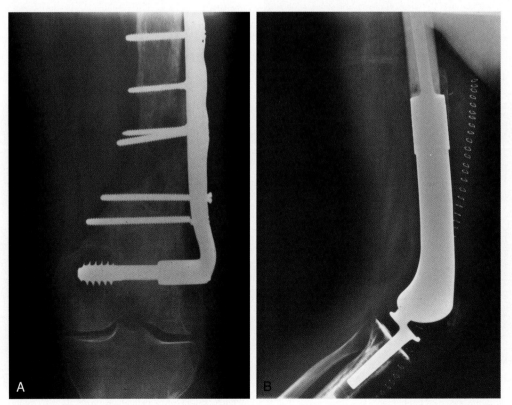

Figure 75–13. *A*, A case of massive osteolysis was treated by internal fixation. Progressive disease resulted in the need for total joint arthroplasty using a custom knee prosthesis, as illustrated in *B*.

CHAPTER 76

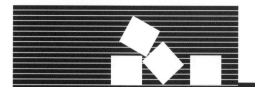

Hemophilia

CLINICAL SIGNS

1. The gene for factor VIII has a high mutation rate, and therefore patients may present with a wide variation in signs and symptoms dependent upon the severity of the factor VIII deficiency.
2. Bloody joint effusion may be seen.
3. Scattered bruises are common.
4. Intramuscular bleeding and hemarthrosis usually do not occur until a child is learning to walk.
5. Young patients may present with limping related to hemarthrosis.
6. Recurrent hemarthroses frequently involve the same joint ("target joint") owing to the synovial proliferation related to prior bleeds and the increased risk of trauma to the hyperplastic synovium.
7. Intramuscular bleeding particularly common in the thigh, calf, forearm, and iliopsoas.
8. Late arthropathy with joint destruction may occur.

CLINICAL SYMPTOMS

1. A warm, painful, swollen joint secondary to hemorrhage into the joint space (most common in knees, ankles, and elbows) may be found.
2. Minor trauma results in joint space hemorrhage.
3. A tingling sensation in the region of the affected joint often precedes painful distention of the joint in hemarthrosis.
4. Occasionally, a large intramuscular hemorrhage in the forearm may cause a compartment syndrome.
5. Secondary contractures of the knees and elbows and equinus of the ankles may be seen.

MAJOR RADIOGRAPHIC FEATURES

1. Narrowing of the joint space may be seen.
2. Cartilage destruction may be evident.
3. Bony erosion may be present.
4. Juxta-articular bony cystic changes may be seen.
5. Osteophyte formation may be evident.
6. Juxtaepiphyseal osteoporosis may be found.
7. Subperiosteal hematomas may be seen to result in subperiosteal lytic pseudotumors.
8. Magnetic resonance imaging (MRI) may define cartilage changes and hypertrophied synovium.

RADIOGRAPHIC DIFFERENTIAL DIAGNOSIS

1. Other causes of recurrent hemarthrosis, e.g., pigmented villonodular synovitis.
2. Arthropathy in advanced disease.

MAJOR PATHOLOGIC FEATURES

1. Grossly, the synovium is mahogany brown secondary to hemosiderin deposition related to joint space hemorrhage.
2. The synovium is hyperplastic and papillary.
3. Numerous hemosiderin-laden macrophages fill the synovium.
4. Loss of articular cartilage and associated pannus-like proliferation may be evident.
5. Degenerative changes in the articular cartilage may be found, including fissuring of the cartilage. (The pannus contains considerable quantities of iron.)

6. Clustering of the chondrocytes in the articular cartilage may be seen.

PATHOLOGIC DIFFERENTIAL DIAGNOSIS

1. Pigmented villonodular synovitis.
2. Rheumatoid arthritis.

TREATMENT

Medical

1. Supportive care is given (e.g., counseling to avoid activities related to increased risk of trauma and subsequent risk of bleeding), as well as physical therapy to maintain joint motion and muscle strength.
2. Factor VIII replacement (factor IX for hemophilia B) is instituted.
3. Radionucleotide synovectomy has been successful in some cases.
4. Desmopressin may be used to treat patients with mild hemophilia.

Surgical

1. Pseudotumors should be recognized and excised.
2. Arthroscopic synovectomy may be done.
3. Total joint replacement may be performed for advanced disease.

References

Barber FA, and Prudich JF: Acute traumatic knee hemarthrosis. Arthroscopy 9(2):174–176, 1993.

Bender JM, Unalan M, Balon HR, et al: Hemophiliac arthropathy. Appearance on bone scintigraphy. Clin Nucl Med 19(5):465–466, 1994.

Idy-Peretti I, Le Balc'h T, Yvart J, and Bittoun J: MR imaging of hemophilic arthropathy of the knee: classification and evolution of the subchondral cysts. Magn Reson Imaging 10(1):67–75, 1992.

Lillicrap D: The molecular pathology of hemophilia A [review]. Transfus Med Rev 5(3):196–206, 1991.

Ljung R: Genetic diagnosis of hemophilia A. Pediatr Hematol Oncol 11(1):9–11, 1994.

Lusher JM, and Warrier I: Hemophilia A. [review]. Hematol Oncol Clin North Am 6(5):1021–1033, 1992.

Magallon M, Monteagudo J, Altisent C, et al: Hemophilic pseudotumor: multicenter experience over a 25-year period. Am J Hematol 45(2):103–108, 1994.

Nuss R, Kilcoyne RF, Geraghty S, et al: Utility of magnetic resonance imaging for management of hemophilic arthropathy in children. J Pediatr 123(3):388–392, 1993.

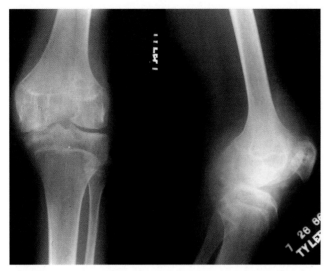

Figure 76–1. This radiograph shows the knee of a patient with hemophilia. The knees, elbows, and ankles are most often affected by hemophilia. Narrowing of the joint space is commonly identified in hemophilic arthropathy.

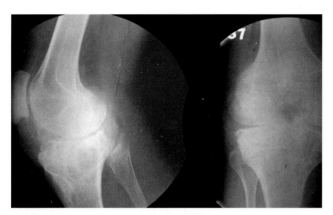

Figure 76–2. This radiograph of the knee of a patient with hemophilia shows joint space narrowing due to loss of articular cartilage after repeated intra-articular bleeds. Other features that may be seen radiographically in patients with hemophilia include bony erosion, juxta-articular cysts, and subperiosteal hematomas.

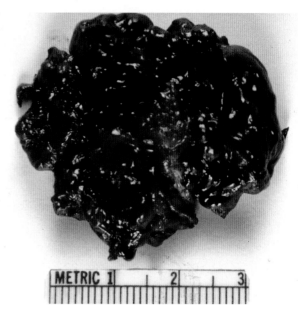

Figure 76–3. This photograph of a gross specimen shows the synovium in a patient with hemophilia who has had multiple intra-articular bleeds. The synovium is dark brown and grossly may mimic the appearance of pigmented villonodular synovitis. Villous hyperplasia of the synovium may be present, but this process is not, in general, tumefacient.

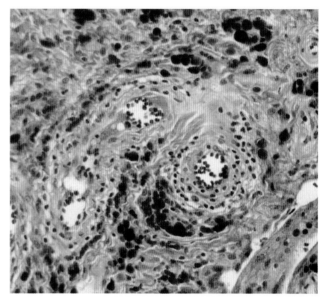

Figure 76–4. This photomicrograph illustrates the numerous hemosiderin-laden macrophages that are seen after an intra-articular bleed. In contrast to pigmented villonodular synovitis, this process lacks multinucleated giant cells and lipid-laden histiocytes.

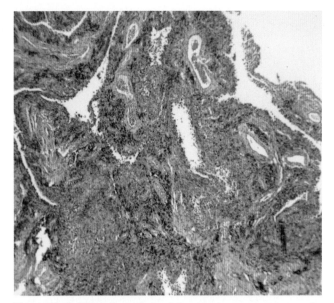

Figure 76–5. Villous hyperplasia of the synovium may accompany the deposition of hemosiderin pigment in hemophilic arthropathy, as shown in this photomicrograph.

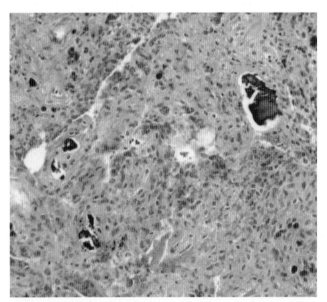

Figure 76–6. As the synovium becomes hyperplastic and the articular cartilage undergoes degenerative changes, bits of cartilage may become embedded in the synovium, as shown in this photomicrograph.

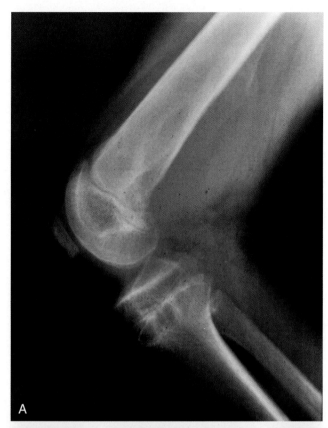

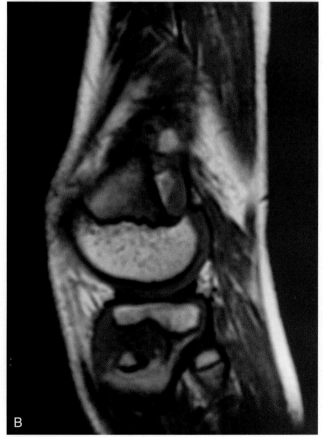

Figure 76–7. This lateral roentgenogram (*A*) and magnetic resonance imaging (MRI) scan (*B*) show the knee of a patient with hemophilia. A pseudotumor is apparent in the proximal tibial metaphysis.

CHAPTER 77

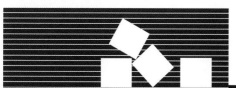

Metastatic Carcinoma

CLINICAL SIGNS

1. Tenderness is noted in the region of the affected bone.
2. A mass lesion is found.
3. Pathologic fracture is present.

CLINICAL SYMPTOMS

1. Pain is the most common symptom; however, metastatic lesions may be asymptomatic and discovered incidentally on radiographic evaluation for an unrelated problem.
2. Swelling may be noticed in the region of the affected bone.

MAJOR RADIOGRAPHIC FEATURES

1. Solitary or, more commonly, multiple lesions arise centrally in a patient with a known primary malignancy.
2. They are usually detected by combined use of radiographic survey and isotope bone scan.
3. Presentations are diverse, with lytic, blastic, or mixed lesions all common.

RADIOGRAPHIC DIFFERENTIAL DIAGNOSIS

1. Multiple myeloma.
2. Lymphoma.
3. "Brown tumor" of hyperparathyroidism.
4. Many primary malignancies of bone, if solitary.

MAJOR PATHOLOGIC FEATURES

Gross

1. The consistency of metastatic lesions varies from firm in those tumors that elicit a desmoplastic stromal reaction to soft in those that do not.
2. The color of the lesions is variable, depending upon the presence or absence of hemorrhage, necrosis, or lipidization of the tumor (as in hypernephroma).
3. The tumors tend to be poorly circumscribed and grow in an invasive, permeative manner.

Microscopic

1. The majority of carcinomas metastatic to bone show obvious glandular or squamous differentiation at low magnification.
2. If obvious glandular or squamous differentiation is lacking, growth in a clustered or organoid pattern is helpful in identifying the lesion as epithelial in origin.
3. Poorly differentiated carcinomas may grow in a sarcomatous pattern and may consist almost entirely of spindled cells. This is particularly common with renal cell carcinomas.
4. Ultrastructural and immunohistochemical investigation of sarcomatous malignancies in patients older than 60 years of age without predisposing factors for developing a primary sarcoma (e.g., Paget's disease and prior radiation) may reveal epithelial characteristics.

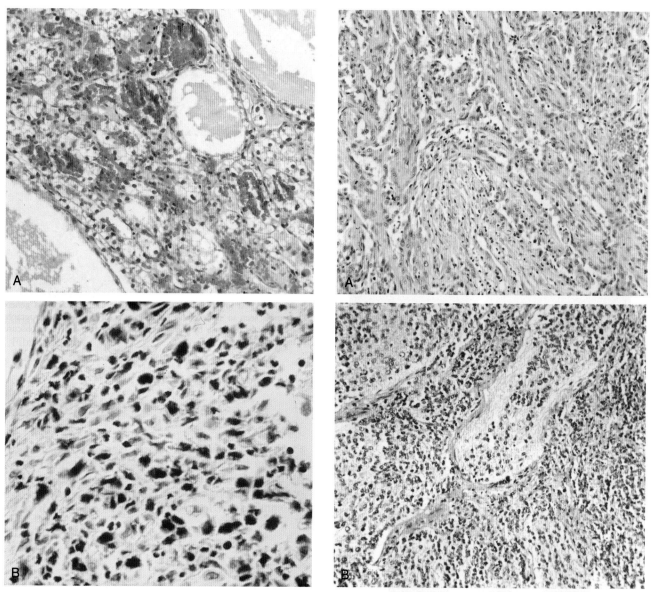

Figure 77–4. Although metastatic renal cell carcinomas generally show a clear cell histologic pattern of differentiation (*A*), metastases from a sarcomatoid renal cell carcinoma may mimic a primary bone tumor (*B*). Fortunately for diagnostic purposes, in general there will be a history of a preceding renal malignancy.

Figure 77–5. *A* shows a metastatic papillary carcinoma that, in some areas, grew in a pattern mimicking that of a vascular tumor. Although uncommon, metastatic neuroblastoma (*B*) can mimic a "small blue cell tumor" if rosettes and neutrophil are not recognized.

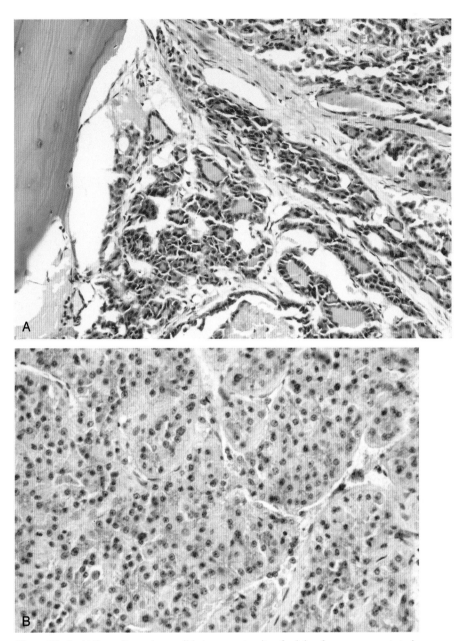

Figure 77–6. At times, it may be possible to suggest a site of origin of an osseous metastasis on the basis of its histologic pattern of growth. *A* shows a metastatic follicular carcinoma of the thyroid; *B* illustrates a metastatic hepatocellular carcinoma in which bile could be seen.

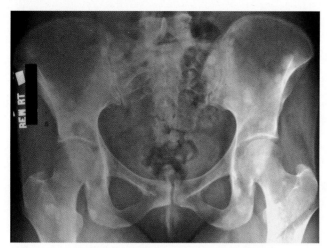

Figure 77–7. Multiple sclerotic metastases are visible in the pelvis of this elderly woman with a prior diagnosis of carcinoma of the breast.

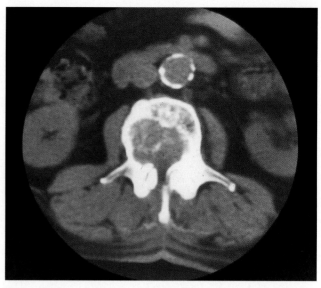

Figure 77–9. A computed tomographic (CT) scan may be helpful in identifying metastasis, as demonstrated by this view showing a mixed lytic and sclerotic metastasis in the lumbar vertebra.

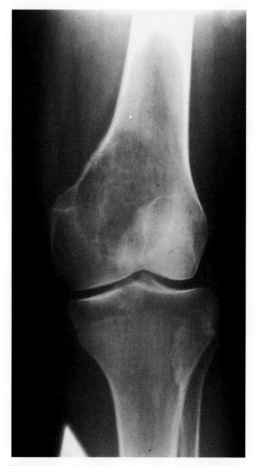

Figure 77–8. This solitary lytic lesion of the distal femur was shown on biopsy to represent metastatic renal cell carcinoma. In this location, a giant cell tumor could also be considered in the differential diagnosis.

Index

Note: Page numbers followed by f refer to illustrations.